CARDIOLOGY RESEARCH AND CLINICAL DEVELOPMENTS

CORONARY ARTERY RESTENOSIS

CAUSES, TREATMENT AND CLINICAL OUTCOMES

Cardiology Research and Clinical Developments

Additional books in this series can be found on Nova's website under the Series tab.

Additional e-books in this series can be found on Nova's website under the e-book tab.

CARDIOLOGY RESEARCH AND CLINICAL DEVELOPMENTS

CORONARY ARTERY RESTENOSIS

CAUSES, TREATMENT AND CLINICAL OUTCOMES

AMIR S. LOTFI, M.D.
EDITOR

New York

Library of Congress Cataloging-in-Publication Data

ISBN: 978-1-63321-346-3

Library of Congress Control Number: 2014942817

Published by Nova Science Publishers, Inc. † New York

Thank you to Danuta, with her all is possible.

Contents

Preface ix

Part I. Definition, Pathophysiology, and Diagnosis 1

Chapter 1 Restenosis: Historical Background and Incidence 3
Justin Maroney, MD and Lloyd W. Klein, MD

Chapter 2 Mechanisms of Restenosis 17
B. Alkhatib, J. DeLeon and S. S. Naidu

Chapter 3 Morphologic Patterns of In-Stent Restenosis 33
Gennaro Giustino, MD, Daniele Giacoppo, MD, Jennifer Yu and Roxana Mehran, MD

Chapter 4 Coronary Restenosis: Clinical Outcomes 69
Hani Kozman, MD and Kan Liu, MD

Chapter 5 Late Phase In-Stent Restenosis after Coronary Stent Implantation 77
Shigenori Ito, MD, PhD

Chapter 6 Stent Sizing Without Intravascular Imaging: Impact on Restenosis 99
Yohan Chacko, J. Kimberly Haladyn and Richard Lim

Part II. Diagnosis of Restenosis –Need Something Here on Angiographic Definition and Their Diagnosis 117

Chapter 7 Physiological Assessment of Coronary Restenosis 119
Mauro Echavarría-Pinto, MD, Tim P. van de Hoef, MD and Javier Escaned, MD, PhD

Chapter 8 The Role of Intravascular Ultrasound in Understanding the Mechanism, Prevention and Management of Restenosis 131
Jaya Mallidi, MD, Ali Haider, MD and Amir S. Lotfi, MD

Chapter 9 Optical Coherence Tomography: Current Utility and Future Potential for Management of In-Stent Restenosis 151
Talla A. Rousan, MD and Faisal Latif, MD

Chapter 10 Coronary CTA for the Evaluation of In-Stent Restenosis **169**
Jaspreet Singh, MD, Amgad N. Makaryus, MD, and Avneet Singh, MD

Part III. Treatment of Restenosis **185**

Chapter 11 Pharmacotherapy of Coronary In-Stent Restenosis **187**
Girish R. Sabnis, MD and Prafulla G. Kerkar, MD

Chapter 12 Interventional Treatment of Restenosis **201**
Larry S. Dean, MD

Chapter 13 Saphenous Vein Graft Restenosis and Management **213**
M. Javed Ashraf MD and James A. Grantham MD

Part IV: Future Strategies in the Treatment of Restenosis **237**

Chapter 14 Prevention of Restenosis with Stent-Based Vascular Gene Delivery: Gene Eluting Stents **239**
Ilia Fishbein, Michael Chorny, Ivan S. Alferiev, Richard F. Adamo and Robert J. Levy

Chapter 15 Future Strategies for Preventing and Treating Coronary Restenosis **263**
Ehrin J. Armstrong and John C. Messenger

Editor Contact Information **285**

Index **287**

Preface

Coronary artery restenosis continues to remain a major limitation to percutaneous coronary intervention. The clinical consequence of restenosis, mainly in the form of repeat intervention, can have significant short and long term clinical sequela. Coronary Artery Restenosis: Causes, Treatment and Clinical Outcomes is aimed at both the general and interventional cardiologist. In this book the authors explore the process of stenosis from mechanism of restenosis to future strategies of treating or preventing restenosis.

I would like to thank the contributors for their time and efforts. Without their dedication and expertise this book would not have been produced.

Part I. Definition, Pathophysiology, and Diagnosis

In: Coronary Artery Restenosis
Editor: Amir S. Lotfi
ISBN: 978-1-63321-346-3

Chapter 1

Restenosis: Historical Background and Incidence

Justin Maroney[1], MD and Lloyd W. Klein[2*], MD
[1] Geisinger Medical Center, Danville, PA, US
[2] Advocate Illinois Masonic Medical Center & Rush Medical College, Chicago, IL, US

Abstract

Coronary restenosis remains a major limitation to percutaneous revascularization. The term restenosis initially was in reference to recurrent valvular heart stenosis and was later applied to renarrowing after open and percutaneous revascularization. The goal of this chapter is to review the definitions and terminology for restenosis. In addition a brief review of the mechanism of restenosis, risk factors, and clinical outcomes will be discussed.

Introduction

Definitions

Restenosis of the coronary arteries results from healing of the arterial wall in response to mechanical injury [1]. Restenosis can manifest by (i) imaging evidence, where quantitative analysis of angiography, CT angiography, intravascular ultrasound (IVUS) and optical coherence tomography (OCT) reveal luminal narrowing, (ii) histologic changes, where elastic recoil, negative remodeling, and neointimal hyperplasia are noted on pathology, and (iii) clinical symptoms of ischemia, which are confirmed by subsequent investigation to have narrowing in the arterial position that suffered the preceding mechanical injury [2].

* Corresponding Author: Lloyd W Klein MD FACC; Advocate Illinois Medical Center Professional Office Building; 3000 North Halsted, Suite #625; Chicago, IL 60657; lloydklein@comcast.net.

Diameter Stenosis (The Emory Definition)

In 1979 Gruntzig described 50 patients treated with percutaneous balloon angioplasty, with a 19% rate of restenosis of treated lesions, diagnosed by clinical symptoms consistent with ischemia followed by repeat angiography revealing target lesion stenosis [3]. Gruntzig and his colleagues at Emory defined restenosis as:

> "a >50% reduction in the diameter of the treated arterial segment compared to a 'normal' reference arterial segment within the same coronary artery, found at repeat angiography 6 months following the initial arterial treatment" [2]

This definition remains the most commonly used definition of restenosis for clinical and research purposes, with the provision that the 6-month timeframe for angiographic follow-up is not strictly adhered to, and is rather more accurately described as "6 months or more" following the initial arterial injury. The >50% luminal narrowing definition also remains unchanged, although with the introduction of stents, the Emory definition was expanded. "In-stent" restenosis was defined as a >50% luminal narrowing *within the stented area.* "In-lesion" restenosis was defined as the same >50% luminal narrowing but included *the vessel segment encompassing both the stent and the 5 mm vessel segments both proximal and distal to the stent.* In-lesion measures can reflect elastic recoil, arterial spasm, and arterial remodeling in the un-stented vessel segments, and thus should not be directly compared to in-stent restenosis for purposes of clinical studies [1].

The Emory definition is derived from compelling physiologic studies that showed that coronary flow reserve becomes impeded when the coronary artery lumen is reduced by 50% or more [4]. The definition is dichotomous; it is either present or absent, and therefore there are certain weaknesses of using this measure. Additionally, the definition is based on luminal assessment and therefore may not reflect diseased reference vessel segments. It does not convey the mechanism of vessel response to injury (elastic recoil vs. negative remodeling vs. neointimal hyperplasia). Lastly, due to the binary nature of the measure, an individual with 49% stenosis would be categorically separate from an individual with 51% restenosis, even though intuitively one would expect both patients to have similar clinical course [2, 5]. Due to the aforementioned weaknesses, several additional definitions of restenosis have been employed since the Emory group posited theirs, and these definitions are discussed below.

Late Loss

Late loss is defined as:

(minimum luminal diameter in the treated arterial segment) – (minimal luminal diameter in the treated segment at subsequent follow-up)

Late loss is a continuous variable, and thus parametric statistical analyses can be performed using this measure, whereas these analyses cannot be performed on a binary measure like the Emory definition. It has been found to have a unimodal, near-normal distribution, suggesting that restenosis is not a dichotomous phenomenon [2]. Late loss is one of the major endpoints employed in studies examining bare metal and drug eluting stents [6].

Stents prevent the elastic recoil and negative remodeling vessel response to injury, and therefore late loss can be viewed as a proxy for neointimal hyperplasia in clinical investigation [2, 7]. A general problem with late loss measures is that the minimum luminal diameters used for the calculation may be obtained from unmatched locations within the treated vessel, and thus may not reflect vessel injury or the degrees of stimulation or inhibition of neointimal hyperplasia, but rather progression of existing disease in the native vessel unrelated to the intervention taken [6, 8]. (This limitation also applies to the Emory definition). Furthermore, the relationship between late loss and the binary Emory definition is non-linear, and one measure cannot be used to infer the other [3].

Loss Index

Loss index is a ratio defined as:

(late loss) ÷ (acute gain in vessel diameter at the initial intervention) [2]

The loss index definition was developed as a continuous variable for the purpose of evaluating suspected biologic factors causing luminal narrowing. Elastic recoil and other mechanical factors were known to contribute only 10% - 20% of diameter stenosis, therefore any narrowing greater than this level was felt to be due to a biologic process. Loss index was the measure that most definitively elucidated diabetes mellitus as a risk factor for restenosis [2].

Rotterdam Definition

Computer assisted measures of the angiographic arterial lumen are commonly used to calculate the degree of arterial narrowing after vessel injury. In 1985 Serruys and colleagues found there was a $\pm$0.36 mm standard deviation in follow-up computer-assisted measurements of treated lesions at 90 days. A threshold of twice the standard deviation (a 95% confidence interval) of the computer-assisted measurement was necessary to define a significant degree of restenosis; therefore this group defined restenosis as:

"a decrease in lumen diameter of $\geq$0.72 mm at follow-up"

This definition is commonly referred to as the "Rotterdam" definition. [2].

Minimum Luminal Area

Newer imaging technologies including intravascular ultrasound and optical coherence tomography have allowed for additional definitions of restenosis, including definitions based on luminal cross-sectional area rather than diameter. A common IVUS-derived definition of restenosis is:

"a minimum luminal area <4 mm^2" [9]

Cross sectional technologies have allowed for various other measures including neointimal volume and thickness [6, 10, 11]. IVUS imaging confirms that neointimal hyperplasia is the dominant factor contributing to restenosis in stented lesions, accounting for approximately >80% of the total degree of restenosis, versus <20% due to pure stent underexpansion [9].

National Heart Lung and Blood Institute Definition

The NHLBI developed a definition for restenosis defined as:

"the loss of half of the acute gain from balloon angioplasty" [2]

This definition is not commonly used in the clinical literature.

Mechanism of Restenosis

Elastic recoil of the arterial wall occurs almost immediately after balloon angioplasty, and results in a 17% - 50% reduction in lumen diameter versus the maximum dilatation diameter attained with the balloon expanded [2]. However, inward displacement of the external elastic lamina ("negative remodeling") is the dominant mechanism of lumen loss after balloon angioplasty, occurring within weeks to months after the initial vessel injury and accounting for approximately 60% of late loss [12]. Restenosis does not appear to progress at a linear rate; most of the degree of restenosis will occur within 6 months of the vessel injury, with a significantly slower rate of progression after that timeframe.

Restenosis rates using the Emory definition in the balloon angioplasty era were as high as 60% when evaluated by repeat angiography, and were less when evaluated clinically. In the stent era, the incidence of restenosis is as high as 40% in bare metal stenting, and 0% - 16% in drug-eluting stenting. The BENESTENT study showed that bare metal stents reduced the rate of restenosis significantly versus balloon angioplasty (22% in the stent group versus 33% in the balloon angioplasty group) [13].

Stenting achieves a larger initial luminal diameter enlargement versus balloon angioplasty, and the stent scaffolding essentially eliminates elastic recoil and negative remodeling, however there is greater late loss due to neointimal hyperplasia [14, 15]. Interestingly, across multiple interventional modalities including balloon angioplasty, bare metal stenting, and laser and directional atherectomy, there will be approximately 0.5 mm of late loss for each 1 mm of acute diameter gain [2].

The benefit of stenting versus balloon angioplasty lies in the attainment of a larger acute gain immediately after the former [2]. Late loss due to neointimal hyperplasia does occur, but the minimum luminal diameter will remain larger due to the larger "starting point." The average late loss after bare metal stenting is 0.8 – 1.0 mm, and this magnitude tends to be conserved regardless of reference vessel size or maximal acute luminal diameter attained at stent deployment. Thus the percentage cross-sectional luminal area lost will be substantially greater in a small reference vessel (e.g. a 2 mm vessel) versus a large vessel (e.g. a 4 mm vessel) [16].

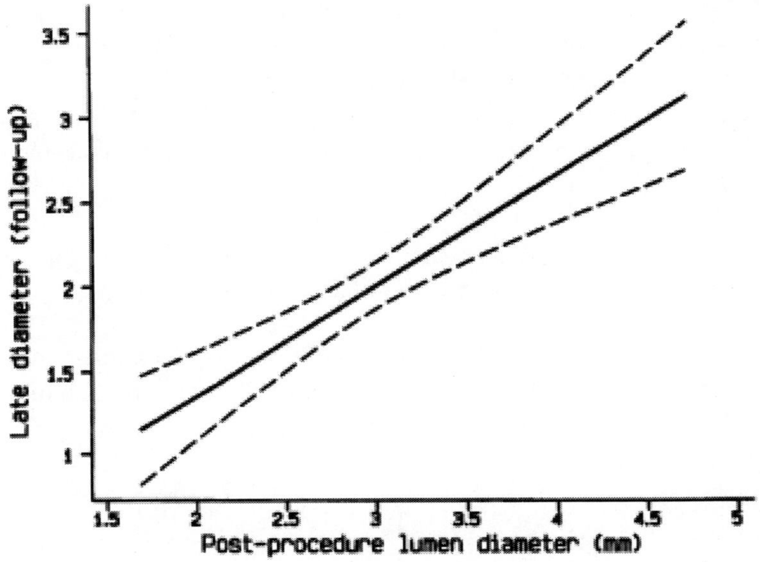

Source: [2].

Figure 1. Plot of a geometric model relating acute post procedure lumen diameter to late luminal diameter. Mean regression line (bold) and the 95% confidence bounds for that regression line (dotted lines) show the tight association between larger post procedure lumen and larger late lumen.

Clinical Sequelae

In addition to quantitative measures, clinical sequelae of ischemia due to restenotic lesions have been used to define restenosis. Death, myocardial infarction, recurrent angina symptoms, target lesion revascularization, and target vessel revascularization have all been used as clinical endpoints defining restenosis. Death as an endpoint is sufficiently rare due to restenosis that most of the literature has adopted "softer" endpoints in order to sufficiently power the studies [2].

The presence of restenosis by the Emory definition has been found to be clinically silent in approximately 50% of patients [17]. Nonetheless, in the bare metal stent era, restenosis >50% presented as unstable angina in 26% – 53% of patients, and as acute myocardial infarction (MI) in 3.5% - 20% [18, 19]. In the drug-eluting stent era, these rates have decreased to approximately 18% for unstable angina, and 2% for acute MI [20]. Nuclear stress testing and echocardiographic stress testing have both been found to be useful in detecting restenosis. Thallium nuclear stress testing has a positive predictive value of 82% [21]. Exercise stress testing without an imaging component is not accurate in detecting restenosis, and CT angiography is limited by the decreased resolution within the stented regions [22, 23].

Restenosis using the Emory definition leads to a 70% increase in the rate of repeat revascularization within 6-12 months after the index procedure versus lesions without restenosis. Furthermore, patients found to have restenosis by this definition have higher 4-year mortality than patients without restenosis [24]. It should be noted that the biologic response to vessel injury appears to occur sooner than its clinical manifestation, which can take months or years [25]. The goal of contemporary drug-eluting stent therapy is to acutely increase arterial luminal patency while also modulating the biologic response to arterial injury in order to reduce or even prevent the clinical sequelae of restenosis.

Target lesion revascularization (TLR) is one of the major endpoints used to evaluate the clinical efficacy of balloon angioplasty and stenting. This endpoint was adopted to evaluate an intervention's ability to maintain absence of ischemia and/or ischemic symptoms after the initial treatment. It is defined as:

> "any repeat percutaneous intervention on the initially treated target segment of artery, or bypass of the vessel containing the initial target lesion" [2].

There is a direct relationship between diameter stenosis after intervention and TLR. Interestingly, very few lesions at the 50% threshold for the Emory definition of restenosis will ultimately require TLR, whereas lesions of 70% diameter stenosis have a 73% TLR rate [26].

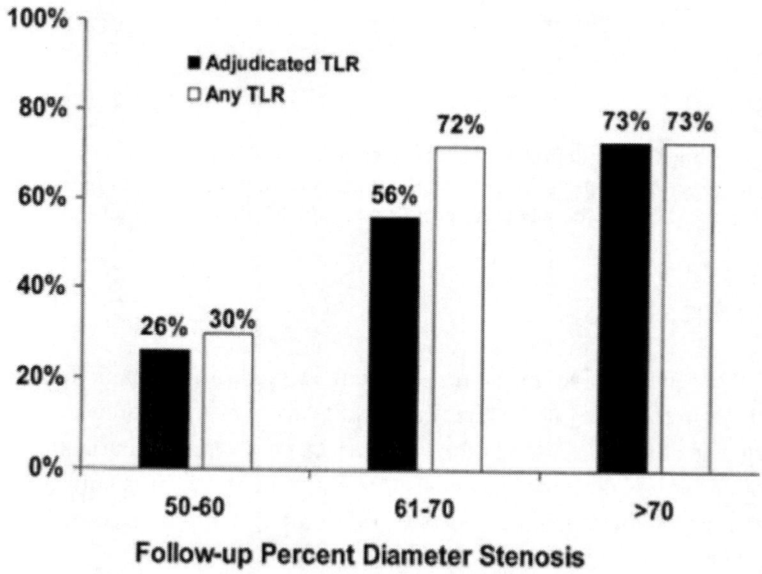

Source: [26].

Figure 2. Target lesion revascularization (TLR) rates according to restenosis severity. Adjudicated TLR rates indicate the Clinical Events Committee determined the TLR was clinically driven.

Late loss has been correlated with the rate of TLR. Lesions having late loss <1 mm have a fairly low rate of TLR, while lesions with late loss >2 mm having a high rate of TLR [3]. Additionally, TLR has been correlated with the pattern of restenosis, both for bare metal and drug-eluting stents. In the drug-eluting stent era, focal areas of in-segment restenosis (<10 mm contiguous lesion length within the treated area of vessel) using the Emory definition have been found to have lower rates of TLR than diffuse restenosis lesions (>10 mm contiguous length), 9.8% versus 23% [27]. These findings are concordant with previous studies showing diffuse lesions having a higher rate of positive nuclear stress findings consistent with ischemia in the target vessel distribution [28].

Target vessel revascularization (TVR), defined as:

> "any repeat percutaneous intervention on or bypass of the initially treated artery"

is a less specific proxy for restenosis. In the drug-eluting stent era, revascularization of the target vessel is more than four times more likely to be due to lesions distant from the initial target lesion (6.3% vs. 1.7%) and unrelated to the degree of restenosis in the treated segment [29]. Its utility is in accounting for restenosis due to edge dissection with healing, and subsequent proliferative response. Similarly, recurrent angina in patients with previous percutaneous coronary intervention has been found to be more commonly associated with progression of disease at a site remote from the previously treated lesion, representing progression of native disease rather than restenosis [2].

Risk Factors for Restenosis

The most important factor determining whether restenosis will occur is the absolute lumen diameter achieved at the end of the index procedure [30, 31]. Three other important risk factors contributing to restenosis are (i) longer stent length, (ii) smaller minimum luminal diameter of the reference vessel, and (iii) the presence of diabetes mellitus [32].

Stent lengths greater than 28 mm increase the incidence of underexpansion at a discrete focal location within the stent, which is significantly less likely to occur with shorter stent lengths [9]. With drug-eluting stents, underexpansion may result in decreased drug delivery and increased neointimal hyperplasia. Furthermore, the angiographic appearance of restenosis differs by which drug is eluted. Restenosis occurring with sirolimus-eluting stents is very commonly found to be focal and at the edge of the stent, while restenosis with paclitaxel-eluting stents tends to occur more diffusely within the entire stented region [33]. Since there is very little neointimal hyperplasia within drug-eluting stents, the DES era has helped reveal the importance of geographic miss as a cause for restenosis, where IVUS evaluation reveals evidence of vessel trauma and/or negative remodeling immediately adjacent to the stented region, suggesting geographic miss with pre-dilatation [34].

A Swedish study of more than 35,000 diabetic patients treated with drug-eluting stents found a significantly higher restenosis rate in patients with diabetes [35]. Moreover, insulin-dependent diabetes was found to have a TLR rate of 28% versus 16.3% in patients without diabetes [36]. Other contributors to restenosis in stented lesions include stent underexpansion, strut thickness, stent fracture, saphenous vein graft stenosis and chronic total occlusion [37, 38]. The ISAR-STEREO-2 study showed that thin-strut stents have a significantly lower rate of restenosis than thick-strut stents (17.9% versus 31.4%) [39]. This is due in part to thin-strut stents having less late loss than thick-strut stents [40]. With stent fracture there is partial or complete separation of a portion of the stent. This phenomenon occurs in 1 – 8% of stents deployed, leading to potential areas for blood to pool between the stent and the vessel wall, and in the case of drug-eluting stents, focal areas of reduced drug delivery [41].

Conclusion

Optimal results for percutaneous coronary intervention can be achieved through understanding the underlying mechanism of restenosis, identifying patient selection with objective evidence of ischemia, and appropriate use of current technology. Future technologies such as bioresorbable vascular scaffold have potential to enhance the durability of coronary intervention and reduce the comorbidity associated with restenosis.

Table 1. Rates of restenosis by modality

Modality	Restenosis Rate
Balloon angioplasty	30-60%
Rotational atherectomy	28-40%
Directional atherectomy	29%
Bare metal stenting	16-40%
Drug eluting stenting	0-16%

Sources: [42 – 45].

Table 2. Drugs studied to prevent restenosis

Study drug	Dosage	No. of patients	Trial result
Anti-platelet agents			
Aspirin	100 mg/day	216	Positive
Aspirin/dipyridamole	330/225 mg/day	376	Neutral
Aspirin/dipyridamole	650/225 mg/day	236	Neutral
Aspirin/Coumadin	325 mg/day, PT >2.5	248	Neutral
Prostacyclin	7 ng/kg/day	286	Neutral
Ciprostene	120 ng/kg/day	270	Neutral
Ticlopidine	750 mg/day	236	Neutral
Sulotroban	3200 mg/day	755	Neutral
Cilostazol	100 mg bid	705	Positive
Anticoagulants			
Heparin	PTT > 1/5 nL	416	Neutral
Coumadin	PT > 2.5 nL	110	Neutral
Enoxaparin	40 mg/day	459	Neutral
Ca channel blockers			
Nifedipine	40 mg/day	241	Neutral
Amlodipine	10 mg/day	635	Neutral
Diltiazem	329 mg/day (mean)	201	Neutral
Verapamil	240 mg bid	700	Neutral
ACE/ARB			
Cilazapril	10 mg/day	693	Neutral
Cilazapril	5/10/20 mg/day	1436	Neutral
Fosinopril	40 mg/day	508	Neutral
Quinapril		100	Neutral
Valsartan	80 mg/day	250	Positive
Corticosteroids			
Methylprednisolone	1 g IV bolus	915	Neutral
Methylprednisolone	125 mg/day	102	Neutral
Antiproliferatives			
Colchicine	1.2 mg/day	197	Neutral

Study drug	Dosage	No. of patients	Trial result
Sirolimus	6 mg load, then 3 mg/day for 14 days	100	Positive
Statins			
Simvastatin	20 mg/day	71	Neutral
Pravastatin	40 mg/day	695	Neutral
Fluvastatin	40 mg bid	1054	Neutral
Thiazolidinediones			
Pioglitazone		54	Positive
Rosiglitazone		95	Positive
Anti-allergens			
Tranilast	300 and 450 mg bid	2018	Neutral
Pemirolast	20 mg/day	205	Positive
Other			
Fish oil	6 g/day	186	Neutral
Fish oil	3.2 g/day	82	Positive
Fish oil	3 g/day	108	Neutral
Folic acid	1.2 mg/day	636	Negative
Probucol	500 mg/day	189	Neutral

Sources: [2, 46 – 61].

References

[1] Topol, E., and P. Teirstein. *Textbook of interventional cardiology.* 6th ed. Philadelphia: Elsevier Saunders, 2012.

[2] Kuntz RE, Baim DS. Defining coronary restenosis. Newer clinical and angiographic paradigms. *Circulation.* 1993;88:1310-1323.

[3] Kern, MJ. *SCAI interventional cardiology board review.* 2nd ed. Philadelphia: Wolters Kluwer Lippincott Williams & Williams, 2014.

[4] Gould KL, Lipscomb K, Hamilton GW: Physiologic basis for assessing critical coronary stenosis. Instantaneous flow response and regional distribution during coronary hyperemia as measures of coronary flow reserve. *Am J Cardiol.* 1974;33:87-94.

[5] Rensing BJ, Hermans WR, Deckers JW, et al.: Which angiographic variable best describes functional status 6 months after successful single-vessel coronary balloon angioplasty? *J Am Coll Cardiol.* 1993;21:317-324.

[6] Costa MA, Sabate M, Angiolillo DJ, et al.: Relocation of minimal luminal diameter after bare metal and drug-eluting stent implantation: incidence and impact of angiographic late loss. *Catheter Cardiovasc Interv.* 2007;69:181-188.

[7] Strauss BH, Serruys PW, de Scheerder IK, et al.: Relative risk analysis of angiographic predictors of restenosis within the coronary wall stent. *Circulation.* 1991;84:1636-1643.

[8] Sabate BH, Costa MA, Kozuma K, et al.: Methodological and clinical implications of relocation of the minimal luminal diameter after intracoronary radiation therapy. Dose finding study group. *J Am Coll Cardiol.* 2000;36:1536-1541.

[9] Kang SJ, Mintz GS, Park DW, et al.: Mechanisms of in-stent *Circ Cardiovasc Interv.* 2011;4(1):9-14.

[10] Garcia-Garcia HM, Shen Z, Piazza N. Study of restenosis in drug eluting stents: new insights from greyscale intravascular ultrasound and virtual histology. *EuroIntervention.* 2009;5 Suppl D:D84-92.

[11] Bezerra HG, Costa MA, Guagliumi G, Rollins AM, Simon DI. Intracoronary optical coherence *JACC Cardiovasc Interv.* 2009;2(11):1035-1046.

[12] Schwartz RS, Topol EJ, Serruys PW, Sangiorgi G, Holmes DR Jr. Artery size, neointima, and remodeling: time for some standards. *J Am Coll Cardiol.* 1998;32(7):2087-2094.

[13] Serruys PW, de Jaegere P, Kiemeneij F, et al.: A comparison of balloon-expandable-stent *N Engl J Med.* 1994;331(8):489-495.

[14] Breeman A, Serruys PW, van den Brand MJ, Deckers JW, van Herwerden LA, Roelandt JR. [Complications shortly after transluminal angioplasty *Ned Tijdschr Geneeskd.* 1994;138(21):1074-1080.

[15] Fischman DL, Leon MB, Baim DS, et al.: A randomized comparison of coronary-stent *N Engl J Med.* 1994;331(8):496-501.

[16] Mehilli J, Kastrati A, Wessely R, et al.: Randomized trial of a nonpolymer-based rapamycin-eluting stent versus a polymer-based paclitaxel-eluting stent for the reduction of late lumen loss. *Circulation.* 2006;113(2):273-279.

[17] Ruygrok PN, Webster MW, de Valk V, van Es GA, Ormiston JA, Morel MA, Serruys PW. Clinical and angiographic factors associated with asymptomatic restenosis after percutaneous coronary intervention. *Circulation.* 2001;104(19):2289-2294.

[18] Bossi I, Klersy C, Black AJ, et al.: In-stent restenosis: long-term outcome and predictors of subsequent target lesion revascularization after repeat balloon angioplasty. *J Am Coll Cardiol.* 2000;35(6):1569-1576.

[19] Chen MS, John JM, Chew DP, Lee DS, Ellis SG, Bhatt DL. Bare metal stent restenosis is not a benign clinical entity. *Am Heart J.* 2006 Jun;151(6):1260-1264.

[20] Rathore S, Kinoshita Y, Terashima M, et al.: A comparison of clinical presentations, angiographic patterns and outcomes of in-stent restenosis between bare metal stents and drug eluting stents. *EuroIntervention.* 2010;5(7):841-6.

[21] Wijns W, Serruys PW, Simoons ML, van den Brand M, de Feijter PJ, Reiber JH, Hugenholtz PG. Predictive value of early maximal exercise test and thallium scintigraphy after successful percutaneous transluminal coronary angioplasty. *Br Heart J.* 1985;53(2):194-200.

[22] Andersen K, Steinthórsdóttir SD, Haraldsdottir S, Gudnason T. Clinical evaluation and stress test have limited value in the diagnosis of in-stent restenosis. *Scand Cardiovasc J.* 2009;43(6):402-407.

[23] Kumbhani DJ, Ingelmo CP, Schoenhagen P, Curtin RJ, Flamm SD, Desai MY. Meta-analysis of diagnostic efficacy of 64-slice computed tomography in the evaluation of coronary in-stent restenosis. *Am J Cardiol.* 2009;103(12):1675-1681.

[24] Schühlen H, Kastrati A, Mehilli J, Hausleiter J, Pache J, Dirschinger J, Schömig A. Restenosis detected by routine angiographic follow-up and late mortality *Am Heart J.* 2004 Feb;147(2):317-322.

[25] Serruys PW, Luijten HE, Beatt KJ, et al.: Incidence of restenosis *Circulation.* 1988;77(2):361-71.

[26] Cutlip DE, Chauhan MS, Baim DS, et al.: Clinical restenosis *J Am Coll Cardiol.* 2002;40(12):2082-2089.

[27] Cosgrave J, Melzi G, Biondi-Zoccai GG, et al.: Drug-eluting stent *J Am Coll Cardiol.* 2006;47(12):2399-2404.
[28] Kang SJ, Cho YR, Park GM, et al.: Predictors for functionally significant in-stent *JACC Cardiovasc Imaging.* 2013(11):1183-1190.
[29] Cutlip DE, Chhabra AG, Baim DS, et al.: Beyond restenosis: five-year clinical outcomes from second-generation coronary stent trials. *Circulation.* 2004;110(10):1226-1230.
[30] De Feyter PJ, Kay P, Disco C, Serruys PW. Reference chart derived from post-stent *Circulation.* 1999;100(17):1777-1783.
[31] Serruys PW, Kay IP, Disco C, Deshpande NV, de Feyter PJ. Periprocedural quantitative coronary angiography *J Am Coll Cardiol.* 1999;34(4):1067-1074.
[32] Kastrati A, Schömig A, Elezi S, et al.: Predictive factors of restenosis *J Am Coll Cardiol.* 1997;30(6):1428-1436.
[33] Corbett SJ, Cosgrave J, Melzi G, et al.: Patterns of restenosis *Eur Heart J.* 2006;27(19):2330-2337.
[34] Castagna MT, Mintz GS, Leiboff BO, et al.: The contribution of "mechanical" problems to in-stent restenosis: An intravascular ultrasonographic analysis of 1090 consecutive in-stent restenosis lesions. *Am Heart J.* 2001;142(6):970-974.
[35] Fröbert O, Lagerqvist B, Carlsson J, Lindbäck J, Stenestrand U, James SK. Differences in restenosis rate with different drug-eluting stents in patients with and without diabetes mellitus: a report from the SCAAR (Swedish Angiography and Angioplasty Registry). *J Am Coll Cardiol.* 2009;53(18):1660-1667.
[36] Aronson D, Bloomgarden Z, Rayfield EJ. Potential mechanisms promoting restenosis in diabetic patients. *J Am Coll Cardiol.* 1996;27(3):528-535.
[37] Kastrati A, Schömig A, Elezi S, et al.: Predictive factors of restenosis *J Am Coll Cardiol.* 1997;30(6):1428-1436.
[38] Kastrati A, Elezi S, Dirschinger J, Hadamitzky M, Neumann FJ, Schömig A. Influence of lesion length on restenosis *Am J Cardiol.* 1999;83(12):1617-1622.
[39] Pache J, Kastrati A, Mehilli J, et al.: Intracoronary stenting and angiographic results: strut thickness effect on restenosis outcome (ISAR-STEREO-2) trial. *J Am Coll Cardiol.* 2003;41(8):1283-1288.
[40] Rittersma SZ, de Winter RJ, Koch KT, et al.: Impact of strut thickness on late luminal loss after coronary artery *Am J Cardiol.* 200415;93(4):477-480.
[41] Umeda H, Gochi T, Iwase M, et al.: Frequency, predictors and outcome of stent *Int J Cardiol.* 2009;133(3):321-326.
[42] Farooq V, Gogas BD, Serruys PW. Restenosis: delineating the numerous causes of drug-eluting stent *Circ Cardiovasc Interv.* 2011;4(2):195-205.
[43] Kiesz RS, Rozek MM, Ebersole DG, Mego DM, Chang CW, Chilton RL. Novel approach to rotational atherectomy results in low restenosis rates in long, calcified lesions: long-term results of the San Antonio Rotablator Study (SARS). *Catheter Cardiovasc Interv.* 1999;48(1):48-53.
[44] Baptista J. [Rotational atherectomy in the drug-eluting stent *Rev Port Cardiol.* 2012 Jan;31(1):7-9
[45] Simonton CA, Leon MB, Baim DS, et al.: 'Optimal' directional coronary atherectomy: final results of the Optimal Atherectomy Restenosis Study (OARS). *Circulation.* 1998;97(4):332-339.

[46] Lange H, Suryapranata H, De Luca G, et al.: Folate therapy *N Engl J Med.* 2004;350(26):2673-2681.

[47] Douglas JS Jr, Holmes DR Jr, Kereiakes DJ, et al.: Coronary stent restenosis in patients treated with cilostazol. *Circulation.* 2005;112(18):2826-2832.

[48] Jørgensen B, Simonsen S, Endresen K, et al.: Restenosis and clinical outcome in patients treated with amlodipine after angioplasty: results from the Coronary AngioPlasty Amlodipine REStenosis Study (CAPARES). *J Am Coll Cardiol.* 2000;35(3):592-599.

[49] Bestehorn HP, Neumann FJ, Büttner HJ, et al.: Evaluation of the effect of oral verapamil on clinical outcome and angiographic restenosis after percutaneous coronary intervention: the randomized, double-blind, placebo-controlled, multicenter Verapamil Slow-Release for Prevention of Cardiovascular Events After Angioplasty (VESPA) Trial. *J Am Coll Cardiol.* 2004;43(12):2160-2165.

[50] O'Keefe JH Jr, Giorgi LV, Hartzler GO, Good TH, Ligon RW, Webb DL, McCallister BD. Effects of diltiazem on complications and restenosis after coronary angioplasty. *Am J Cardiol.* 1991;67(5):373-376.

[51] Okumura K, Sone T, Kondo J, et al.: Quinapril prevents restenosis after coronary stenting in patients with angiotensin-converting enzyme D allele. *Circ J.* 2002;66(4):311-316.

[52] Bertrand ME, McFadden EP, Fruchart JC, et al.: Effect of pravastatin on angiographic restenosis after coronary balloon angioplasty. The PREDICT Trial Investigators. Prevention of Restenosis by Elisor after Transluminal Coronary Angioplasty. *J Am Coll Cardiol.* 1997 Oct;30(4):863-869.

[53] Rodés J, Côté G, Lespérance J, et al.: Prevention of restenosis after angioplasty in small coronary arteries with probucol. *Circulation.* 1998;97(5):429-436.

[54] Holmes DR Jr, Savage M, LaBlanche JM, et al.: Results of Prevention of REStenosis with Tranilast and its Outcomes (PRESTO) trial. *Circulation.* 2002;106(10):1243-1250.

[55] Peters S, Götting B, Trümmel M, Rust H, Brattström A. Valsartan for prevention of restenosis after stenting of type B2/C lesions: the VAL-PREST trial. *J Invasive Cardiol.* 2001;13(2):93-97.

[56] Rodriguez AE, Granada JF, Rodriguez-Alemparte M, et al.: Oral rapamycin after coronary bare-metal stent implantation to prevent restenosis: the Prospective, Randomized Oral Rapamycin in Argentina (ORAR II) Study. *J Am Coll Cardiol.* 2006;47(8):1522-1529.

[57] Petronio AS, Amoroso G, Limbruno U, et al.: Simvastatin does not inhibit intimal hyperplasia and restenosis but promotes plaque regression in normocholesterolemic patients undergoing coronary stenting: a randomized study with intravascular ultrasound. *Am Heart J.* 2005;149(3):520-526.

[58] Serruys PW, Foley DP, Jackson G, et al.: A randomized placebo-controlled trial of fluvastatin for prevention of restenosis after successful coronary balloon angioplasty; final results of the fluvastatin angiographic restenosis (FLARE) trial. *Eur Heart J.* 1999;20(1):58-69.

[59] Nishio K, Sakurai M, Kusuyama T, et al.: A randomized comparison of pioglitazone to inhibit restenosis after coronary stenting in patients with diabetes mellitus type. *Diabetes Care.* 2006;29(1):101-106.

[60] Choi D, Kim SK, Choi SH, et al.: Preventative effects of rosiglitazone *Diabetes Care.* 2004;27(11):2654-2660.

[61] Ohsawa H, Noike H, Kanai M, et al.: Preventive effects of an antiallergic drug, pemirolast potassium, on restenosis after percutaneous transluminal coronary angioplasty. *Am Heart J.* 1998;136(6):1081-1087.

In: Coronary Artery Restenosis
Editor: Amir S. Lotfi
ISBN: 978-1-63321-346-3

Chapter 2

Mechanisms of Restenosis

B. Alkhatib, J. DeLeon and S. S. Naidu*
From the Division of Cardiology, Department of Medicine,
Winthrop University Hospital, Mineola, NY, US

Abstract

Binary restenosis is defined as greater than 50% luminal narrowing over the intermediate term after coronary intervention. Regardless of the endovascular treatment for coronary stenosis, restenosis, which is a distinct pathophysiology rather than an accelerated form of atherosclerosis, can occur and limits the long-term effectiveness of coronary intervention. Despite progress in interventional techniques and changes in stent design and technology specifically aimed at restenosis, it has continued to be an important clinical concern. In fact, these technological advances themselves have also brought about new mechanisms of restenosis. In this chapter we discuss the mechanisms and pathophysiologic conditions contributing to restenosis, specifically acute vessel wall injury, elastic recoil, thrombogenesis, negative remodeling, neointimal hyperplasia and neoatherosclerosis.

Introduction

Since the first balloon angioplasty performed on a coronary artery in 1977 by Dr. Andreas Gruentzig, cardiologists have been noting vessel wall damage and associated clinical sequelae. [1] In particular, a phenomenon of accelerated vessel closure was observed at an alarmingly high rate. The term coronary restenosis was thereby coined. Regardless of the endovascular treatment for coronary stenosis, restenosis, which is a distinct pathophysiology rather than an accelerated form of atherosclerosis, can occur and limits the long-term effectiveness of coronary intervention. However, the time frame and mechanism differs with

*Corresponding Author: Srihari S. Naidu, MD, FACC, FAHA, FSCAI. Associate Professor of Medicine. SUNY – Stony Brook School of Medicine. Director, Cardiac Catheterization Laboratory. Winthrop University Hospital. 120 Mineola Blvd, Suite 500. Mineola, NY 11501. 516-663-9696. ssnaidu@winthrop.org

each treatment method. Binary restenosis is defined as greater than 50% luminal narrowing over the intermediate term after coronary intervention, whereas clinical restenosis is defined as symptoms or abnormal stress test findings followed by documented angiographic binary restenosis [2]). In this chapter we discuss the mechanisms and pathophysiologic conditions contributing to restenosis, specifically acute vessel wall injury, elastic recoil, thrombogenesis, negative remodeling, neointimal hyperplasia and neoatherosclerosis.

Despite progress in interventional techniques and changes in stent design and technology specifically aimed at restenosis, it has continued to be an important clinical concern. In fact, these technological advances themselves have brought about new mechanisms of restenosis. Using a historical perspective, this chapter will discuss the mechanisms of restenosis over time, the understanding of which has led to both incremental advancements in treating coronary artery disease and entirely new stent platforms. Current restenosis rates and processes, as well as future directions and stent platforms, will be discussed.

Coronary Artery Anatomy

Understanding the pathogenesis of restenosis first requires knowledge of the structure, indigenous cell types, and function of a normal artery. Coronary arteries have a trilaminar structure made up of the tunica intima, tunica media, and tunica adventitia. The innermost layer, the intima, in adult humans is made up of endothelial cells resting on a basement membrane containing collagen, laminin, fibronectin, and other extracellular molecules. The middle layer, tunica media of elastic arteries, has well-developed concentric layers of smooth muscle cells (SMC) with elastin-rich extracellular matrix (ECM). The SMCs in normal arteries seldom proliferate. Rates of both cell division and cell death are low. The tunica media is also bordered by an internal and external elastic lamina separating it from the intimal and adventitial layers, respectively. The adventitia is the outermost layer of elastic arteries, made up of a loose array of collagen fibrils and very few cells as compared to other arterial vessel layers. The cell types include fibroblasts and mast cells. Historically, the adventitia received little attention, but now is thought to play a major role in restenosis and in particular a phenomenon known as negative remodeling [3].

Risk Factors

The biologic mechanism of restenosis is independent of patient co-morbidities and of lesion type, but there are several factors that render patients more susceptible to initiation and propagation of the process. These factors may be divided into 3 categories: 1) Patient characteristics: diabetes mellitus, chronic renal failure, Class IV angina, restenosis after prior angioplasty, and inflammatory states, 2) Angiographic characteristics: Chronic occlusion, lesion location (Ostia LAD or vein graft), small vessel diameter (<3mm), bifurcation or long lesions, and 3) Procedure characteristics: smaller post stent diameter (<3mm), multiple stent placement, suboptimal stent apposition and/or stent under expansion, and stent fracture (4,5). The mechanism of restenosis varies based on intervention, however, with different mechanisms predominating after balloon angioplasty, bare metal stenting and drug-eluting stenting. Accordingly, type of intervention is a risk factor for various forms and amounts of restenosis.

Balloon Angioplasty Restenosis

Elastic recoil and negative remodeling are the two primary processes leading to restenosis after balloon angioplasty and will be the focus of this discussion. Initially, neointimal formation due to SMC proliferation was thought to be the cause of restenosis after balloon angioplasty. This was because initial animal studies using rat carotid artery models demonstrated extensive SMC proliferation at sites of balloon expansion [3, 6]. However, observations of cadaveric human specimens showed relatively minimal SMC proliferation and called into question the therapeutic targeting of this process. Moreover, intravascular ultrasound (IVUS) studies in humans suggested that a substantial portion of the loss of luminal caliber after balloon angioplasty resulted from a constriction of the vessel due to adventitial changes. This difference was likely due to the fact that the substrate of animal studies was normal arteries rather than atherosclerotic disease [3]. Such observations led to further studies evaluating adventitial inflammation and response to injury, including scar formation and wound contraction, as a mechanism of arterial constriction after balloon angioplasty.

Elastic Recoil

Balloon angioplasty achieves gain in luminal caliber by cracking and compressing atherosclerotic plaque, but in the process it stretches and disrupts the tunica intima and tunica media, thereby expanding the outer diameter of the vessel [7]. Initial restenosis after this type of intervention is caused by acute prolapse of the disrupted plaque and also the fact that the outward expansion leads to a rebound contraction defined by the elastic properties of the vessel wall. This rebound is likely determined by the density of elastin in ECM. This process occurs almost immediately after balloon angioplasty, constitutes the phenomenon of elastic recoil, and has been observed both clinically and with angiographic studies [8].

Positive and Negative Remodeling

In a variety of clinical settings, blood vessels react with expansion or constriction to physiologic or pathophysiologic conditions. These compensatory changes in vessel size and structure are termed vascular remodeling. In certain vascular disease entities, for example abdominal aortic aneurysms, a change in vessel size is a disease –initiating event rather than a compensatory response. During the formation of an atheromatous lesion in coronary arteries, however, as plaque grows there is compensatory vascular outward growth and enlargement that serves to minimize the percent stenosis until no further vascular enlargement is possible. This is a compensatory mechanism seen early in the atherogenic process and prevents luminal loss despite significant plaque development and accumulation. This compensatory mechanism is termed positive remodeling and is defined as an expansion of the external elastic membrane (EEM), and occurs by turnover of EEM molecules to accommodate the circumferential growth of the artery [9]. This outward growth leads to an increase in the caliber of the artery and no significant lumen loss until the plaque burden exceeds roughly 40% of the cross-sectional area of the artery. Studies using epicardial ultrasound and intravascular ultrasound (IVUS) reported that EEM area of atherosclerotic segments was significantly larger than the proximal non-diseased segments, despite no loss in lumen size, confirming this pathophysiology in vivo [10,11].

Negative remodeling, in contrast, is now thought of as the mechanism that leads to restenosis and substantial loss of luminal caliber after balloon angioplasty. It results from constrictive remodeling due to fibrotic healing of the injured vessel and scar-related tissue contraction, predominantly from the adventitia [3].

The pathophysiology of this remodeling is not fully understood. However, available data suggests that negative remodeling is initiated by vascular injury, inflammation, and changes in hemodynamic conditions (flow, shear stress, and wall stretch) leading to release of humeral factors. It is hypothesized that these signals are initiated in the endothelium and relayed to adjacent cells. Release of these factors leads to several biochemical pathways that influence cell growth, apoptosis, migration, and altered composition of the ECM [10].

The ECM therefore appears to play a central role in this remodeling process. Matrix-metalloproteinases (MMP) regulate the composition of the ECM by selective degradation of its components and by formation of collagen, leading to negative remodeling. Clinically, restenosis increases markedly between 1 and 3 months after balloon angioplasty, but rarely occurs after 3 months. In clinical studies of angioplasty, resultant binary restenosis rates have averaged 30-40%. [7]. See table 1.

Table 1. Comparison of restenosis in balloon angioplasty, BMS, and DES

	Balloon Angioplasty	Bare Metal Stent	Drug Eluting Stent
Mechanism of restenosis	Elastic recoil Negative remodeling	Neointimal hyperplasia	Neointimal hyperplasia Neoatherosclerosis
Timing of restenosis	<1hr 1-3 months	6-12 months	>6months-5yrs
Rates	~40%	~20%	3-5%

Bare Metal Stent Restenosis

With the advent of the bare metal stent (BMS), rates of restenosis decreased from 40% to approximately 20% [12]. BMS with their associated radial strength prevented early elastic recoil and limited late negative remodeling, the two biggest mechanisms of restenosis seen in the balloon angioplasty era, as discussed above. However, a new mechanism emerged, known as neointimal hyperplasia, resulting in observed clinical restenosis rates.

Neointimal Hyperplasia

The pathophysiology of stent restenosis in the bare metal stent era was attributed to neointimal hyperplasia, a reparative process whereby various coagulation, inflammatory factors and cells stimulate SMC proliferation and extracellular matrix formation, usually as a consequence of severe injury and exaggerated inflammatory response, thought related to the foreign body. In BMS, peak neointimal growth is observed at 6-12 months, and in particular is contributed to by thrombogenesis, inflammation, growth factors and SMC migration and proliferation. See figure 1.

Thrombogenesis: In humans, in response to coronary stent implantation, partial to complete destruction of the endothelial cell layer is observed. This initiates platelet adherence and aggregation on stent struts and exposed injured vascular surface components. As a result, thrombus formation is observed on stent struts within 10 days after stent deployment [13]. Thrombus formation is stimulated by tissue factor (TF), a procoagulant upregulated in balloon-injured vessels. TF initiates the extrinsic coagulation pathway, resulting in thrombin production. Thrombin stimulates release of platelet-derived growth factor (PDGF), proliferation of SMCs and alteration of ECM composition (14). This then leads to upregulating the gene expression of TF, perpetuating a thrombogenic cycle. Regenerated endothelial cells after stent implantation promote mobilization of bone marrow derived endothelial progenitor cells to accelerate vascular repair, which also manifests in the development of neointimal hyperplasia [15].

Inflammation: Many studies have shown the importance of inflammation as an early event after stenting in different animal studies using specific antibodies to leukocytes (CD45), macrophages (CD14), and monocytes (CD115). Endothelial injury leads to activation of platelets and their deposition at the site of the lesion recruits circulating leukocytes [16]. The exact mechanism is thought to be upregulation of selectins, integrins, and vascular cellular and intracellular adhesion molecules (VCAM-1 and ICAM-1) on the remaining endothelium of the injured artery, resulting in leukocyte adhesion [14]. Leukocyte-platelet interaction is critical in the initiation and progression of neointimal formation. Coronary stenting is associated with a persistent increase in ICAM-1 (receptor that mediates adhesion of leukocytes to endothelial cells) levels, which may explain the mechanism of increased neointimal formation after stenting as compared with balloon angioplasty alone [17]. It was also noted that leucopenia decreases neointimal formation and adventitial fibrosis, further corroborating the relationship of persistent inflammation to restenosis in patients undergoing stent placement.

Along with ICAM-1, a neutrophil integrin called MAC-1 correlated with late restenosis and lumen loss post BMS placement. Inhibition of MAC-1 diminishes leukocyte accumulation, SMC proliferation, and neointimal formation. Further, single nucleotide polymorphisms of the MAC-1 gene, causing dysfunction, are associated with lower incidence of angiographic restenosis [18, 19]. Neutrophils also promote PDGF and cell proliferation through oxygen free radical production (20). These observations suggest neutrophil activation plays a critical role in the pathogenesis of neointimal formation.

Mononuclear leukocytes, which make up 20% of coronary plaque cells in human atherectomy tissue, also appear to play a major role in neointimal formation. Monocytes convert to activated macrophages when recruited by the injured vessel after BMS placement. Disruption of the monocyte adhesion process by inhibiting monocyte chemoattractant protein

(MCP-1) decreases neointimal formation in injured rat carotid arteries [21]. The development of neointima is also mediated by various inflammatory cytokines such as IL-1 and TNF alpha; both IL-1 and TNF alpha stimulate SMC proliferation by inducing PDGF [22].

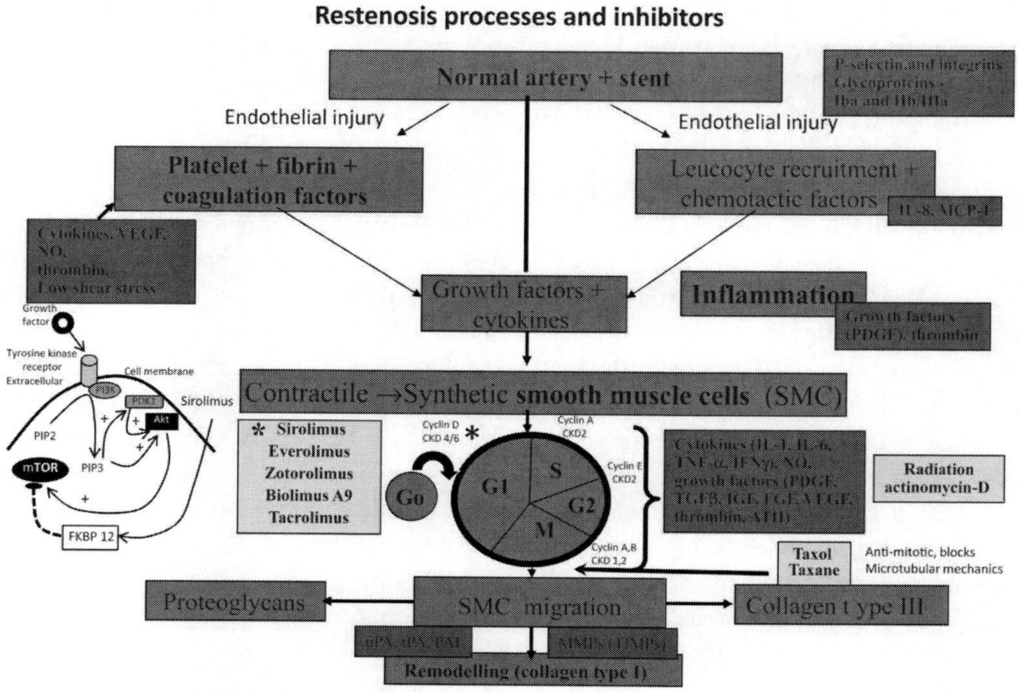

Chaabane C et al. Cardiovasc Res 2013;99:353-363

Figure 1. Overview of the molecular mechanisms of restenosis and their inhibitors. The normal coronary artery is injured secondarily from ballooning and stenting resulting in endothelial cells (EC) loss followed by mural thrombus consisting of platelet aggregation with fibrin deposition. The platelets within the thrombus release a number of chemokines essential for the initiation of inflammation. This includes activation of P-selectin and integrins such as β2-integrin Mac-1 and thrombin. Local production of chemokines like interleukin (IL)-1, IL-6, interferon (IFN)γ, and tumour necrosis factor-alpha (TNF-α) by macrophages result in the induction of inflammation at the injury site. The injury is not only to the endothelium but also to the underlying medial wall. There is an imbalance between stimulatory growth factors (PDGF, FGF, TGF-β, and IGF-1) and chemokines and the inhibitory factors like endothelial-derived nitric oxide and heparin sulfate proteoglycans that results in the activation of smooth muscle cells (SMCs). The SMCs within the media transform from a quiescent contractile state to a synthetic cell which not only proliferate but also migrate into the intima. Within the intima they further proliferate but also secrete extracellular matrix. SMC proliferation involves cell division with different cyclins that are required at different steps of the cell cycle. CDK (cyclin-dependent kinase) activity is also regulated by cell-cycle inhibitory proteins called cyclin-dependent kinase inhibitors (CKIs), which counteract CDK activity. SMC membranes are also stimulated by several classes of tyrosine kinase receptors (TKR). One of the intracellular signalling pathways involves the phosphatidylinositol (PI)3-kinase (PI3K) pathway. PI3K is a lipid kinase that phosphorylates PI. The dominant lipid product generated by PI3K—PI 3,4-biphosphate (PIP2) and PI 3,4,5-triphosphate (PIP3), the latter recruits phosphoinositide-dependent kinase-1 and Akt. Akt is then capable of phosphorylating the mammalian target of rapamycin (mTOR). The yellow squares show the various inhibitors and at which site of the cell cycle they are involved, especially sirolimus and its analogues which inhibit mTOR, whereas paclitaxel blocks microtubular mechanisms. Reproduced with permission from Chaabane et al. [15].

Growth Factors: Macrophages enhance the inflammatory response, and along with platelets and endothelial cells serve to secrete growth factors. These growth factors, including PDGF, fibroblast growth factor (FGF), insulin-like growth factor (IGF), and transforming growth factor beta (TGF-B), work in a synergistic and interdependent fashion resulting in SMC proliferation and migration [23,24], promoting restenosis through neointimal hyperplasia.

Smooth muscle cells: In order for SMCs to undergo proliferation and migration, they must be transformed from a contractile to a synthetic phenotype. SMCs in the media of normal arteries are predominantly contractile phenotype (quiescent and non-proliferative) in the normal state [25]. Once injury to the vessel occurs, however, there is an imbalance between stimulatory growth factors (PDGF, FGF, IGF, and TGF-B) and chemokines (cyclin dependent kinases (CDKs) and inhibitory factors such as endothelial-derived nitric oxide, heparin sulfate proteoglycans, and cyclin dependent kinase inhibitors (CKDIs); this imbalance serves to induce SMC activation (and conversion from quiescent contractile phase to synthetic phenotype) and migration from media to intima. Unlike SMCs in media, which normally exist in phase G0 of cell cycle, the SMCs in the intima enter into the cell cycle and undergo proliferation. This SMC cell cycle is the final common pathway that leads to intimal hyperplasia. Indeed, understanding this mechanism is what has led to the discovery that inhibiting the cell cycle of the SMC with various agents could decrease intimal hyperplasia and resultant restenosis. Sirolimus and its analogues, for example, work by inhibiting two steps in this mechanism. First, they inhibit degradation of CDKIs, and second, they block tyrosine kinase, which prevents SMC stimulation. Once in the intima the SMCs not only proliferate but secrete ECM. The matrix also traps inflammatory cells that release MMPs. Through the action of MMPs, the SMC are able to remodel the ECM by digesting the hyaluronase such that collagen type I and III production occurs, ultimately leading to wound healing and fibrosis [15].

Taken together, while bare metal stents prevent elastic recoil and eliminate negative remodeling, the sequence of injury, thrombogenesis, inflammation, and the resultant growth factors and smooth muscle cell migration, proliferation and activity, cause significant neointimal formation that persists for roughly 6-12 months. Since the final common pathway for tissue growth appeared to be SMC proliferation and matrix production, the next iteration of stent technology, drug-eluting stents, aimed to inhibit the cell cycle and thereby markedly reduce neointimal hyperplasia.

Drug-Eluting Stent Restenosis

Drug-eluting stents (DES) were the next evolutionary step as they combined properties of radial vessel support similar to BMS with the possibility of local anti-proliferative drug delivery. The drug is delivered on permanent polymer coatings with most of the drug being delivered in 3-6 months. Accordingly, DES have further decreased the incidence of restenosis [12], with recent studies showing rates less than 10% in real world practice.

Initial clinical trials reported near undetectable rates of restenosis following DES implantation in short term follow-up. However, both long term follow-up and "real-world" application and analysis have determined that both angiographically and clinically significant in-stent restenosis does occur and remains a clinical challenge. Rates of DES restenosis are now thought to be roughly 5-10% at 2 years out [26], a marked improvement over BMS but problematic when it occurs. As in balloon angioplasty and BMS, shear stress and mechanical stretch play a role in causing platelet activation, thrombus formation, and resultant inflammatory reaction. To further understand the mechanism of in-stent restenosis specific to DES, however, it is imperative to first understand the mechanism of action of the drugs they contain.

The immunosuppressant drugs include Sirolimus, Tacrolimus, Everolimus, Zotrolimus, and BiolimusA9. They are delivered (eluted) from within durable polymers, and work on both SMCs and endothelial cells. On SMCs they work by inhibiting the mammalian target of repamycin and preventing the degradation of pk27ip1, a CDKI that plays an important role in regulating vascular SMC migration and proliferation [27]. They are also potent inhibitors of endothelial cells by deactivating the p70 S6 kinase pathway, an essential step for cell-cycle interaction and arterial healing [28].

Human autopsy studies and clinical trials have shown the high efficiency of DES in comparison with BMS in preventing restenosis (neointimal hyperplasia) at the cost of delayed arterial healing of the stented segment, including delayed endothelialization [29]. Angiographic studies show peak neointimal formation at 6 months for BMS, whereas in DES neointimal formation was delayed but remained a dynamic process with late lumen loss seen even at five years out [12, 30]. A recent autopsy study of DES restenosis found that restenosis was more frequently found in distal regions of coronary vessels, which exhibited more pronounced vessel injury or uneven strut distribution. This lead to drug being concentrated in some areas of the stent, and other areas where inter-strut distance was greatest were associated with less drug concentration and higher rates of restenosis [31, 32]. Histological examination of these restenotic DES lesions demonstrated greater proteoglycan deposition, and fewer SMCs when compared with duration-matched BMS lesions [7, 31]. The exact mechanism of increased proteoglycan deposition in restenotic DES lesions is not well understood, but is at the crux of the problem of DES restenosis. Indeed, medicated stents work by inhibiting SMC infiltration and proliferation but do not affect proteoglycan deposition.

High resolution optical coherence tomography (OCT) and IVUS have noted BMS restenosis to have a predominantly homogenous high-signal tissue echogenicity, while DES restenosis has exhibited a heterogeneous tissue composition, consistent with uneven strut distribution [33]. Therefore, DES neointimal hyperplasia, leading to restenosis, occurs due to several reasons. First, absent or uneven drug distribution from a myriad of causes such as uneven struts, malapposition, stent fracture or medication dissipation is a contributor. Second a persistent inflammatory response is present, mainly due to permanent polymer, although incomplete drug delivery has been thought to play a small role as well. Third, and most importantly delayed arterial healing from antiproliferative effects of medicated stents leads to delayed but dynamic and persistent neointimal growth (late luminal creep) [7]. In addition to causing delayed neointimal hyperplasia, delayed arterial healing leads to accelerated in-stent neoartherosclerosis in DES, and will be the focus of the next section of this chapter.

Although there are differences in rates of restenosis among different DES, it is unlikely due to different mechanisms and more likely due to second generation stents each having distinct technology, such as thinner struts and flexible cell geometry. These advancements have led to a decreased inflammatory response than was seen with the thicker more rigid first generation stents, and consequently lower restenosis rates [34]. An exception may be seen in diabetics, as higher rates of restenosis were seen in first-generation Zotarolimus eluting stents compared to Paclitaxel and Sirolimus eluting stents in a national registry study comparing drug-eluting stents in patients with and without diabetes mellitus [26]. However this was felt to be due to inadequate duration of drug delivery, which did not adequately cover the period of maximal restenotic response. It was also hypothesized that a difference in the mechanism of action of paclitaxel and sirolimus in diabetics exists [35]. However, the differences are likely due to differential abilities of the two distinct anti-proliferative agents among patients with hyperglycemia, and not due to differences in the underlying mechanisms of restenosis. Accordingly, no studies to date have shown a difference in the underlying mechanism of restenosis with different DES.

Neoatherosclerosis

Neoatherosclerosis is a relatively new term, characterized as infiltration of foamy macrophage clusters within the neointima. The appearance is similar to de novo atherosclerosis, hence the term. Traditionally, intimal hyperplasia after BMS implantation has been considered a stable and confined process, with peak activity between 6 months and 1 year and relative quiescence thereafter. However, further long-term follow-up studies demonstrated a 3 phase luminal response after BMS placement: early restenosis (neointimal formation), followed by regression, then a late luminal re-narrowing likely related to neoatherosclerosis beyond 4 years [36]. In one OCT study comparing early neointima in BMS (<6 months) with late phase (>5 years), early phase neointima exhibited a homogenous OCT appearance, and there was a lack of lipid-laden intima. Conversely, lipid-laden intima and intimal disruption were more frequently observed in the late phase when compared with early phase (67% vs. 0%, 38% vs. 0%, respectively, $p<0.05$) [37]. Further, a histologic study looked at new restenotic lesions that developed beyond 5 years in 14 BMS lesions. These restenotic tissues retrieved by directional coronary atherctomy were composed of newly developed atherosclerosis overlaying the previously healed intima [38]. This was an important finding as prior studies suggested that chronic inflammation induced late de novo neoatherosclerosis inside BMS and DES. This hypothesis is less likely as there is a significant difference in the timing of neoatherosclerosis development between BMS and DES, likely due to different pathogenesis. This difference in timing was seen in an autopsy study which compared 66 DES lesions with 77 BMS lesions [39]. Neoatherosclerotic change, including the presence of lipid-laden foamy macrophages was more frequently identified in DES lesions than in BMS (35% vs. 10% $p<0.001$). A significant difference in the timing of neoatherosclerosis development was also noted; the earliest atherosclerotic change was seen 4 months after DES implantation, whereas the same change in BMS occurred beyond 2 years and remained a rare occurrence until 4 years [40].

The theory underlying accelerated in-stent neoatherosclerosis after DES placement is not well understood, but is thought to be due to DES-induced delayed arterial healing. This delay in healing, leads to an absence or dysfunctional arrangement of endothelial cells, which may predispose to early migration of lipid particles into the intima and resultant neoatherosclerosis, whereas the same does not occur when an intact endothelium is present earlier in the pathophysiology, as seen for BMS. Further validating this theory is the fact that clinical studies have shown endothelial dysfunction to be a well-documented phenomenon with DES as compared to BMS [40,41,42], consistent with their anti-proliferative mechanism of action. Other histopathological and autopsy studies have confirmed these findings of neoatherosclerosis occurring at a greater rate and earlier in DES as compared to BMS (6 months vs. 5 years, respectively), [41] contributing to clinical restenosis. See Table 2.

Table 2. Comparison of neointimal hyperplasia and neoatherosclerosis in BMS and DES

	Neointimal Hyperplasia	Neoatherosclerosis
Timing	Early in BMS Late in DES	Late in BMS Early in DES
Composition	Marked reparative process leading to homogenous neointima, made up of SMC and ECM, in BMS Minimal reparative process, leading to less homogenous neointima made up of predominantly of ECM and less SMC, in DES.	Lipid-laden foamy macrophages in clusters within the neointima, in both BMS and DES.

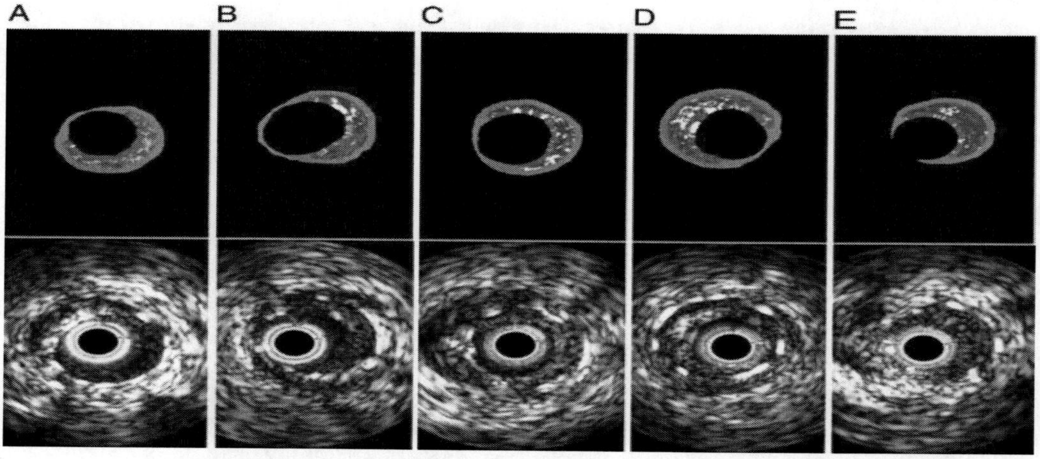

(A) Six-month follow-up of paclitaxel-eluting stent [percent necrotic core [%NC] 10%, percent dense calcium [%DC] 2%); (B) 9-month follow-up of paclitaxel-eluting stent (%NC 28%, %DC 8%); (C) 22-month follow-up of paclitaxel-eluting stent (%NC 39%, %DC 20%); (D) 48-month follow-up of bare-metal stent (%NC 40%, %DC 25%); and(E) 57-month follow-up of bare-metal stent (%NC 57%, %DC 15%). Reprinted with permission from Park SJ et al. [41].

Seung-Jung Park, Soo-Jin Kang, Renu Virmani, Masataka Nakano, Yasunori Ueda. In-Stent Neoatherosclerosis: A Final Common Pathway of Late Stent Failure. Journal of the American College of Cardiology Volume 59, Issue 23 2012 2051 – 2057.

Figure 2.

In addition to histopathological and autopsy studies, angiographic, IVUS, OCT, and near infrared light-based imaging studies have all confirmed the presence of in-stent neoatherosclerosis in both BMS and DES. It is clear that neoatherosclerosis plays an important role in restenosis after both BMS and DES, but more relevant and to a larger extent in DES, as it occurs earlier in the process (see figure2) [42]. Thus, while DES results in a marked reduction in neointimal hyperplasia through inhibition of SMC activity, the endothelial dysfunction likely results in neoatherosclerosis that begins early. While overall a major advance, especially with second generation DES, future platforms aim to rectify these new findings and contributors to both early and late clinical events.

Conclusion

Coronary artery restenosis after percutaneous intervention has been the bane of interventional cardiology since the advent of balloon angioplasty. Over the last 35 years significant advancements have been made to treat this problem. Unfortunately, with each breakthrough in technology has come a new process by which restenosis could still occur, albeit at lower rates each time. Restenosis in balloon angioplasty is mainly due to elastic recoil and negative remodeling. Because of these mechanisms the BMS was invented, which reduced restenosis markedly. However, the tissue reacted to the foreign body of the BMS by producing neointimal hyperplasia over the stent. Once we understood the mechanism behind neointimal hyperplasia we invented the DES to treat it, by incorporating a durable polymer and anti-proliferative drugs. DES leads to delayed arterial healing (including delayed endothelialization and SMC activity) which reduced restenosis overall, but delayed neointimal hyperplasia and caused early neoatherosclerosis from endothelial dysfunction. While rates of restenosis have continued to decline to almost clinically irrelevant rates, new problems such as neoatherosclerosis may prove more problematic and will need to be addressed.

Future Directions

With the above understanding, it would appear that the best way to combat restenosis might be to utilize stents with thin struts that minimize vessel injury, polymers that are inert and do not cause any inflammatory reaction, and drugs that target SMCs but not endothelial cells. In addition, stents that disappear over time (bioabsorbable stents) and drugs that target SMCs and then are completely eluted (no residual) would be ideal. Accordingly, clinical trials are ongoing to evaluate bio-absorbable polymer coated stents. The EVOLVE and DISSOLVE trials showed safety of bio-absorbable polymer stents and non-inferiority to current DES [43, 44]. In the DISSOLVE trial the MiStent used very thin 64 micron struts coated with Sirolimus in a fully absorbable polymer. Deposition of the drug into the surrounding tissue occurred at a controlled rate through 6 months and the polymer is then fully absorbed into tissue within 90 days, leaving an inert BMS. In this study they observed decreased neointimal formation up to 8 months, followed by no further progression up to 18 months. Using IVUS they hypothesized that this was due to absence of late in-stent neointimal "catch-up" phenomenon [44], presumably due to the lack of any pro-inflammatory polymer. Despite the promise shown with these new stents, long-term and post-marketing studies need to be conducted, to evaluate restenosis rates and any other potential new problems.

More recently, the ABSORB trial is evaluating a fully absorbable stent, polymer and drug-delivery system. In this trial, a bioabsorbable everolimus eluting stent (BVS) system was used. The BVS stent has a bioabsorbable poly-L-lactic acid (PLLA) backbone with a bioabsorbable poly-D, L-lactide (PDLLA) coating that contains everolimus. Both PLLA and PDLLA are fully bioabsorbable. During bioabsorption the long chains of PLLA and PDLLA are broken down into small particles less than 2 um in diameter and phagocytosed by macrophages. Finally, PLLA and PDLLA are degraded to lactic acid, which in turn is metabolized by the Krebs cycle into carbon dioxide and water [45]. Subsequent studies using multiple imaging modalities evaluated the 30 patients enrolled in the ABSORB trial. The multi-imaging approach has shown several important findings. Echogenicity, IVUS-virtual histology and OCT showed that by 2 years the stent was completely absorbed, leaving behind proteoglycan with translucent appearance by OCT. IVUS also showed at 2 years late enlargement of the lumen, likely because the vessel was not adherent to a stent with fixed diameter, and thereby can continue to undergo positive remodeling. Coronary angiograms did not corroborate late lumen enlargement but did show stable lumen size between 6 months and 2 years [46].

This study also alluded to the return of normal endothelial function. Nine patients received acetylcholine, an endothelium dependent vasoactive agent at two years post stent placement to evaluate vasomotor function. 5 of the 9 patients showed vasodilatation suggesting a response to acetylcholine and presence of functionally active endothelium at the site of stent implantation [46]. If these results, specifically homogenous vessel wall structure and restoration of vasomotor function, can be duplicated with large multi-center trials, it would be a significant advancement in combating restenosis because they suggest healing of the artery with a return to normal, protective functioning.

References

[1] Mueller R. and Sanborn T. The History of Interventional Cardiology, *Am Heart J* 1995; 129:146-72.

[2] Hamid H, Coltart J. 'Miracle stents" – a future without restenosis. *Mcgill J Med.* 2007;10(2):105-11.

[3] Libby P. *The Vascular Biology of Atherosclerosis.* In: Bonow RO, Mann DL, Zipes DP, Libby P, Ed. Braunwald's Heart Disease: A textbook of Cardiovascular Medicine 9th Ed. Vol 1 Ch. 43: *The Vascular Biology of Atherosclerosis*. 2012. 897-913.

[4] Kastrati A, Schomig A, Elezi S, et al. Predictive factors of restenosis after coronary stent placement. *J Am Coll Cardiol* 1997; 30: 1428-1436.

[5] Berenguer A, Mainar V, Bordes P, Valencia J et al. Incidence and predictors of restenosis after sirolimus-eluting stent implantation in high-risk patients. *Am Heart J* 2005; 150: 536-542.

[6] Casscells W, Engler D, Willerson JT. *Mechanisms of Restenosis*. Texas Heart Institute Journal 1994; 21: 68-77.

[7] Byrne RA, Joner M, Tada T, Kastrati A. Restenosis in bare metal and drug-eluting stents: distinct mechanistic insights from histopathology and optical intravascular imaging. *Minerva Cardioangiol*. 2012; 60: 473-89.

[8] Rensing BJ, Hermans WRM, Beatt KJ, et al. Quantitative angiographic assessment of elastic recoil after percutaneous transluminal coronary angioplasty. *Am J Cardiol* 1990; 66: 1039-44.

[9] Berglund H, Luo H, Niskioka T, et al. Highly Localized Arterial Remodeling in Patients With Coronary Atherosclerosis: An Intravascular Ultrasound Study. *Circulation*. 1997; 96:1470-1476.

[10] Schoenhagen P, Ziada KM, et al. Arterial Remodeling and Coronary Artery Disease: The Concept of "Dilated" versus "Obstructive" Coronary Atherosclerosis. *J Am Coll Cardiol.* 2001; 38 (2): 297-306.

[11] McPherson DD, Sirna SJ, Hiratzka LF, et al. Coronary arterial remodeling studied by high-frequency epicardial echocardiography. *J Am Coll Cardiol* 1991; 17: 79-86.

[12] Kim MS, Dean LS. In-Stent Restenosis. *Cardiovascular therapeutics*. 2011; 29: 190-198.

[13] Grewe PH, Deneke T, Machraoui A et al. Acute and chronic tissue response to coronary stent implantation: Pathologic findings in human specimens. *J Am Coll Cardiol* 2000; 35:157-163.

[14] Ashikaga H, Ben-Yehuda O, *Chien KR. Coronary Restenosis*. In: Chien KR, Ed. *Molecular Basis of Cardiovascular Disease: a companion to Braunwald's heart disease*. 2nd. Ed. 2004 Ch. 25; 455-469.

[15] Chaabane C, Otsuka, F. et al. Biological responses in stented arteries. *Cardiovascular Research* 2013; 99:353-363.

[16] Virmani R, Kolodgie FD, Farb A, Lafont A. Drug eluting stents: are human and animal studies comparable?. *Heart* 2003;89:133-138.

[17] Inoue T, Sohma R, Miyazaki T, et al.: Comparison of activation process of platelets and neutrophils after coronary stent implantation versus balloon angioplasty for stable angina pectoris. *Am J Cardiol* 2000; 86: 1057-1062.

[18] Yasukawa H, Imaizumi T, Matsuoka H, et al. Inhibition of intimal hyperplasia after balloon injury by antibodies to intercellular adhesion molecule-1 and lymphocyte function-associated antigen-1. *Circulation* 1997;95:1515-1522.

[19] Simon DI, Dhen Z, Seifert P, et al. Decreased neointimal formation in Mac-1(-/-) mice reveals a role for inflammation in vascular repair after angioplasty. *J clin Invest* 2000;105:293-300.

[20] Rao GN, Berk BC. Active oxygen species stimulate vascular smooth muscle growth and proto-oncogene expression. *Circ Res* 1992; 70: 593-599.

[21] Furukawa Y, Matsumori A, Ohashi N, et al.: Anti-monocyte chemoattractant protein-1/monocyte chemotactic and activating factor antibody inhibits neointimal hyperplasia in injured rat carotid arteries. *Circ Res*. 1999; 84: 306-314.

[22] Ikeda U, Ikeda M, Oohara T, et al. Mitogenic action of interleukin-1 alpha on vascular smooth muscle cells mediated by PDGF. *Atherosclerosis* 1990; 84: 183-188.

[23] Delafontaine P, Lou H, Alexander RW. Regulation of insulin-like growth factor I messenger RNA levels in vascular smooth muscle cells. *Hypertension* 1991; 18: 742-747.

[24] Grant MB, Wargovich TJ, Ellis EA, et al. Localization of insulin-like growth factor I and inhibition of coronary smooth muscle cell growth by somatostatin analogues in human coronary smooth muscle cells: A potential treatment for restenosis? *Circulation* 1994; 89: 1511-1517.

[25] Campbell JH, Campbell GR. Smooth muscle phenotypic modulation- a personal experience. *Arterioscler Thrombo Vasc Biol* 2012;32: 1784-1789.

[26] Frobert O, Lagerqvist B, Carlsson J et al. Differences in Restenosis Rate With Different Drug-Eluting Stents in Patients With and Without Diabetes Mellitus. *J Am Coll Cardiol* 2009; 53:1660-7.

[27] Grewe PH, Deneke T, Machraoui A, et al. Acute and chronic tissue response to coronary stent implantation: Pathologic findings in human specimen. *J Am Coll Cardiol* 2000; 35: 157-163.

[28] CharronT, Nili N, Strauss BH. The cell cycle: a critical therapeutic target to prevent vascular proliferative disease. *Can J Cardiol* 2006; 22 (Suppl. B):41B-55B.

[29] Joner M, Finn AV, Farb A, et al. Pathology of Drug-Eluting Stents in Humans: Delayed Healing and Late Thrombotic Risk. *J Am Coll Cardiol* 2006;48:193-202.

[30] Byrne RA, Joner M, et al. Restenosis in bare metal and drug-eluting stents: distinct mechanistic insights from histopathology and optical intravascular imaging. *Minerva Cardioangiol.* 2012; 60 (5):473-89.

[31] Von Zur Muhlen C, Kahlert P, Bode C. Coronary stent restenosis and occlusion: messages from the dead. *Eur Heart J* 2013; First published online 0ct 2.

[32] Nakano M, Otsuka F, Yahagi K et al. Human autopsy study of drug-eluting stents restenosis: histomorphological predictors and neointimal characteristics. *Euro Heart Journal* 2013; 34 3304-3313.

[33] Ando H, Amano T, Takashima H, et al. Differences in tissue characterization of restenotic neointima between sirolimus-eluting stent and bare-metal stent: integrated backscatter intravascular ultrasound analysis for in-stent restenosis. *European Heart Journal – Cardiovascular Imaging* 2013;14: 996-1001.

[34] Stone GW, Rizvi A, Newman W, et al. Everolimus-eluting versus paclitaxel-eluting stents in coronary artery disease. *N Engl J Med* 2010; 362:1663-1674.

[35] Mahmud E, Bromberg-Marin G, Palakodeti V, et al. Clinical efficacy of drug-eluting stents in diabetic patients: a meta-analysis. *J Am Coll Cardiol* 2008; 51: 2385-95.

[36] Kang SJ, Song HG, Ahn JM et al. OCT-Verified Neotherosclerosis in BMS Restenosis at 10 years. J Am Coll Cardiol: Cardiovascular Imaging. 2012; 5 (12): 1267-68.

[37] Gonzalo N, Serruys PW, Okamura T, et al. Optical coherence tomography patterns of stent restenosis. *Am Heart J* 2009; 158:284-93.

[38] Hasegawa K, Tamai H, Kyo E, et al. Histopathological findings of new in-stent lesions developed beyond five years. *Catheter Cardiovasc Interv* 2006;68:554-8.

[39] Nakazawa G, Vorpahl M, Finn AV et al. One step forward and two steps back with drug-eluting stents. *J Am Coll Cardiol Img* 2009; 2:623-628.

[40] Yonetsu T, Kim JS, Kato K, Kim SJ et al. Comparison of incidence and Time Course of Neoatherosclerosis Between Bare Metal Stents and Drug-Eluting Stents Using Optical Coherence Tomography. *Am J Cardiol* 2012;110: 933-939.

[41] Park SJ, Kang SJ, Viramani R, et al. In-Stent Neoatherosclerosis: A Final Common Pathway of Late Stent Failure. *J Am Coll Cardiol.* 2012; 59(23): 2051-7

[42] Nakazawa G, Otsuka F, Nakano M, et al. The pathology of neoatherosclerosis in human coronary implants bare-metal and drug-eluting stents. *J Am Coll Cardiol* 2011; 57:1314-22.

[43] Meredith I, Verheye S, Dubois C, et al. Primary Endpoint Results of the EVOLVE Trial: A Randomized Evaluation of a Novel Bioabsorbable Polymer-Coated, Everolimus-Eluting Coronary Stent. *J Am Coll Cardiol* 2012; 59: 1362-70.

[44] Ormiston J, Webster M, Stewart J, et al. First-in-Human Evaluation of a Bioabsorbable Polymer-coated Sirolimus-Eluting Stent: Imaging and Clinical Results of the DESSOLVE I Trial (DES with Sirolimus and a Bioabsorbable Polymer for the Treatment of Patients With De Novo Lesion in the Native Coronary Arteries). *J Am Coll Cardiol: Cardiovascular Interventions* 2013; 6: 1026-34.

[45] Ormiston JA, Serruys PW, Regar E, et al. A bioabsorbable everolimus-eluting coronary stent system for patients with single de-novo coronary artery lesions (ABSORB): a prospective open-label trial. *Lancet* 2008; 371:899-907.

[46] Serruys PW, Ormiston JA, Onuma Y, et al. A bioabsorbable everolimus-eluting coronary stent system (ABSORB): 2-year outcomes and results from multiple imaging methods. *Lancet* 2009;373: 897-910.

[47] Charron T, Nili N, Strauss BH. The cell cycle: a critical therapeutic target to prevent vascular proliferative disease. *Can J Cardiol* 2006; 22(suppl.B): 41B-55B.

In: Coronary Artery Restenosis
Editor: Amir S. Lotfi

ISBN: 978-1-63321-346-3

Chapter 3

Morphologic Patterns of In-Stent Restenosis

Gennaro Giustino, MD[1], Daniele Giacoppo, MD[2], Jennifer Yu, MBBS[2] and Roxana Mehran, MD[2*]
[1]Ospedale San Raffaele, Milan, Italy
[2]Mount Sinai Medical Center,
New York, New York, US

Abstract

In-stent restenosis (ISR), first described as a major limitation of percutaneous coronary intervention with bare-metal stents (BMS), continues to occur albeit at a reduced rate after the introduction of drug-eluting stents (DES). The pathogenesis of ISR is multifactorial and involves clinical, biological, mechanical and technical factors. Specific underlying mechanisms of ISR can often manifest in its morphological pattern and this has led to attempts in ISR morphology classification. In turn, the ISR pattern classification has been demonstrated to correlate with mid- and long-term outcomes following treatment.

The predominant observed pattern of ISR differs between BMS and DES and reflects differences in the causative mechanisms of BMS- and DES- ISR. The most common ISR pattern in BMS is diffuse. Conversely the most common ISR pattern in DES is focal, with a higher prevalence of diffuse ISR associated with paclitaxel-eluting stents (PES) as compared to sirolimus-eluting stents (SES). In the DES era, the morphologic pattern of DES-ISR remains an important predictor of clinical outcomes. Finally, recent advances in intravascular imaging technology such as intravascular ultrasound virtual histology and optical coherence tomography have improved our understanding of the pathophysiology and morphologic patterns of ISR.

---

* Corresponding Author: Roxana Mehran MD, The Zena and Michael A. Wiener Cardiovascular Institute. The Icahn School of Medicine at Mount Sinai. One Gustave L. Levy Place, Box 1030. New York, NY 10029-6574. Roxana.Mehran@mountsinai.org

1. Introduction

In this chapter we will discuss in-depth the morphology of in-stent restenosis (ISR) observed by coronary angiography and endovascular imaging following PCI with different stents, and examine the associations between ISR morphology, pathogenesis and treatment outcomes. The other aspects of ISR including definition, etiology and treatment will be covered in other chapters in this book.

The advent of percutaneous coronary intervention (PCI) with bare-metal stents (BMS) gave rise to the new phenomenon of in-stent restenosis. Although stent delivery system design evolved over the following decade, ISR remained the “Achilles’ heel” of coronary stenting procedures resulting in repeated revascularizations of target (treated) lesions [1, 2]. The morphologic patterns of ISR relate to multiple biological, mechanical, and technical factors and clinical outcomes [3]. Furthermore, the morphology of ISR can hint toward the specific underlying pathophysiological mechanism involved, which in turn may impact on clinical and procedural outcomes [4].

The ISR pattern can be classified in general as focal (≤ 10 mm in length) or diffuse (> 10 mm in length). In addition, the Mehran classification provides information regarding the geographic position of the lesion relative to stent landmarks[5]. This classification was shown in the same and subsequent studies, to be correlated with long-term clinical outcomes, specifically, the need for repeat revascularization. These initial studies were carried out in the BMS era. The most common morphologic pattern of BMS ISR was diffuse neointimal hyperplasia, distributed uniformly over the length of the stent (diffuse pattern) with or without involvement of the proximal and distal edges [6, 7]

The introduction of the drug-eluting stent (DES) led to the significant reduction in the occurrence of ISR and target lesion revascularization (TLR) after PCI compared to BMS [8-10]. However, with the progressive expansion of PCI performance to high-risk patients as well as more complex coronary lesions, TLR continues to be a limitation of PCI today [11, 12]. Furthermore, the specific morphologic pattern associated with coronary stenting shifted from a relatively high incidence of diffuse pattern with BMS to a highly prevalent focal pattern with DES, in particular most commonly situated at the proximal stent edge [13].

On histopathological analyses, the in-stent neointimal hyperplasia (NIH) which comprises ISR, bears close resemblance between BMS- and DES-ISR [6, 14-16]. While some differences at the cellular level were present, histologically the NIH with both BMS and DES was characterized by smooth muscle cell proliferation and areas rich in neo-synthesized collagen and reticular fibers. The observed differences in the morphologic patterns of ISR between BMS and DES, and amongst different types of DES, were therefore attributed biological, technical and device-related pathogenic factors, for example focal DES-ISR related to local failure of drug delivery [17].

Finally, recent advances in intracoronary imaging technologies including virtual histology intravascular ultrasound (VH-IVUS), optical coherence tomography (OCT) and near-infrared spectroscopy (NIRS) has added further insight to the characterization of ISR morphology and pathophysiology and resulted in new classifications based on observed morphologic patterns.

2. Classification of Angiographic Patterns of In-Stent Restenosis

Although various ISR classifications have been proposed, the most widely used and accepted is the classification by Mehran and colleagues [5]. The 288 ISR lesions observed in 245 patients post PCI with BMS were classified according to the angiographic morphological pattern (Figure 1):

- Class I, "Focal ISR group": Lesions are ≤10 mm in length and are sub-classified according to location in the unscaffolded segment (the articulation or gap between two stents, Type IA), the proximal or distal margin (Type IB), the body of the stent (Type IC), or a combination of these sites ("multifocal ISR", Type ID).
- Class II, "Diffuse ISR": Lesions are > 10 mm in length and are confined to the stented segment, without extending outside the margins.
- Class III, "Diffuse proliferative" ISR: Lesions are > 10 mm in length and extend beyond the margin(s) of the stented segment.
- Class IV, "ISR with total occlusion": Lesions associated with a Thrombolysis in Myocardial Infarction (TIMI) flow grade of 0.

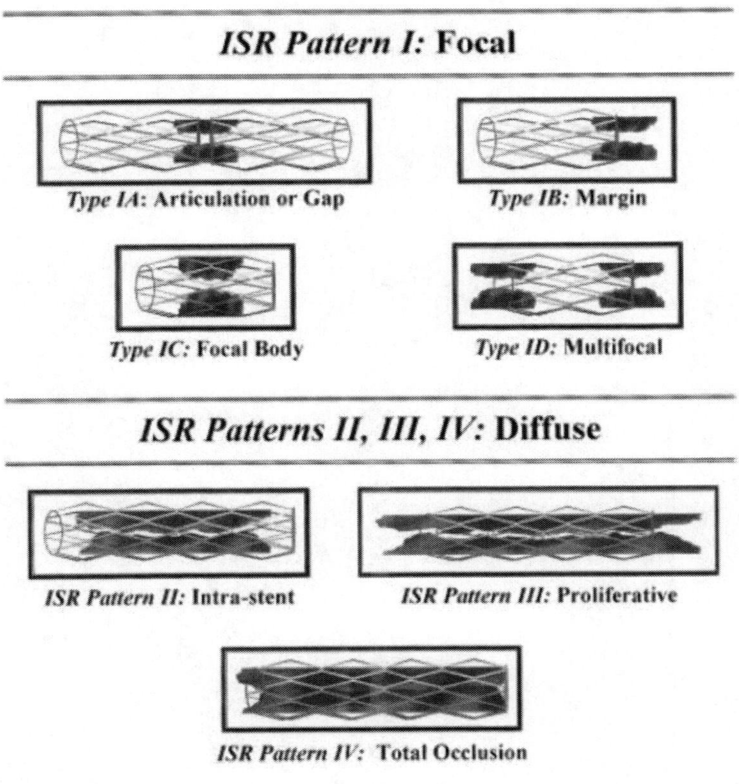

Figure 1. ISR angiographic patterns. Pattern I (Focal-Type) is ≤ 10 mm in length and contains 4 subtypes (Type IA – Type ID). Patterns II – IV (Diffuse-Type) are > 10 mm in length and are distinguished according to the relation with the stent and the vessel lumen. Reproduced with permission from Mehran et al.

Examples of ISR as seen by coronary angiography are illustrated in Figure 2. Before the introduction of this classification, patterns of ISR were grossly described as focal (< 10 mm in length) or diffuse (> 10 mm in length). The Mehran classification added information regarding the topographic relationship between the NIH and the coronary stent.

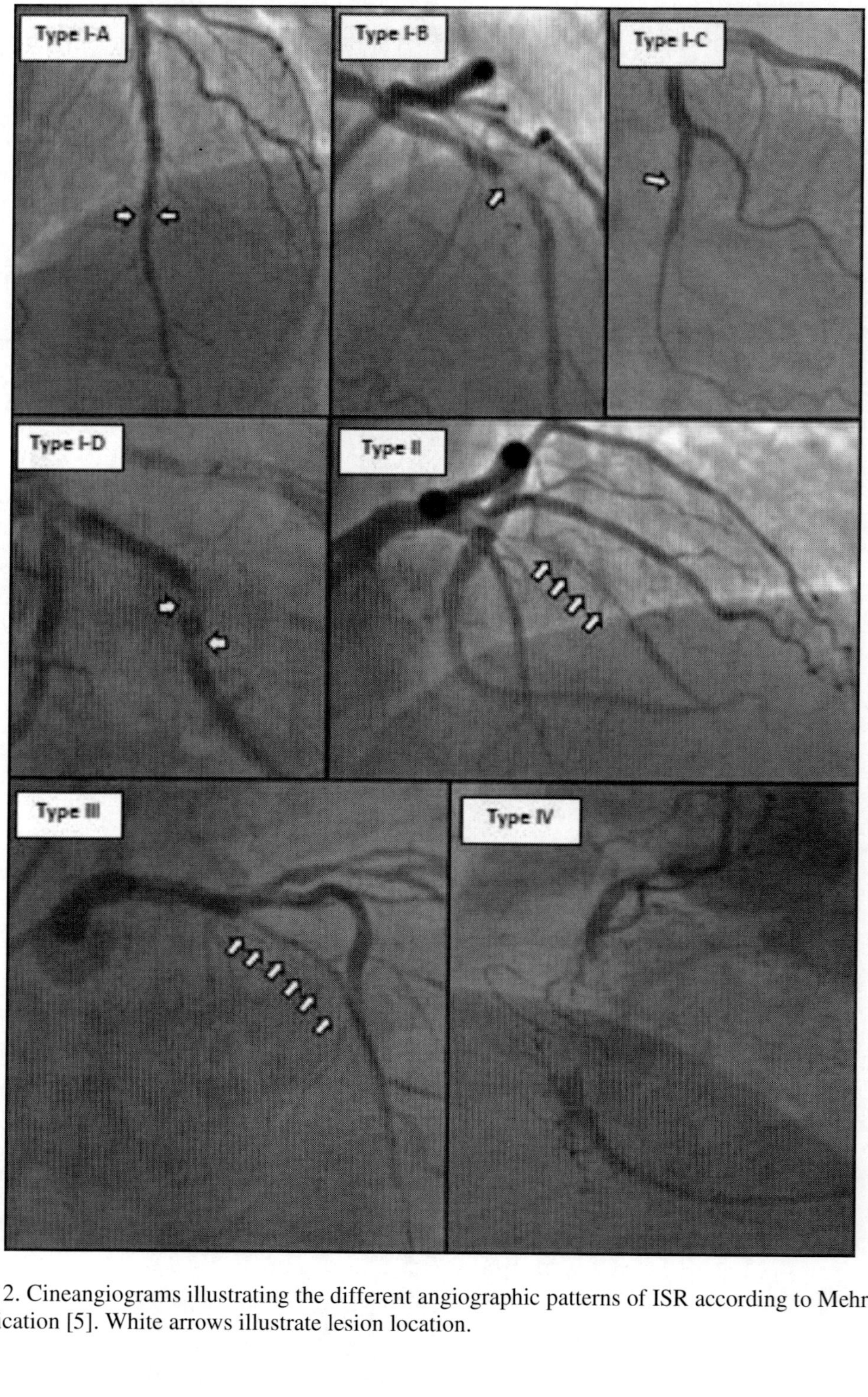

Figure 2. Cineangiograms illustrating the different angiographic patterns of ISR according to Mehran classification [5]. White arrows illustrate lesion location.

Mehran et al. validated their angiographic classification of ISR using intravascular ultrasound (IVUS). IVUS imaging showed that focal-type ISR were shorter and associated with greater luminal and stent cross sectional area (CSA) when compared to higher grade ISR. Interestingly they found that the burden of NIH was similar between the focal-, diffuse intrastent- and diffuse proliferative-ISR.

3. Impact of ISR Pattern on Clinical Outcomes

The angiographic classification of ISR introduced by Mehran and colleagues is not exclusively descriptive but also has prognostic significance [5]. Diffuse intra-stent, proliferative and ISR with total occlusion represent a spectrum of increased ISR severity linked to an exaggerated NIH response. Significantly higher rates of TLR (percutaneous or surgical), were associated with progressively increasing levels of ISR classification (Class I, 19%; Class II, 35%; Class III, 50%; Class IV, 83%; P = 0.0001). In the same study, multivariable hazard regression analysis identified ISR angiographic pattern among factors independently associated with TLR (OR 1.7, P = 0.038).

The morphologic pattern is also a significant predictor of outcomes following treatment of DES-ISR [4, 18]. Cosgrave et al. demonstrated a significantly higher rate of recurrent ISR following percutaneous revascularization (with either DES or POBA) of non-focal versus focal ISR in 1st generation DES (51.1% vs. 17.8%; p = 0.001). Focal-type ISRs were associated with lower late lumen loss (LLL) as compared to non-focal type and lower TLR rates (9.8% vs. 23%, p = 0.007). Following multivariate adjustment they found a robust, independent relationship between ISR non-focal pattern and TLR (OR 3.61, p = 0.02). The same authors also compared DES-ISR in paclitaxel-eluting stents (PES) and sirolimus-eluting stents (SES) treated with the same versus different type of DES (with respect to the drug eluted). Again, non-focal pattern of ISR was associated with higher rates of restenosis as compared to focal type regardless of the DES strategy used (47.1% vs. 20% receiving the same DES, and 40% vs. 13.9% receiving different DES) [4].

Latib et al. observed in a large group of consecutive patients with DES-ISR treated with PCI with stents or POBA that recurrent ISR occurred in 29.1% of the focal-type (Class I), 45.8% (p = 0.007) of the diffuse-type (Class II and III), and 65.6% (p < 0.001) of the occlusive-type (Class IV) ISR. Accordingly, diffuse ISR was associated with a significant increase in TLR compared to focal ISR (27.1% vs. 15.8%; p = 0.008). Diffuse DES-ISR was a strong independent predictor of TLR (HR 2.05, p = 0.02) and recurrent angiographic restenosis (HR 2.19, p < 0.001) at multivariable analysis. Occlusive-type DES-ISR was another strong predictor of recurrent angiographic restenosis (HR: 4.86, p < 0.001). However, the authors attributed the relatively low TLR rate of 22% among patients with occlusive-type ISR to the medical management of recurrent occlusive restenosis in these patients[18]. Rates from several studies of TLR after treatment of BMS- and DES-ISR according to ISR morphologic pattern are reported in Figure 3.

Beyond TLR, other cardiovascular outcomes such as death, myocardial infarction and stent thrombosis, seem to be similar across ISR morphology patterns in both BMS and DES [4,5]. The morphologic pattern of ISR also predicts the pattern of ISR recurrence [18].

Latib et al. demonstrated that the initial pattern of DES-ISR was associated with the same or worse pattern with respect to recurrent ISR (Figure 4): occlusive ISR recurred as a re-occlusion in 66.7%, diffuse ISR (Class II and III) recurred as diffuse or occlusive in 57.9%, and focal ISR (Class I) as recurrent focal ISR in 67.2% of cases [18].

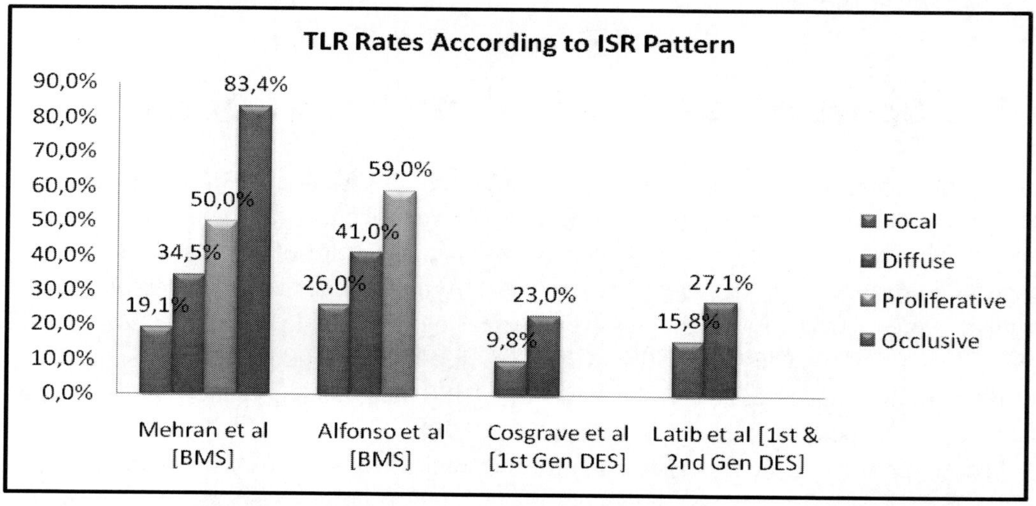

Figure 3. Morphological patterns of ISR predicts treatment outcomes: rates of target lesion revascularization (TLR) according to ISR pattern. Adapted from Mehran et al. [5], Alfonso et al.[21], Cosgrave et al. [19] and Latib et al. [18].

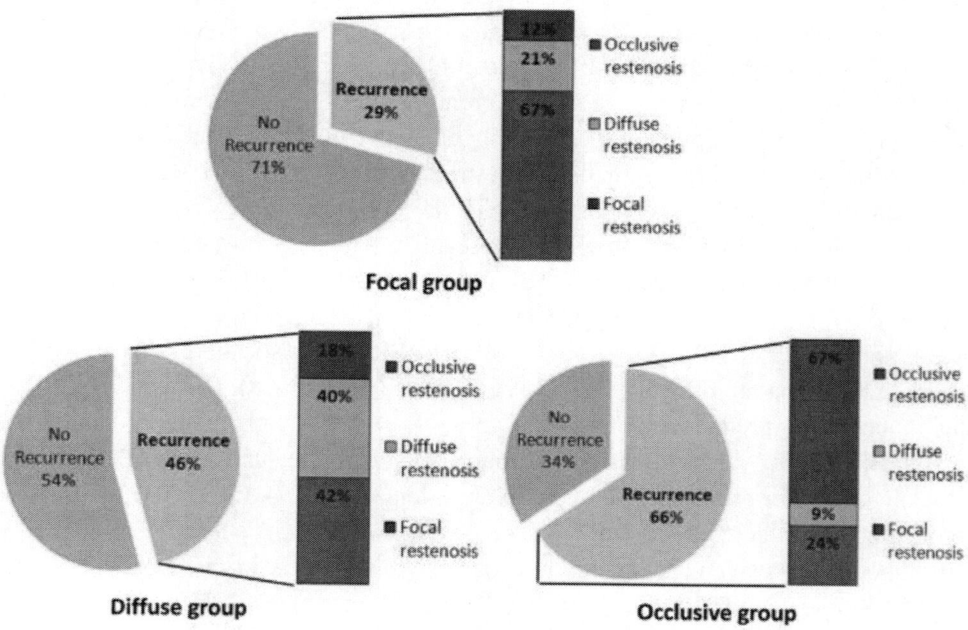

Figure 4. Patterns of Recurrent Angiographic DES-ISR According to the Initial Pattern of Restenosis. Focal-type ISR was associated with the lowest rate of recurrence after ISR treatment. Diffuse-type ISR recurred more commonly as the same or as an occlusive-type ISR. Focal and occlusive ISR recurred more commonly with the same initial pattern of restenosis. Reproduced with permission from Latib et al. [18].

Cosgrave et al. in a study on 250 DES-ISR lesions (treated with POBA or restenting) reported that the pattern of recurrent ISR remained the same as the first ISR in 50% of patients, became worse in 26.2% and improved in 23.8% [19]. Notably, the authors found that one of the most important risk factors for developing recurrent ISR in the non-focal group was the treatment with POBA instead of restenting. Finally, no differences were found in clinical outcomes between groups. However patients with non-focal ISR had a non-significant, numerically higher rate of major adverse cardiac events (focal 18.9% vs. non-focal 29.6%; $p = 0.11$).

Rathore et al. studied 344 patients that underwent treatment for SES-ISR and found that patients with focal versus non-focal ISR treated with repeated stenting or POBA, had lower rate of recurrent ISR (32.4% vs. 49.2%; $p = 0.012$) and target vessel revascularization (TVR, 30.6 vs. 42.9; $p=0.06$) [20]. Furthermore, while restenosis rates were similar after repeated stenting or POBA in focal-type ISR (28% vs. 23%), repeated stenting showed better outcomes than POBA in non-focal-type ISR (36% vs. 60%), suggesting that stenting could be the preferred treatment for non-focal-type SES-ISR. Interestingly, unstable angina was the strongest independent predictor of recurrent ISR after treatment in multivariable analysis (OR: 3.764, $p = 0.014$). Therapeutic implications of ISR patterns will be further discussed in the section "Patterns of In-Stent Restenosis: Therapeutic Implications" in this chapter.

The value of various ISR classification schemes was examined by Alfonso et al. [21]. The authors compared the Mehran, the American College of Cardiology / American Heart Association (ACC/AHA) lesion, and dichotomous focal vs. diffuse classifications as well as an ISR "index" (lesion length to stent length ratio) for the prediction of an acute unsatisfactory result (early angiographic result), recurrent restenosis, and long-term clinical outcomes following ISR treatment. Although the distribution of suboptimal postprocedural results presented good agreement with the original angiographic pattern severity, showing a rise of unsatisfactory results across ISR classes, the highest predictive value was provided by ACC/AHA classification ($p = 0.001$). Additionally, the ACC/AHA classification, designed specifically to predict acute procedural success after percutaneous coronary intervention, when inserted together with Mehran classification in the same logistic regression model, emerged as the only independent factor. Conversely, the Mehran classification, designed to predict recurrent ISR in the long term, emerged as an independent predictor of recurrent ISR ($p = 0.001$) while the ACC/AHA classification was not useful in the long term. None of the aforementioned classification systems were significant predictors of clinical events long-term after multivariable adjustment for other clinical and procedural factors.

4. Histopathology of ISR

The histopathology of BMS-ISR has been studied from post-mortem [22, 23] and endarterectomy [24, 25] specimens. As opposed to the response after POBA, smooth muscle cell proliferation is one of the dominant pathologic processes leading to restenosis after coronary stent implantation. Restenotic tissue in BMS-ISR is generally composed of α-smooth muscle actin-positive cells embedded in a collagen-rich, extra-cellular matrix. In the early stages, greater cellular proliferation and proteoglycan-rich extracellular matrix are characteristic whereas in the later stages, restenosis is composed mainly by large amounts of proteoglycan-rich and collagen-rich extra-cellular matrix with a relatively small number of proliferative smooth muscle cells [25]. In particular, collagen-rich extra-cellular matrix was prevalent in cellular-depleted areas. Interestingly, the composition and burden extra-cellular matrix, but not the extent of cellular proliferation, were correlated to ISR severity.

Van Bausekom and colleagues compared the pathologic features of atherectomy specimens obtained from BMS-ISR, DES-ISR and *de novo* atherosclerotic lesions [26]. They observed that *de novo* atherosclerotic lesions were more commonly collagen-rich whereas ISR tissue with both BMS and DES was more commonly proteoglycan-rich. In both BMS- and DES-ISR the cellular component mainly comprised proliferated smooth muscle cells. Compared to BMS-ISR, DES-ISR was richer in fibrinoid tissue, indicating a persistent incomplete vascular healing response. Furthermore, PES-ISR tissue had a greater fibrinoid component than SES. The percentage of fibrotic tissue in BMS-ISR and PES-ISR were similar, but higher than that found in SES-ISR. The authors also observed that specimen quantity after DES-ISR atherectomy was significantly less when compared to BMS specimens. This difference was most probably due to higher prevalence of focal ISR in DES. These histopathologic differences between BMS- and DES-ISR, as well as the different DES subtypes, may account for the different morphologic patterns of ISR observed with each of these stents.

Later, Chieffo et al. compared the histopathology of ISR with DES and BMS using light microscopy specimens obtained through directional coronary atherectomy [14]. The DES included in this study were SES, PES, zotarolimus-eluting stents (ZES) and tacrolimus-eluting stents (TES). In both BMS- and DES-ISR, specimens were composed mainly of proteoglycan-rich smooth muscle cells, scarce macrophages and a fibrolipidic stroma composed of collagen and reticular fibers. However, differences in smooth muscle cell phenotypes were observed between the restenotic tissue of BMS and DES. Specifically, BMS-, PES-ISR was mainly composed of smooth muscle cell of the intermediate-synthetic phenotype, in ZES of the intermediate phenotype, in SES-ISR of the contractile-intermediate phenotype and TES-ISR mostly of the contractile phenotype. These differences in smooth muscle cell phenotype reflect the differential responses and adaptation to both stent struts and, in the case of DES, to the delivered drug. The association between BMS, PES and intermediate-synthetic phenotype smooth muscle cells may explain in part the higher degree of NIH observed with these stents.

The inflammatory reaction occurring after arterial stenting is a critical factor that influences the burden of ISR. Farb et al. demonstrated that features of acute inflammation at the stent-arterial wall interface were almost always present early after stent implantation [22]. However, the persistence of an inflammatory response at long-term follow-up was associated with greater NIH thickness and subsequent ISR. Importantly, NIH thickness was greater when damage to the arterial tunica media (laceration or rupture) occurred [22].

More recently, in-stent neoatherosclerosis was described as another potential mechanism of stent failure, being associated with both ISR and stent thrombosis (ST) [27, 28]. Neoatherosclerosis is defined as the presence of atherosclerotic plaque elements such as foamy macrophages in clusters with or without calcification, and thin- and thick-cap fibroatheromas within the neointima. An OCT study by Takano et al. assessed the neointimal characteristics after PCI with BMS at early (< 6 months) and very late (> 5 years) follow-up [29]. They observed that the neointima often transformed into lipid-laden tissue with luminal narrowing.

Table 1. Morphologic patterns of ISR with BMS, SES, PES, ZES and EES

Study/ 1° Author (Ref.)	Year	SES		PES		R-ZES		EES		BMS	
		Focal	Non-Focal	Focal	Non-Focal	Focal	Non-Focal	Focal	Non-Focal	Focal	Non-Focal
Mehran et al. [5]	1999	-	-	-	-	-	-	-	-	42%	58%
Lemos et al. [45]	2003	75%	25%	-	-	-	-	-	-	-	-
Colombo et al. [17]	2003	100%	0	-	-	-	-	-	-	-	-
SIRIUS [51]	2004	84%	16%	-	-	-	-	-	-	43%	57%
TAXUS IV [34]	2004	-	-	62.5%	17.5%	-	-	-	-	31%	69%
ISAR-DIABETIC [59]	2005	100%	0%	76.4%	23.6%	-	-	-	-	-	-
ISAR-SMART [60]	2006	80%	20%	69.6%	30.4%	-	-	-	-	-	-
Iakovou et al. [53]	2005	-	-	50%	50%	-	-	-	-	-	-
Corbett et al. [52]	2006	71.3%	28.7%	51.7%	48.3%	-	-	-	-	-	-
Park et al. [31]	2007	76.3%	23.7%	51.3%	48.7%	-	-	-	-	-	-
Solinas et al. [40]	2008	73%	27%	58%	42%	-	-	-	-	-	-
Kitahara et al. [129]	2009	79%	21%	-	-	-	-	-	-	-	-
Rathore et al. [30]	2010	47%	53%	-	-	-	-	-	-	19.3%	80.7%
Lee et al. [88]	2012	84.7%	15.3%	50.5%	49.5%	85%	15%	84.6%	15.4%	-	-

Neovascularization processes expanded from the peri-stent area to intima with associated neoatherosclerosis. As it is well established that neoangiogenesis is closely associated with plaque progression, it is feasible that it could also play a role in in-stent neoatherosclerosis. Finally the authors found that lipid-laden intima was highly associated with ISR as compared to non-lipid-laden intima (86% vs. 14%, p = 0.001). This study reinforces the hypothesis that in very late stages following PCI, ISR can be due to in-stent neoatheroma formation. Neoatherosclerosis and its role in ISR will be further discussed in the section "OCT Assessment of ISR" in this chapter.

5. Patterns of ISR in BMS and DES

5.1. Comparison between BMS and 1st generation DES

ISR in BMS is generally characterized by a diffuse pattern while in DES ISR a focal pattern is more commonly seen [9, 30-35]. The incidence of various ISR morphologic patterns with BMS and DES are illustrated in Table 2. The rate of development, clinical presentation and risk varies by ISR morphology.

Table 2. Predictors of ISR (any pattern), non-focal ISR and TLR in BMS and DES

	ISR (Any Pattern)	Non-Focal ISR	TLR
Predictors in BMS			
Clinical	DM	DM Female Gender	DM Female Gender
Angiographic	Vessel size Complex lesion (B2/C) Baseline MLD Plaque burden	Lesion length Baseline MLD Coronary artery remodeling index	Multivessel Disease Complex lesion (B2/C) Small vessels ISR lesion
Procedural	Stented length vessel Post-procedure MLD	Coil stents Post-procedure MLD Stent length / lesion length ratio	Post-procedure MLD Coil stents Longer stented lesions
Predictors in DES			
Clinical	DM	DM Female Gender Unstable angina	DM Female Gender
Angiographic	ISR lesion Vessel size LAD artery Complex lesion (B2/C) Multiple lesions	Reference vessel diameter	ISR lesion Lesion length Saphenous graft Complex lesion (B2/C) Multiple lesions Vessel size
Procedural	Post-procedure MLD PES or E-ZES	Overlapping stents PES	ISR Treatment PES or E-ZES Post-procedure MLD Total implanted stent length

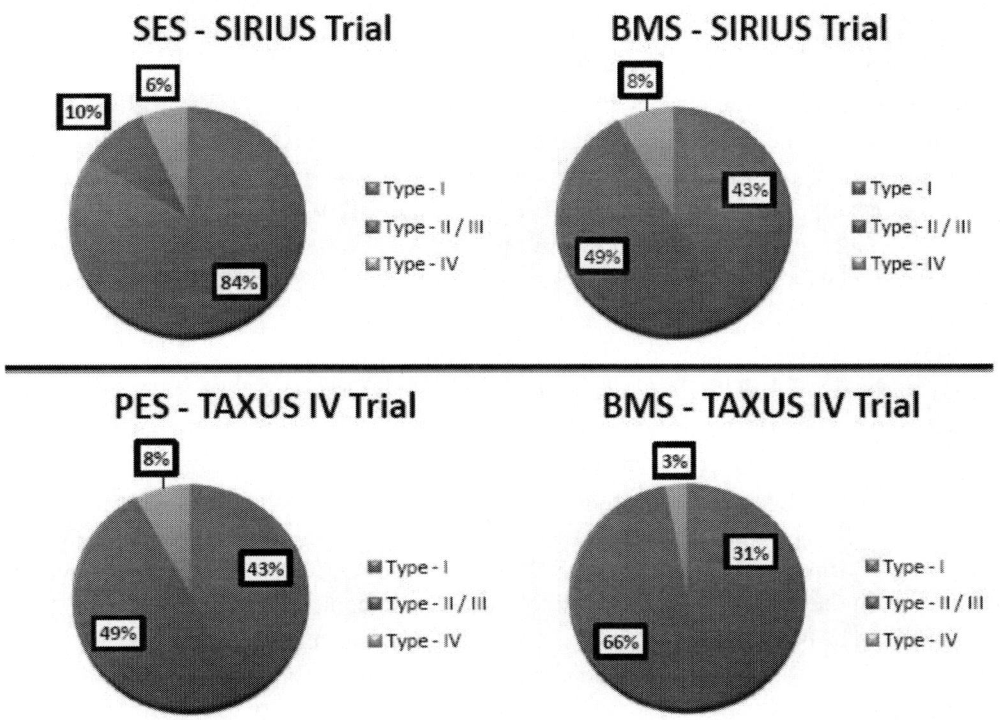

Figure 5. Relative incidence of morphological patterns of ISR with bare metal stents (BMS), sirolimus-eluting stents (SES) and paclitaxel-eluting stents (PES). Data reported from Stone GW [34] et al. and Popma JJ et al. [51].

After BMS-ISR implantation, for example, the NIH is uniform and more commonly distributed along the stent length, as a result of the vascular response to stent implantation. ISR usually develops 5-6 months after stent implantation[36]. In a single-center registry, Kini et al. reported a diffuse pattern in 78% of patients with ISR after receiving early generation BMS [37]. Although later BMS platforms are associated a lower rate of ISR, a diffuse pattern remains the most commonly observed morphology. Moreover, diffuse ISR usually presents with stable angina or troponin negative acute syndromes [38, 39].

Conversely, DES-ISR is characterized by delayed development and a predominantly focal pattern. Park et al. described focal ISR in approximately 65% of 177 consecutive first-generation DES-ISR, while Solinas et al. reported a prevalence of 69.5% focal ISR in 182 lesions [31, 40]. The different pattern of ISR between BMS and DES is consistent with different rates of neointimal accumulation between the stent platforms and reflects the delayed arterial healing after DES implantation [41-44].

The predominantly focal pattern of DES-ISR is likely related to non-uniform drug delivery and subsequent local failure of the anti-restenotic effect [43, 44]. Underlying reasons for this phenomenon may be attributable to mechanical PCI related factors such as stent under-expansion, vessel barotrauma, repeated balloon post-dilatation, extremely tortuous lesions and stent fracture [13, 45, 46]. A larger reference plaque burden and a larger ratio of stent-edge cross sectional area to reference vessel minimum lumen area (MLA) have been associated with edge stenosis in DES (Class IC and ID) [47, 48]. ISR Class IA is observed when adjacent lesions are treated separately with two stents separated by a short gap. The negative remodeling and exuberant hyperplasia not suppressed by antiproliferative drug at this gap results in this subtype of focal ISR [49, 50].

The RAVEL (RAndomised study with the Sirolimus coated BX™ VElocity balloon expandable stent in the treatment of patients with De Novo native coronary artery Lesions) trial was the first randomized study to demonstrate the angiographic superiority of DES over BMS, reporting a greater mean lumen diameter (MLD) and lower LLL and ISR rates with SES at 6 months [9]. The SIRIUS (Sirolimus-Eluting Stent in Coronary Lesions) trial reported an incidence of in-segment ISR of 8.9% in SES versus 36.3% in BMS [51]. Of all patients who had ISR, non-focal ISR comprised 16.1% of SES ISR as opposed to 57% of BMS ISR [51].

Conversely the TAXUS IV (Treatment of De Novo Coronary Disease Using a Single Paclitaxel-Eluting Stent) trial, which reported a restenosis rate of 7.9% and 26.6% in PES and BMS respectively, showed that the proportion which was non-focal in morphology was 37.5% with PES while the proportion in BMS was significantly higher at 69.2% [34]. Interestingly, both randomized studies reported higher rates of focal ISR (83.9% of SES ISR in the SIRIUS trial and 62.5% of PES ISR in the TAXUS IV trial) as compared to observational studies. These differences likely reflect the complexity of the baseline lesions that were treated. While these randomized controlled trials recruited patients with single-vessel disease, no ostial lesions, no left main involvement, no bifurcation and no occluded lesions were, in the real-world observational registries the complexity of the treated lesions is significantly higher. For example, Rathore et al. reported that 47% of SES ISR was focal in pattern (as opposed to 83.9% in the SIRIUS trial) and 19.3% of BMS ISR (as opposed to 43% in the SIRIUS trial and 30.8% in the TAXUS IV trial) [30], while Corbett et al. observed focal ISR in 71.3% and 51.7% of SES-ISR and PES-ISR respectively (as opposed to 62.5% in the TAXUS IV trial) [52].

Possible down-stream effects of DES may explain observations of increased involvement of the proximal versus distal stent edge in DES-ISR [45, 53]. Lemos et al. examined the morphological patterns of ISR after SES implantation using IVUS [45]. They found that 30% of restenotic lesions were located at the proximal 5-mm segment of the proximal stent edge, while 70% were intra-stent. Local injury outside the stent was observed in 83% of cases of edge restenosis, suggesting that incomplete lesion coverage and local trauma during implantation, as well as increased drug effect in the outflow stent play a role in the pathogenesis of edge restenosis. Conversely among the in-stent lesions, 86% were focal with a very localized stenotic site bordered by segments with no evidence of lumen involvement. Among lesions evaluated by IVUS, the presence of stent discontinuity was observed in 36% of lesions, suggesting that a decrease in local drug availability may be responsible for the restenosis.

5.2. ISR Morphology in 1st Generation DES

The pattern of ISR also varies within 1st generation DES [54-56]. Comparisons involving patients treated with first generation SES and PES, for example, have shown that focal ISR was more common in SES whereas diffuse instar-stent ISR was more common in PES treated patients, occurring in up to 50% of lesions [31, 40]. No differences in the prevalence of proliferative (type III) and occlusive (type IV) patterns between SES and PES have been documented [31, 52].

A meta-analysis by Kastrati and colleagues reported an overall incidence of ISR with SES of 9.3% and 13.1% with PES (OR: 0.68; $p = 0.001$) [57]. No differences were found in other outcomes. The superiority of SES over PES with respect to the ISR incidence was explained by the almost constant finding, both with angiography and IVUS, of a lower degree of LLL and a higher MLD with SES at follow up. These findings were confirmed later in another larger meta-analysis [54].

Recently, Raber et al. reported in the SIRTAX LATE (Sirolimus-Eluting Versus Paclitaxel-Eluting Stents for Coronary Revascularization) study, where 293 patients treated with PES or SES underwent serial angiography at 8 months and 5 years, an ongoing reduction of the MLD between 8 months and 5 years [58, 59]. While SES was superior in terms of late loss at 8 months, no differences were found at 5 years. This was explained by a late catch-up phenomenon and a higher delayed lumen loss observed with SES. While SES guarantees a superior suppression of NIH and lower risk of ISR as compared to PES at mid-term, these results suggest that this advantage is no longer achieved at more long-term of follow-up, most probably due to ongoing neointimal proliferation.

The ISAR-DIABETES (Paclitaxel-Eluting Stent Versus Sirolimus-Eluting Stent for the Prevention of Restenosis in Diabetic Patients With Coronary Artery Disease) trial compared SES and PES in patients affected by DM [59]. Again PES was associated with higher rates of LLL and higher incidence of angiographic ISR (16.5% vs. 6.8%). All patients with ISR in the SES group had a (Mehran classification) type I pattern (100%). Among all patients with PES-ISR, 76.4% had type I, 5.8% had type II, 5.8% had type III and 11.7% had type IV ISR.

Differences between SES and PES were also compared in small coronary vessels[60]. The ISAR-SMART 3 (Sirolimus- and Paclitaxel-Eluting Stents for Small Vessels) randomized trial reported a lower LLL, ISR incidence and TLR rates with SES. In particular, angiographic ISR was found in 19% in the PES group compared with 11.4% in the SES group. Regarding the pattern of ISR in the PES group, ISR type-I was observed in 69.6%, type-II in 9%, type-III in 6% and type-IV in 15%. In the SES group, 80% of lesions presented with type-I pattern; of the remainder 5% had type-III and 15% had type-IV ISR.

Several observational studies have also reported a higher incidence of non-focal ISR with PES as compared to SES, ranging from 24-27% with SES and 42-49% with PES [31, 40, 52]. Furthermore, patients with focal ISR had significantly higher 1-year survival free from TLR as compared to patients with diffuse ISR patterns [41].

Differences between SES- and PES-ISR patterns may be related to several factors. Firstly, the cellular mechanism of the 2 drugs is different. Sirolimus is a mammalian target of rapamycin (mTOR) inhibitor, while paclitaxel is a microtubule-stabilizing agent leading to reduced cell division and mobility [61-64]. In-vitro studies show that smooth muscle cells adopt a differentiated contractile phenotype under sirolimus and a synthetic phenotype under paclitaxel. Accordingly, a smooth muscle cell synthetic phenotype is more frequent in both PES- and BMS-ISR as compared to SES, which may in turn influence the ISR pattern [14]. Conversely, SES has been demonstrated to be associated with higher inhibition of NIH [65]. Differences in the inflammatory response following PCI with PES and SES may also contribute to differences in ISR patterns. SES is more commonly associated with a granulomatous and eosinophilic reaction starting at 28 days while PES is characterized by a lower inflammation burden but higher amounts of fibrin deposition, a powerful trigger for cellular proliferation [43, 66, 67].

5.3. ISR Morphology in 2nd Generation *DES*

Everolimus-eluting stents (EES) and zotarolimus-eluting stents (ZES) are the most commonly used commercially available 2nd-generation DES. In general, both generations of DES most commonly present with focal-type ISR. However specific differences between 1st- and 2nd-generation DES exist. Firstly, EES were associated with lower LLL, ISR and TLR rates compared with PES [68-72]. Comparisons of EES and SES suggest similar performance with respect to LLL, ISR (including focal-ISR) and TLR [73, 74]. In contrast, the Endeavor ZES (E-ZES, Medtronic, Santa Rosa, California) demonstrated higher rates of ISR and TLR compared to SES [75, 76]. Also, while the most common pattern of ISR was focal with both types of DES, E-ZES was associated with higher restenosis length (12.9 mm with ZES vs. 6.46 mm with SES; $p < 0.001$), higher percentage of volume obstruction (16.1% with ZES vs. 2.7% with SES; $p < 0.001$) and mean neointimal thickness (0.19 +/- 0.07 mm vs. 0.10 +/- 0.06 mm, $p < 0.001$). Compared to PES, E-ZES again showed a higher rate of ISR, higher in-segment LLL, NIH volume and percent volume obstruction [77, 78]. These findings were attributed the intrinsic drug release kinetics of the E-ZES (95% eluted in the first 2 weeks after implantation) [76].

On the other hand, E-ZES were associated with lower rate of death or myocardial infarction beyond 3 years, mainly due to lower rates of late stent thrombosis and late MI events [79-81].

Results of E-ZES from clinical trials drove to the production of the Resolute ZES (R-ZES, Medtronic, Santa Rosa, California) which has an extended delivery of zotarolimus, with 85% of release within 2 months and the remainder by 6 months. The initial results of the RESOLUTE clinical trial showed that R-ZES were associated with lower LLL, ISR rates and TLR as compared to E-ZES [82]. An IVUS-based study comparing E-ZES, R-ZES, ZoMaxx and Driver (all zotarolimus eluting-stents with different polymer and drug elution times) demonstrated lower NIH volume, percent neointimal obstruction and LLL with the R-ZES [83]. Interestingly, after multivariable adjustment R-ZES correlated with neointimal suppression.

Finally several randomized trials reported that EES and R-ZES are similar in terms of clinical outcomes. The RESOLUTE All-comers trial showed no differences in primary endpoint showing the non-inferiority of R-ZES respect to EES [84-86]. However R-ZES was associated with higher LLL at 13 month, but no significant difference in target lesion failure at 2 and 4 years (2 years, 12.6% R-ZES vs. 12.2% EES; 4 years, 15.2% R-ZES vs. 14.6% EES). An OCT-based substudy showed no differences in MLA, NIH volume and percent neointimal volume obstruction between R-ZES and EES [87].

Observational studies related to patterns of ISR in 1st and 2nd generation DES are scarce. Lee et al. reported an incidence of focal ISR of 50.5% with PES, 84.7% with SES, 84.6% with EES and 85% with R-ZES, with a much lower incidence of diffuse intra-stent ISR with 2nd generation DES (5.6% vs. 40%) [88]. Of note, the proportion and distribution of margin-type focal ISR was similar between different generations of DES.

New therapeutic prospects are emerging after the recent introduction of bioabsorbable DES[89]. The LEADERS (Limus Eluted From A Durable Versus ERodable Stent Coating) trial compared the biodegradable polymer biolimus-eluting stent (BES) with SES [90]. No differences were found in ISR rates, percentage stenosis, LLL, TLR and TVR at 9 months. An OCT-based substudy of the LEADERS trial demonstrated that while the quantity of neointimal tissue was similar, BES was associated with improved stent strut coverage [91]. Long-term results (1-4 years) have demonstrated a significant reduction in very late definite stent thrombosis and TLR with BES compared with SES [92, 93].

Early results with the bioresorbable vascular scaffold (BVS) stents have been promising. The ABSORB trial, which 101 patients, reported 2 cases of early ISR (< 6 months; 2%), 1 case of late ISR (6-12 months; 1%) and 3 cases of very late ISR (> 12 months; 3%) [94, 95]. Two of the later cases of ISR were focal and located at the proximal stent edge, suggesting that edge vascular response may play a potential critical role in ISR with this class of stents. An OCT-based comparison at 1 year of BVS and EES showed similar rates of LLL, NIH thickness and NIH composition [96]. However, these studies to date have been small and the processes leading to ISR in these devices warrant further investigation [95, 97]. Moreover, whether bioabsorbable stents have a role in treating ISR remains unknown [98].

6. Edge Vascular Response and In-Stent Restenosis

Edge vascular response (EVR) can be defined as the pathophysiological changes in the vascular tissue adjacent to the segment of stent implantation [99]. In general, it consists of a focal and sometimes significant LLL which can result in restenosis and subsequent TLR. The mechanisms underlying EVR can be clinical (patient related propensity for ISR), procedural (plaque shift, vascular injury) and device-related (eluted drug and stent polymer). The TAXUS-II, -IV, -V and -VI trials documented comparable luminal loss at both the proximal and distal stent edges with PES and BMS [100-102]. The SIRIUS trial showed ISR with SES was more commonly focal and located at the proximal stent edge [47, 103, 104]. The SPIRIT III US trial reported a significant reduction in lumen volume at the proximal edge with EES [105, 106]. Luminal loss at both stent edges was evident in an IVUS substudy of the ENDEAVOR-IV trial at 8 months[78]. The ABSORB cohort B1 showed significant lumen loss with BVS at 2 years at the proximal scaffold edge [107]. In summary, DES seem to improve EVR compared to BMS, particularly at the distal edge likely due to down-stream drug effects.

7. ISR Morphology in Patients with Diabetes Mellitus

Clinical, anatomical and procedural predictors of ISR have been studied extensively. An overview of the predictors of ISR with BMS and DES is illustrated in Table 1. Among other factors, diabetes mellitus (DM) has been established as a strong ISR clinical predictor [108]. ISR in diabetic patients is usually characterized by a relatively high-risk morphologic pattern with a significant number of proliferative (type III) and occlusive ISR (type IV) [5]. An accentuated neo-intimal response in diabetics versus non-diabetics after stent implantation appears to be an important contributor to observed differences in ISR development in the setting of DM. For example, an IVUS-based analysis of ISR in patients treated with BMS showed substantial differences in the degree of neointimal hyperplasia among diabetics (5.1 ± 2.8 mm²) compared to non-diabetics (2.1 ± 2.0 mm²) [109]. These findings were further validated by a separate IVUS study in which, in addition to a trend toward a larger overall amount of neointimal hyperplasia, a more heterogeneous neointimal pattern was observed among diabetics [110].

DES implantation appears to be effective in attenuating the neo-intimal response leading to ISR in diabetic patients. After PES implantation, for example, no differences were observed between diabetic and non-diabetic patients in the volume of neointimal hyperplasia (22.8 vs. 16.3 mm³, $p = 0.35$) or percentage of neointimal hyperplasia (9.1% vs. 9.2%, $p = 0.27$) [111]. Notwithstanding, it is important to note that other reports have shown that the presence of DM may attenuate other benefits associated with newer versus first-generation DES [11, 112].

8. Endovascular Imaging and ISR

8.1. IVUS Assessment of ISR

Intravascular imaging technologies have imparted greater understanding regarding coronary pathology and vascular response to stent implantation. IVUS has provided further insight into vascular remodeling, stent under-expansion and the distribution of NIH. A classification system for DES-ISR according to intravascular ultrasound (IVUS) findings has been proposed [113]:

- Focal ISR, defined as lumen area < 4 mm2 and length ≤ 10 mm, subcategorized by the location within the stent,
  - "Focal body type", confined to the body of stent.
  - "Focal marginal type", extending to the margins of stent
- Multifocal ISR, multiple focal lesions, with subcategories
  - "Multifocal body type", confined to the body of the stent
  - "Multifocal marginal type", involving stent margins
- Diffuse ISR, defined as MLA < 4 mm^2 and length > 10 mm, with subcategories
  - "Diffuse body type": confined to the stent body
  - "Diffuse marginal type": associated with stent involvement

The same study reported that stent underexpansion was the underlying etiology of ISR in 21% of cases, and of NIH in 88% of cases. Again, focal ISR was the most common pattern of ISR encountered (47%). Of note, patients with diffuse ISR had longer total stent length and higher rate of stent underexpansion (39%) at the minimum lumen site compared with focal (6%) and multifocal (22%) ISR ($p = 0.004$). However the amount of NIH was similar across the IVUS categories of ISR (diffuse 90% vs. focal 89% vs. multifocal 78%, $p = 0.58$). In the comparison of SES, PES and ZES, no differences in the angiographic or IVUS patterns of restenosis were observed but a higher rate of significant NIH was found with PES (p = 0.04). Also, PES and ZES were more commonly associated with > 10 mm of significant NIH when compared to SES (32% vs. 33% vs. 9%, p = 0.04).

Kang et al. reported findings from 70 DES-ISR and 47 BMS-ISR lesions assessed by VH-IVUS [114]. DES-ISR featured more fibrous NIH, while necrotic core and dense calcium were more prevalent in BMS-ISR. Older ISR lesions irrespective of stent type had higher prevalence of necrotic core and dense calcium, suggestive of neoatheroma.

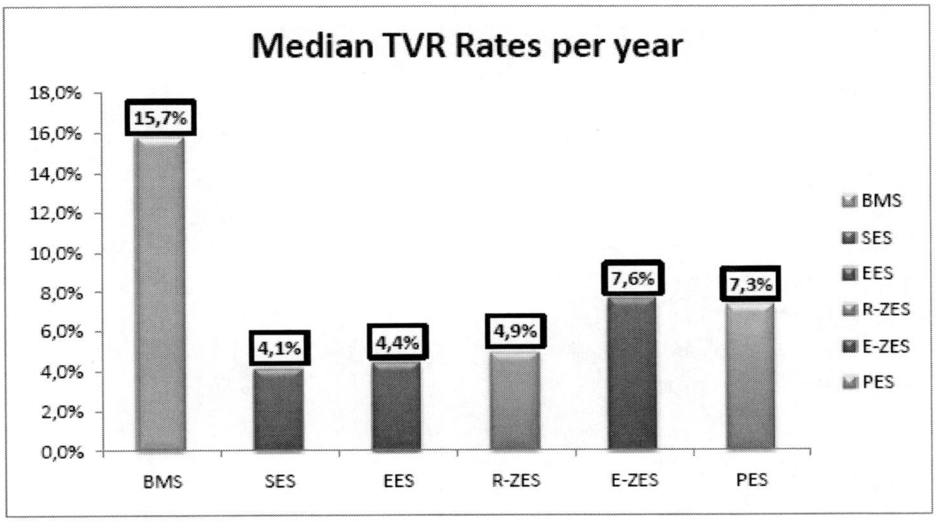

Figure 6. Median rates of target vessel revascularization (TVR) per year of follow-up with bare metal stents (BMS), 1st- and 2nd-generation drug-eluting stents (DES): sirolimus-eluting stents (SES), everolimus-eluting stents (EES), Resolute zotarolimus-eluting stents (R-ZES), Endeavor zotarolimus-eluting stents (E-ZES) and paclitaxel-eluting stents (PES). Results from Bangalore et al., a meta-analysis on 117.762 patient-year of follow-up [130].

8.2. OCT Assessment of ISR

OCT has led to better characterization of the morphologic characteristics of ISR. Gonzalo et al. classified morphologic and structural characteristics of ISR according to quantitative and qualitative OCT parameters (Figure 7) [115]:

- Restenotic tissue structure:
  a. Homogeneous: uniform optical proprieties without focal variation in backscattering pattern
  b. Heterogeneous: focal changes in optical properties and various backscattering pattern
  c. Layered: concentric layers with adluminal high scattering layer and abluminal low scattering layer
- Restenotic tissue backscatter:
  - High: predominant bright tissue with backscatter

  - Low: predominant dark tissue with low backscatter
- Lumen shape:
  - Irregular: sharp delineation of lumen border which appears smooth and circular
  - Regular: irregular border with tissue protrusion from the vessel wall into the lumen
- Intraluminal material:
  - Presence: visible material within the vessel lumen
  - Absence: of same
- Microvessels:
  - Presence: well delineated structures < 200 μm in diameter with a course within the vessel.
  - Absence: of same

OCT quantitative analysis assessed:

- o Mean lumen area (mm^2)
- o Minimal lumen area (MLA; mm^2)
- o Mean stent area (mm^2)
- o Mean restenotic tissue area (mm^2)
- o Restenotic tissue burden (%)

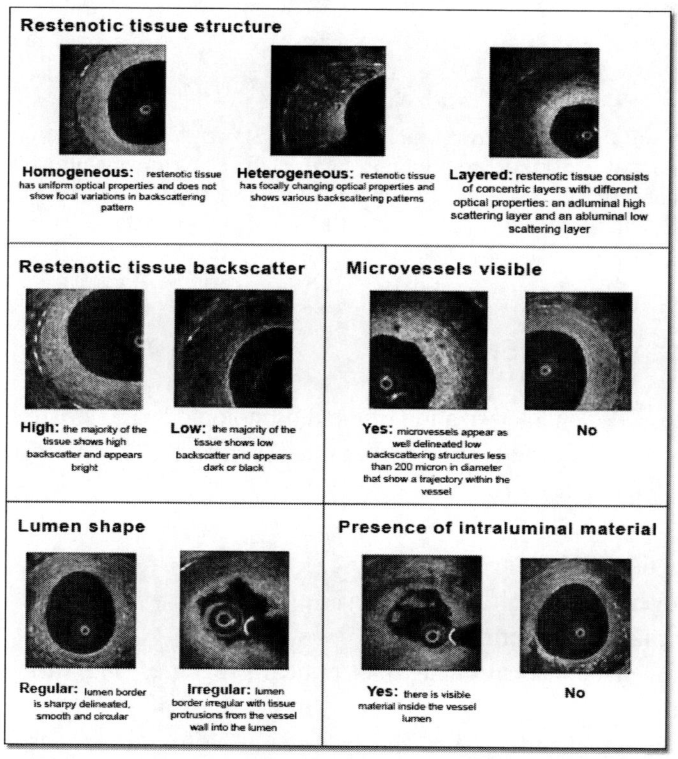

Figure 7. OCT qualitative characterization of ISR lesions. Reproduced with permission from Gonzalo et al. [115].

The relationship between OCT and angiographic ISR assessment was also evaluated (Figure 8). The tissue coverage structure pattern at OCT was most commonly layered in diffuse ISR, homogeneous in margin ISR and similarly layered or heterogeneous in focal ISR. High backscatter was associated with diffuse ISR, while focal ISR was more likely to have low backscatter. Although not statistically significant (probably due to small sample size), irregular lumen shape, intraluminal material and microvessels were all more common in focal ISR. Irregular lumen shape and higher neointima symmetry ratio were also associated with unstable angina at clinical presentation whereas long ISR was associated with stable presentation.

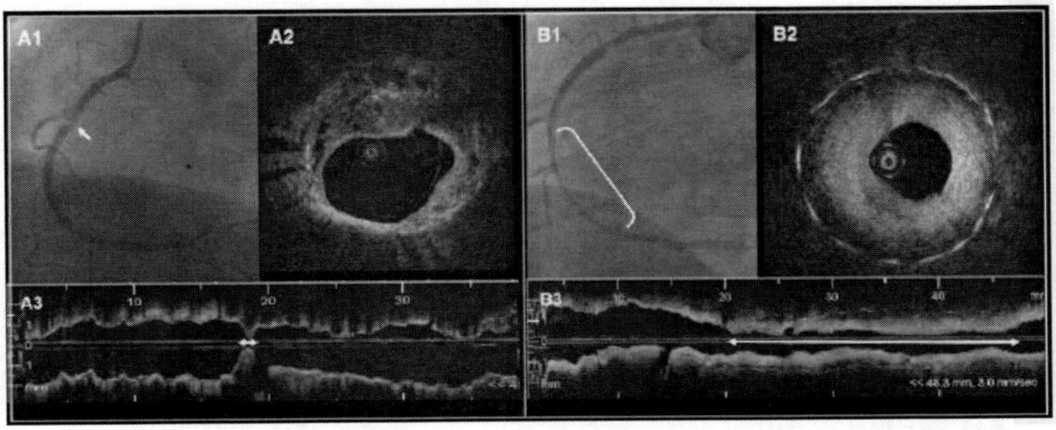

Figure 8. ISR morphology by OCT and angiographic appearance. A) Patient with angiographic focal ISR (A1, white arrow). A cross-section imaging by OCT shows heterogeneous tissue with low backscatter (A2). The longitudinal OCT image shows a very focal restenosis (A3, white arrows). B) Patient with angiographic diffuse ISR (B1, white bracket). Cross-sectional OCT shows restenotic tissue with layered structure with high backscatter (B2). OCT longitudinal view demonstrates the diffuse restenosis (B3). Reproduced with the permission from Gonzalo et al. [115].

Stratifying the lesions according to the time from stent implantation also revealed differences in the OCT pattern of ISR. Early ISR (≤ 12 months) was primarily a layered pattern (84.3%) while later ISR (> 12 months) showed a homogeneous pattern in 50% and a heterogeneous pattern in 33.3%. Mean lumen area was smaller in more early compared to later ISR (3.9 ± 1.3 vs. 5.3 ± 1.7, p = 0.03).

Habara et al. also investigated the temporal relationships between DES-ISR (1st generation) and OCT features [116]. A total of 43 early (< 1 year), 22 late (1 – 3 years) and 21 very late (> 3 years) ISR were compared. Angiography alone did not detect any differences between the groups. However, quantitative OCT analysis showed differences in mean stent area, with lowest area in the late ISR group, and the highest in the very late ISR group (p = 0.08). On, qualitative OCT analysis, heterogeneous intima with thin-cap fibroatheroma-like (TCFA) pattern, intra-intimal microvessels, peri-stent ulcer-like appearance, disrupted intima with visible cavity and intraluminal material were most commonly found in very late ISR. These changes suggest a continuous remodeling of ISR lesions and the possible superimposition of neoatherosclerosis. Neoatherosclerosis has been proposed as a possible pathway for late DES failure and may account for the "late catch-up phenomenon" observed in DES trials at long-term follow-up. Pathologically, neoatherosclerosis in DES-ISR represents a form of accelerated atherosclerosis secondary to delayed re-endothelization and severe endothelial dysfunction. A histopathologic study conducted by Nakazawa et al. reported that neoatherosclerosis was more frequently observed in DES than BMS ISR (31% vs. 16%, $p < 0.001$) [27]. The median stent duration with neoatherosclerosis was shorter in DES than BMS (DES: 420 days; BMS: 2160 days; $p < 0.001$), suggesting that this process begins earlier in DES. Interestingly, SES was associated with a greater neoatherosclerosis change compared to PES for implant durations of 2 years or less (SES 37% vs. PES 21%, $p = 0.021$). The earlier development of neoatherosclerosis in DES may be due to incomplete (delayed) stent endothelization and reduced cell-to-cell contact with increased lipidic and macrophage intimal infiltration.

Kang et al. reported a high prevalence of in-stent neoatherosclerosis in an OCT DES-ISR study of 50 patients, especially in very-late DES ISR (> 20 months post PCI) [117]. 52% of lesions had at least 1 site containing thin-cap fibroatheroma (TCFA), 58% had at least 1 site of in-stent neointimal rupture and 58% had evidence of thrombus. According to the interval time (< 20 vs. > 20 months post-PCI) patients with DES-ISR > 20 months had higher incidence of single TFCA (33% vs. 69%, $p = 0.012$) and multiple TFCA (0% vs. 23%, $p = 0.014$). Using receiver operator curve analysis, DES-ISR presenting more than 20 months after PCI was the best predictor of TFCA-containing neointima, with a sensitivity of 73% and a specificity of 67%.

Ali et al. characterized in-stent neoatheroma with OCT and near-infrared spectroscopy (NIRS) in consecutive patients with BMS- and DES-ISR [118]. Neoatherosclerosis was defined at OCT as a signal-poor region with diffuse borders. The authors morphologically classified neoatherosclerosis through OCT assessment as the following:

- Type I Thin-Cap Neo-Atheroma (TCNA): ≥ 1 area of thin cap, neoatherosclerosis located between the lumen and the stent struts
- Type II Thick-Cap Neo-Atheroma (ThkNA): absence of thin cap, neoatherosclerosis located between the lumen and the stent struts.
- Type III (Peri-Strut Neo-Atheroma; PSNA): neoatherosclerosis located around the stent struts.
- Type IV (Pre-Existing Fibro-Atheroma; PEFA): native pre-existing atherosclerosis displaying as poor region signals with diffuse border between the stent struts and the adventitia.

The authors observed that neoatherosclerosis was significantly more common in DES vs. BMS (68% vs. 36%, $p = 0.02$). DES-ISR had more TCNA finding and lower minimal cap thickness. On NIRS assessment, DES-ISR had greater total lipid burden and density. Neoatherosclerosis was more common at sites of culprit lesions in DES but not in BMS. There were no differences among DES stent types in the incidence of neoatherosclerosis, however PES was associated with a higher proportion of type III neoatherosclerosis. The interval time since PCI was significantly shorter in neoatherosclerosis in DES compared with BMS.

Interestingly, the authors reported a correlation between the occurrence of periprocedural myocardial infarction (MI) and neoatherosclerosis type. Periprocedural MI occurred exclusively in DES, with almost half of the events attributable to luminal-type (I / II) neoatherosclerosis within the culprit ISR.

The speckled pattern and peri-strut low intensity areas (PLIA) observed in early ISR reflects the phenomenon of delayed endothelization observed with DES [117, 119]. More than 10 years ago, Chung et al. reported that myxoid tissue containing proteoglycan-rich extra-cellular matrix was prevalent in patients with early BMS-ISR and decreased over time, with an expansion of the collagen-rich component [25]. DES however suppress the immune response delaying arterial healing, resulting in the replacement of extracellular matrix by proliferating smooth muscle cells or neo-synthesized collagen, which contributes to the observed speckled pattern. Teramoto et al., reported that PLIA was more commonly encountered in DES than BMS [119]. PLIA corresponded to hypocellular regions containing fibrinoid or proteoglycans, considered to reflect areas of delayed arterial healing following PCI with DES. Otake et al. compared the PLIA between SES and PES implantation. PLIA was more commonly encountered after PES implantation (PES 86% vs. SES 58%, $p = 0.005$) [120]. Importantly stents with PLIA showed a significantly greater neointimal thickness.

Recently, Kilickesmez et al. compared OCT findings in 1st generation DES (SES and PES) vs. 2nd generation DES (ZES, EES and BES) ISR at early and late follow up (before or after 1-year) [121]. The homogeneous OCT pattern was most common in 1st generation DES whereas the heterogeneous pattern was more common in 2nd generation stents. Neoatherosclerosis and neovascularization was more prevalent in 1st generation DES in the early period (< 1 year follow up) and after 1 year follow-up in 2nd generation DES.

In summary, the study of ISR morphology with OCT has greatly increased our understanding of the etiology and pathogenesis of ISR and TLR, particularly with respect to the nature and time-course of neoatherosclerosis with various stents. The relationship between ISR morphology determined at OCT and clinical outcomes is an ongoing area of investigation.

10. Fractional Flow Reserve and ISR Morphology

There is limited data on the use of FFR in ISR lesions. In a study of 62 patients, Lopez-Palop and colleagues reported a poor correlation between angiographic quantification of ISR and fractional flow reserve (FFR) assessment [122]. In this study, there was poor correlation between the various angiographic measures of ISR such as MLD, lesion length and percent stenosis and significant vs. non-significant (≥ 0.75) FFR.

11. Patterns of ISR: Therapeutic Implications

The pattern of ISR may influence therapeutic decisions by affording insight into the underlying mechanism of ISR. Focal DES-ISR where mechanical factors such as stent fractures, non-uniform strut distribution and edge effects play a determinant role may be effectively treated with balloon angioplasty or drug-eluting balloon. Diffuse DES-ISR where exaggerated NIH plays a central role may instead benefit from repeat stent implantation. Drug resistance is another potential mechanism of DES failure, therefore in this case patients may benefit of repeated stenting with different DES [13]. Pate et al. in a study of 363 patients reported that the choice of therapy was related to ISR pattern [38]. Patients treated with medical therapy more often had total occlusion, those with PCI / PCI + brachytherapy more often had diffuse ISR and those selected for coronary-artery by-pass graft (CABG) had proliferative ISR. CABG was also more commonly associated with multiple ISR lesions.

As previously discussed in this chapter, the angiographic pattern of ISR also has an important impact on percutaneous revascularization outcomes. Diffuse ISR has been shown to be associated to higher rates of TLR (up to 85%) after successful intervention. While most of these studies included patients treated with POBA or PCI, some data is available for other percutaneous treatment modalities. Among patients treated for ISR with rotational coronary atherectomy, directional coronary atherectomy and excimer laser, Kini et al. reported TLR rates of 46% in diffuse-type ISR and 14% in focal-type ISR [37].

Edge ISR represent a small subgroup of ISR lesions that can have benign angiographic appearance but are associated with high rates of TLR. A substudy from the RIBS (Restenosis Intra-stent: Balloon angioplasty vs. elective Stenting) trial demonstrated that the use of stents in this type of ISR significantly reduce the need for TLR when compared to balloon angioplasty [124]. After multivariable adjustment, stent implantation was the only independent predictor of freedom from TVR (HR: 0.15, p = 0.003). The recent RIBS V trial that compared treatment with EES and paclitaxel-eluting balloon (PEB) in BMS-ISR, found that even if both techniques provided excellent results, EES appeared superior to PEB in terms of acute and late angiographic results [125]. This result was also consistent in patients with diffuse ISR.

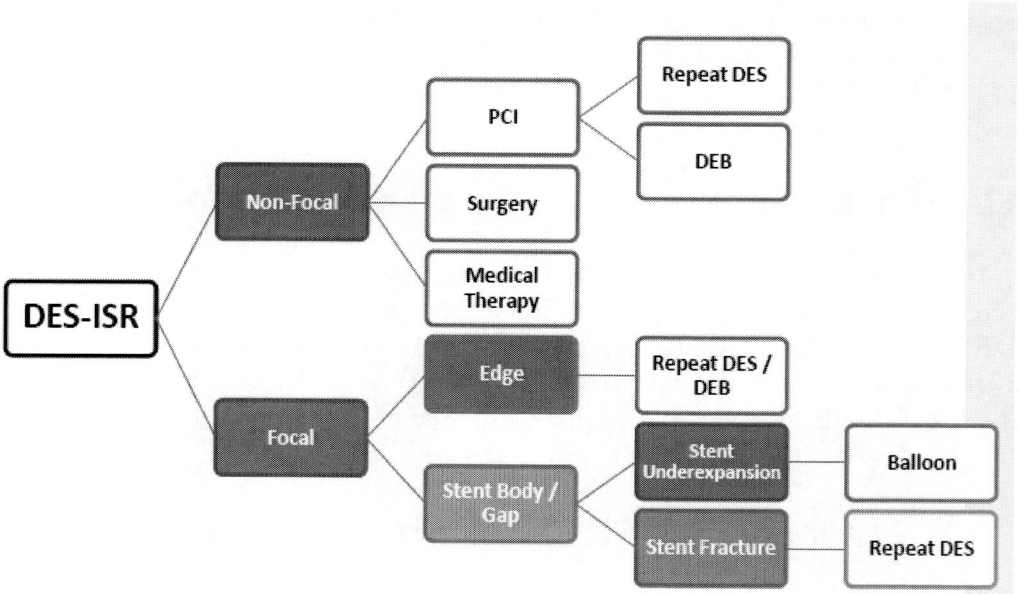

Figure 9. A proposed treatment algorithm for DES-ISR according to morphologic pattern presentation. DEB: Drug-Eluting Balloon; DES: Drug-Eluting Stent; PCI: Percutaneous Coronary Intervention.

Regarding DES-ISR (SES, PES, ZES and BES), the recent ISAR-DESIRE (Intracoronary Stenting and Angiographic Results: Drug Eluting Stents for In-Stent Restenosis) III trial showed that, independent of the baseline pattern of ISR, paclitaxel-eluting balloons and PES were markedly superior to POBA in preventing recurrent TLR [126]. Of note, POBA was more commonly associated with a higher incidence of recurrent ISR with diffuse pattern (POBA 39% vs. PES 21% vs. PEB 21%). Conversely, PES and PEB were more commonly associated with a focal type recurrent ISR (POBA 31% vs. PES 41% vs. PEB 46%), however these differences. Previously, the ISAR-DESIRE II trial demonstrated no differences in the treatment of SES-ISR with SES or PES[127]. No statistically differences were observed in the pattern of recurrent ISR between the 2 types of DES. The similar efficacy of SES and PES was also confirmed in diabetic and non-diabetic patients by Kufner et al. [128].

In summary, higher grade patterns of ISR are more likely to present with recurrent ISR and TLR following percutaneous revascularization. Furthermore, higher grade patterns of ISR are at increased risk of developing similarly higher grade patterns of recurrent ISR. These findings suggest treatment of diffuse, proliferative and occlusive ISR treatment with DES, which have been shown to superior in reducing TLR in this setting. Patients who develop recurrent advanced ISR patterns following an initial ISR revascularization may require surgical treatment. Figure 9 illustrates a theoretical treatment algorithm for DES-ISR.

Conclusion

The study of ISR morphology has provided valuable understanding regarding this complex, multifactorial complication of PCI with stents. With recent advances in intravascular imaging technologies and new stent designs, this field is rapidly changing with new insights into the pathophysiologic mechanisms and clinical implications. These important developments ultimately help to inform clinical practice regarding the optimal treatment of patients who develop ISR, and to design improved stent systems with respect to long-term patient safety and efficacy.

References

[1] Stettler C, Wandel S, Allemann S, Kastrati A, Morice MC, Schomig A, Pfisterer ME, Stone GW, Leon MB, de Lezo JS, Goy JJ, Park SJ, Sabate M, Suttorp MJ, Kelbaek H, Spaulding C, Menichelli M, Vermeersch P, Dirksen MT, Cervinka P, Petronio AS, Nordmann AJ, Diem P, Meier B, Zwahlen M, Reichenbach S, Trelle S, Windecker S, Juni P. Outcomes associated with drug-eluting and bare-metal stents: A collaborative network meta-analysis. *Lancet*. 2007;370:937-948.

[2] Dangas G, Fuster V. Management of restenosis after coronary intervention. *Am Heart J*. 1996;132:428-436.

[3] Farooq V, Gogas BD, Serruys PW. Restenosis: Delineating the numerous causes of drug-eluting stent restenosis. *Circ Cardiovasc Interv*. 2011;4:195-205.

[4] Cosgrave J, Melzi G, Biondi-Zoccai GG, Airoldi F, Chieffo A, Sangiorgi GM, Montorfano M, Michev I, Carlino M, Bonizzoni E, Colombo A. Drug-eluting stent restenosis the pattern predicts the outcome. *Journal of the American College of Cardiology*. 2006;47:2399-2404.

[5] Mehran R, Dangas G, Abizaid AS, Mintz GS, Lansky AJ, Satler LF, Pichard AD, Kent KM, Stone GW, Leon MB. Angiographic patterns of in-stent restenosis: Classification and implications for long-term outcome. *Circulation*. 1999;100:1872-1878.

[6] Hoffmann R, Mintz GS, Dussaillant GR, Popma JJ, Pichard AD, Satler LF, Kent KM, Griffin J, Leon MB. Patterns and mechanisms of in-stent restenosis. A serial intravascular ultrasound study. *Circulation*. 1996;94:1247-1254.

[7] Abizaid A, Costa JR, Jr., Banning A, Bartorelli AL, Dzavik V, Ellis S, Gao R, Holmes DR, Jr., Jeong MH, Legrand V, Neumann FJ, Nyakern M, Orlick A, Spaulding C, Worthley S, Urban PM. The sirolimus-eluting cypher select coronary stent for the treatment of bare-metal and drug-eluting stent restenosis: Insights from the e-select (multicenter post-market surveillance) registry. *JACC Cardiovasc Interv*. 2012;5:64-71.

[8] Moses JW, Leon MB, Popma JJ, Fitzgerald PJ, Holmes DR, O'Shaughnessy C, Caputo RP, Kereiakes DJ, Williams DO, Teirstein PS, Jaeger JL, Kuntz RE. Sirolimus-eluting stents versus standard stents in patients with stenosis in a native coronary artery. *N Engl J Med*. 2003;349:1315-1323.

[9] Morice MC, Serruys PW, Sousa JE, Fajadet J, Ban Hayashi E, Perin M, Colombo A, Schuler G, Barragan P, Guagliumi G, Molnar F, Falotico R, Lesions RSGRSwtS-CBVB-ESitToPwdNNCA. A randomized comparison of a sirolimus-eluting stent with a standard stent for coronary revascularization. *N Engl J Med*. 2002;346:1773-1780.

[10] James SK, Stenestrand U, Lindback J, Carlsson J, Schersten F, Nilsson T, Wallentin L, Lagerqvist B. Long-term safety and efficacy of drug-eluting versus bare-metal stents in sweden. *N Engl J Med*. 2009;360:1933-1945.

[11] Stone GW, Kedhi E, Kereiakes DJ, Parise H, Fahy M, Serruys PW, Smits PC. Differential clinical responses to everolimus-eluting and paclitaxel-eluting coronary stents in patients with and without diabetes mellitus. *Circulation*. 2011;124:893-900.

[12] Kedhi E, Genereux P, Palmerini T, McAndrew TC, Parise H, Mehran R, Dangas GD, Stone GW. Impact of coronary lesion complexity on drug-eluting stent outcomes in patients with and without diabetes mellitus: Analysis from 18 pooled randomized trials. *J Am Coll Cardiol*. 2014.

[13] Dangas GD, Claessen BE, Caixeta A, Sanidas EA, Mintz GS, Mehran R. In-stent restenosis in the drug-eluting stent era. *Journal of the American College of Cardiology*. 2010;56:1897-1907.

[14] Chieffo A, Foglieni C, Nodari RL, Briguori C, Sangiorgi G, Latib A, Montorfano M, Airoldi F, Michev I, Carlino M, Colombo A, Maseri A. Histopathology of clinical coronary restenosis in drug-eluting versus bare metal stents. *Am J Cardiol*. 2009;104:1660-1667.

[15] Mehran R, Mintz GS, Hong MK, Tio FO, Bramwell O, Brahimi A, Kent KM, Pichard AD, Satler LF, Popma JJ, Leon MB. Validation of the in vivo intravascular ultrasound measurement of in-stent neointimal hyperplasia volumes. *J Am Coll Cardiol*. 1998;32:794-799.

[16] Dussaillant GR, Mintz GS, Pichard AD, Kent KM, Satler LF, Popma JJ, Wong SC, Leon MB. Small stent size and intimal hyperplasia contribute to restenosis: A volumetric intravascular ultrasound analysis. *J Am Coll Cardiol*. 1995;26:720-724.

[17] Colombo A, Orlic D, Stankovic G, Corvaja N, Spanos V, Montorfano M, Liistro F, Carlino M, Airoldi F, Chieffo A, Di Mario C. Preliminary observations regarding

angiographic pattern of restenosis after rapamycin-eluting stent implantation. *Circulation*. 2003;107:2178-2180.

[18] Latib A, Mussardo M, Ielasi A, Tarsia G, Godino C, Al-Lamee R, Chieffo A, Airoldi F, Carlino M, Montorfano M, Colombo A. Long-term outcomes after the percutaneous treatment of drug-eluting stent restenosis. *JACC. Cardiovascular interventions*. 2011;4:155-164.

[19] Cosgrave J, Melzi G, Biondi-Zoccai GG, Airoldi F, Chieffo A, Sangiorgi GM, Montorfano M, Michev I, Carlino M, Bonizzoni E, Colombo A. Drug-eluting stent restenosis the pattern predicts the outcome. *J Am Coll Cardiol*. 2006;47:2399-2404.

[20] Rathore S, Kinoshita Y, Terashima M, Katoh O, Tanaka N, Kimura M, Tsuchikane E, Nasu K, Ehara M, Asakura K, Asakura Y, Suzuki T. Sirolimus eluting stent restenosis: Impact of angiographic patterns and the treatment factors on angiographic outcomes in contemporary practice. *Int J Cardiol*. 2011;146:390-394.

[21] Alfonso F, Cequier A, Angel J, Marti V, Zueco J, Bethencourt A, Mantilla R, Lopez-Minguez JR, Gomez-Recio M, Moris C, Perez-Vizcayno MJ, Fernandez C, Macaya C, Seabra-Gomes R, Restenosis Intra-stent Balloon angioplasty versus elective Stenting I. Value of the american college of cardiology/american heart association angiographic classification of coronary lesion morphology in patients with in-stent restenosis. Insights from the restenosis intra-stent balloon angioplasty versus elective stenting (ribs) randomized trial. *Am Heart J*. 2006;151:681 e681-681 e689.

[22] Farb A, Sangiorgi G, Carter AJ, Walley VM, Edwards WD, Schwartz RS, Virmani R. Pathology of acute and chronic coronary stenting in humans. *Circulation*. 1999;99:44-52.

[23] Komatsu R, Ueda M, Naruko T, Kojima A, Becker AE. Neointimal tissue response at sites of coronary stenting in humans: Macroscopic, histological, and immunohistochemical analyses. *Circulation*. 1998;98:224-233.

[24] Arbustini E, De Servi S, Bramucci E, Porcu E, Costante AM, Grasso M, Diegoli M, Fasani R, Morbini P, Angoli L, Boscarini M, Repetto S, Danzi G, Niccoli L, Campolo L, Lucreziotti S, Specchia G. Comparison of coronary lesions obtained by directional coronary atherectomy in unstable angina, stable angina, and restenosis after either atherectomy or angioplasty. *Am J Cardiol*. 1995;75:675-682.

[25] Chung IM, Gold HK, Schwartz SM, Ikari Y, Reidy MA, Wight TN. Enhanced extracellular matrix accumulation in restenosis of coronary arteries after stent deployment. *J Am Coll Cardiol*. 2002;40:2072-2081.

[26] van Beusekom HM, Saia F, Zindler JD, Lemos PA, Swager-Ten Hoor SL, van Leeuwen MA, de Feijter PJ, Serruys PW, van der Giessen WJ. Drug-eluting stents show delayed healing: Paclitaxel more pronounced than sirolimus. *Eur Heart J*. 2007;28:974-979.

[27] Nakazawa G, Otsuka F, Nakano M, Vorpahl M, Yazdani SK, Ladich E, Kolodgie FD, Finn AV, Virmani R. The pathology of neoatherosclerosis in human coronary implants bare-metal and drug-eluting stents. *J Am Coll Cardiol*. 2011;57:1314-1322.

[28] Park SJ, Kang SJ, Virmani R, Nakano M, Ueda Y. In-stent neoatherosclerosis: A final common pathway of late stent failure. *J Am Coll Cardiol*. 2012;59:2051-2057.

[29] Takano M, Yamamoto M, Inami S, Murakami D, Ohba T, Seino Y, Mizuno K. Appearance of lipid-laden intima and neovascularization after implantation of bare-

metal stents extended late-phase observation by intracoronary optical coherence tomography. *J Am Coll Cardiol.* 2009;55:26-32.

[30] Rathore S, Kinoshita Y, Terashima M, Katoh O, Matsuo H, Tanaka N, Kimura M, Tsuchikane E, Nasu K, Ehara M, Asakura K, Asakura Y, Suzuki T. A comparison of clinical presentations, angiographic patterns and outcomes of in-stent restenosis between bare metal stents and drug eluting stents. *EuroIntervention: journal of EuroPCR in collaboration with the Working Group on Interventional Cardiology of the European Society of Cardiology.* 2010;5:841-846.

[31] Park CB, Hong MK, Kim YH, Park DW, Han KH, Lee CW, Kang DH, Song JK, Kim JJ, Park SW, Park SJ. Comparison of angiographic patterns of in-stent restenosis between sirolimus- and paclitaxel-eluting stent. *International journal of cardiology.* 2007;120:387-390.

[32] Escolar E, Mintz GS, Popma J, Michalek A, Kim SW, Mandinov L, Koglin J, Stone G, Ellis SG, Grube E, Dawkins KD, Weissman NJ. Meta-analysis of angiographic versus intravascular ultrasound parameters of drug-eluting stent efficacy (from taxus iv, v, and vi). *Am J Cardiol.* 2007;100:621-626.

[33] Weissman NJ, Koglin J, Cox DA, Hermiller J, O'Shaughnessy C, Mann JT, Turco M, Caputo R, Bergin P, Greenberg J, Kutcher M, Wong SC, Strickland W, Mooney M, Russell ME, Ellis SG, Stone GW. Polymer-based paclitaxel-eluting stents reduce in-stent neointimal tissue proliferation: A serial volumetric intravascular ultrasound analysis from the taxus-iv trial. *J Am Coll Cardiol.* 2005;45:1201-1205.

[34] Stone GW, Ellis SG, Cox DA, Hermiller J, O'Shaughnessy C, Mann JT, Turco M, Caputo R, Bergin P, Greenberg J, Popma JJ, Russell ME, Investigators T-I. A polymer-based, paclitaxel-eluting stent in patients with coronary artery disease. *N Engl J Med.* 2004;350:221-231.

[35] Stone GW, Ellis SG, Cox DA, Hermiller J, O'Shaughnessy C, Mann JT, Turco M, Caputo R, Bergin P, Greenberg J, Popma JJ, Russell ME, Investigators T-I. One-year clinical results with the slow-release, polymer-based, paclitaxel-eluting taxus stent: The taxus-iv trial. *Circulation.* 2004;109:1942-1947.

[36] Nayak AK, Kawamura A, Nesto RW, Davis G, Jarbeau J, Pyne CT, Gossman DE, Piemonte TC, Riskalla N, Chauhan MS. Myocardial infarction as a presentation of clinical in-stent restenosis. *Circ J.* 2006;70:1026-1029.

[37] Kini A, Marmur JD, Dangas G, Choudhary S, Sharma SK. Angiographic patterns of in-stent restenosis and implications on subsequent revascularization. *Catheter Cardiovasc Interv.* 2000;49:23-29.

[38] Pate GE, Lee M, Humphries K, Cohen E, Lowe R, Fox RS, Teskey R, Buller CE. Characterizing the spectrum of in-stent restenosis: Implications for contemporary treatment. *The Canadian journal of cardiology.* 2006;22:1223-1229.

[39] Appleby CE, Khattar RS, Morgan K, Clarke B, Curzen N, Neyses L, Fath-Ordoubadi F. Drug eluting stents for the treatment of bare metal in-stent restenosis: Long-term outcomes in real world practice. *EuroIntervention: journal of EuroPCR in collaboration with the Working Group on Interventional Cardiology of the European Society of Cardiology.* 2011;6:748-753.

[40] Solinas E, Dangas G, Kirtane AJ, Lansky AJ, Franklin-Bond T, Boland P, Syros G, Kim YH, Gupta A, Mintz G, Fahy M, Collins M, Kodali S, Stone GW, Moses JW, Leon MB, Mehran R. Angiographic patterns of drug-eluting stent restenosis and one-

year outcomes after treatment with repeated percutaneous coronary intervention. *The American journal of cardiology*. 2008;102:311-315.

[41] Kimura T, Yokoi H, Nakagawa Y, Tamura T, Kaburagi S, Sawada Y, Sato Y, Hamasaki N, Nosaka H, et al. Three-year follow-up after implantation of metallic coronary-artery stents. *N Engl J Med*. 1996;334:561-566.

[42] Byrne RA, Iijima R, Mehilli J, Pinieck S, Bruskina O, Schomig A, Kastrati A. Durability of antirestenotic efficacy in drug-eluting stents with and without permanent polymer. *JACC Cardiovasc Interv*. 2009;2:291-299.

[43] Finn AV, Nakazawa G, Kolodgie FD, Virmani R. Temporal course of neointimal formation after drug-eluting stent placement: Is our understanding of restenosis changing? *JACC Cardiovasc Interv*. 2009;2:300-302.

[44] Takebayashi H, Mintz GS, Carlier SG, Kobayashi Y, Fujii K, Yasuda T, Costa RA, Moussa I, Dangas GD, Mehran R, Lansky AJ, Kreps E, Collins MB, Colombo A, Stone GW, Leon MB, Moses JW. Nonuniform strut distribution correlates with more neointimal hyperplasia after sirolimus-eluting stent implantation. *Circulation*. 2004;110:3430-3434.

[45] Lemos PA, Saia F, Ligthart JM, Arampatzis CA, Sianos G, Tanabe K, Hoye A, Degertekin M, Daemen J, McFadden E, Hofma S, Smits PC, de Feyter P, van der Giessen WJ, van Domburg RT, Serruys PW. Coronary restenosis after sirolimus-eluting stent implantation: Morphological description and mechanistic analysis from a consecutive series of cases. *Circulation*. 2003;108:257-260.

[46] Sianos G, Hofma S, Ligthart JM, Saia F, Hoye A, Lemos PA, Serruys PW. Stent fracture and restenosis in the drug-eluting stent era. *Catheter Cardiovasc Interv*. 2004;61:111-116.

[47] Sakurai R, Ako J, Morino Y, Sonoda S, Kaneda H, Terashima M, Hassan AH, Leon MB, Moses JW, Popma JJ, Bonneau HN, Yock PG, Fitzgerald PJ, Honda Y. Predictors of edge stenosis following sirolimus-eluting stent deployment (a quantitative intravascular ultrasound analysis from the sirius trial). *Am J Cardiol*. 2005;96:1251-1253.

[48] Ichimoto E, Fujimoto Y, Kubo K, Miyayama T, Iwata Y, Kitahara H, Kobayashi Y. Mechanism of edge restenosis after sirolimus-eluting stent implantation. *J Invasive Cardiol*. 2012;24:55-57.

[49] Hecht HS, Polena S, Jelnin V, Jimenez M, Bhatti T, Parikh M, Panagopoulos G, Roubin G. Stent gap by 64-detector computed tomographic angiography relationship to in-stent restenosis, fracture, and overlap failure. *J Am Coll Cardiol*. 2009;54:1949-1959.

[50] Zhang X, Yang L, Ju H, Zhang F, Wu J, He B, Chen Y. Prevalence and prognosis of coronary stent gap detected by multi-detector ct: A follow-up study. *Eur Radiol*. 2012;22:1896-1903.

[51] Popma JJ, Leon MB, Moses JW, Holmes DR, Jr., Cox N, Fitzpatrick M, Douglas J, Lambert C, Mooney M, Yakubov S, Kuntz RE, Investigators S. Quantitative assessment of angiographic restenosis after sirolimus-eluting stent implantation in native coronary arteries. *Circulation*. 2004;110:3773-3780.

[52] Corbett SJ, Cosgrave J, Melzi G, Babic R, Biondi-Zoccai GG, Godino C, Morici N, Airoldi F, Michev I, Montorfano M, Sangiorgi GM, Bonizzoni E, Colombo A. Patterns of restenosis after drug-eluting stent implantation: Insights from a contemporary and

comparative analysis of sirolimus- and paclitaxel-eluting stents. *European heart journal*. 2006;27:2330-2337.

[53] Iakovou I, Schmidt T, Ge L, Sangiorgi GM, Stankovic G, Airoldi F, Chieffo A, Montorfano M, Carlino M, Michev I, Corvaja N, Cosgrave J, Gerckens U, Grube E, Colombo A. Angiographic patterns of restenosis after paclitaxel-eluting stent implantation. *Journal of the American College of Cardiology*. 2005;45:805-806.

[54] Schomig A, Dibra A, Windecker S, Mehilli J, Suarez de Lezo J, Kaiser C, Park SJ, Goy JJ, Lee JH, Di Lorenzo E, Wu J, Juni P, Pfisterer ME, Meier B, Kastrati A. A meta-analysis of 16 randomized trials of sirolimus-eluting stents versus paclitaxel-eluting stents in patients with coronary artery disease. *J Am Coll Cardiol*. 2007;50:1373-1380.

[55] Morice MC, Colombo A, Meier B, Serruys P, Tamburino C, Guagliumi G, Sousa E, Stoll HP, Investigators RT. Sirolimus- vs paclitaxel-eluting stents in de novo coronary artery lesions: The reality trial: A randomized controlled trial. *Jama*. 2006;295:895-904.

[56] Windecker S, Remondino A, Eberli FR, Juni P, Raber L, Wenaweser P, Togni M, Billinger M, Tuller D, Seiler C, Roffi M, Corti R, Sutsch G, Maier W, Luscher T, Hess OM, Egger M, Meier B. Sirolimus-eluting and paclitaxel-eluting stents for coronary revascularization. *N Engl J Med*. 2005;353:653-662.

[57] Kastrati A, Dibra A, Eberle S, Mehilli J, Suarez de Lezo J, Goy JJ, Ulm K, Schomig A. Sirolimus-eluting stents vs paclitaxel-eluting stents in patients with coronary artery disease: Meta-analysis of randomized trials. *Jama*. 2005;294:819-825.

[58] Raber L, Wohlwend L, Wigger M, Togni M, Wandel S, Wenaweser P, Cook S, Moschovitis A, Vogel R, Kalesan B, Seiler C, Eberli F, Luscher TF, Meier B, Juni P, Windecker S. Five-year clinical and angiographic outcomes of a randomized comparison of sirolimus-eluting and paclitaxel-eluting stents: Results of the sirolimus-eluting versus paclitaxel-eluting stents for coronary revascularization late trial. *Circulation*. 2011;123:2819-2828, 2816 p following 2828.

[59] Dibra A, Kastrati A, Mehilli J, Pache J, Schuhlen H, von Beckerath N, Ulm K, Wessely R, Dirschinger J, Schomig A, Investigators I-DS. Paclitaxel-eluting or sirolimus-eluting stents to prevent restenosis in diabetic patients. *N Engl J Med*. 2005;353:663-670.

[60] Mehilli J, Dibra A, Kastrati A, Pache J, Dirschinger J, Schomig A, Intracoronary Drug-Eluting Stenting to Abrogate Restenosis in Small Arteries Study I. Randomized trial of paclitaxel- and sirolimus-eluting stents in small coronary vessels. *Eur Heart J*. 2006;27:260-266.

[61] Marx SO, Marks AR. Bench to bedside: The development of rapamycin and its application to stent restenosis. *Circulation*. 2001;104:852-855.

[62] Poon M, Marx SO, Gallo R, Badimon JJ, Taubman MB, Marks AR. Rapamycin inhibits vascular smooth muscle cell migration. *J Clin Invest*. 1996;98:2277-2283.

[63] Rowinsky EK, Donehower RC. Paclitaxel (taxol). *N Engl J Med*. 1995;332:1004-1014.

[64] Drachman DE, Edelman ER, Seifert P, Groothuis AR, Bornstein DA, Kamath KR, Palasis M, Yang D, Nott SH, Rogers C. Neointimal thickening after stent delivery of paclitaxel: Change in composition and arrest of growth over six months. *J Am Coll Cardiol*. 2000;36:2325-2332.

[65] Lemos PA, Moulin B, Perin MA, Oliveira LA, Arruda JA, Lima VC, Lima AA, Caramori PR, Medeiros CR, Barbosa MR, Brito FS, Jr., Ribeiro EE, Martinez EE, investigators Pt. Randomized evaluation of two drug-eluting stents with identical metallic platform and biodegradable polymer but different agents (paclitaxel or

sirolimus) compared against bare stents: 1-year results of the paint trial. *Catheter Cardiovasc Interv*. 2009;74:665-673.

[66] Joner M, Finn AV, Farb A, Mont EK, Kolodgie FD, Ladich E, Kutys R, Skorija K, Gold HK, Virmani R. Pathology of drug-eluting stents in humans: Delayed healing and late thrombotic risk. *J Am Coll Cardiol*. 2006;48:193-202.

[67] Finn AV, Kolodgie FD, Harnek J, Guerrero LJ, Acampado E, Tefera K, Skorija K, Weber DK, Gold HK, Virmani R. Differential response of delayed healing and persistent inflammation at sites of overlapping sirolimus- or paclitaxel-eluting stents. *Circulation*. 2005;112:270-278.

[68] Stone GW, Midei M, Newman W, Sanz M, Hermiller JB, Williams J, Farhat N, Mahaffey KW, Cutlip DE, Fitzgerald PJ, Sood P, Su X, Lansky AJ, Investigators SI. Comparison of an everolimus-eluting stent and a paclitaxel-eluting stent in patients with coronary artery disease: A randomized trial. *Jama*. 2008;299:1903-1913.

[69] Applegate RJ, Yaqub M, Hermiller JB, Sood P, Yu S, Doostzadeh J, Williams JE, Farhat N, Caputo R, Lansky AJ, Cutlip DE, Sudhir K, Stone GW. Long-term (three-year) safety and efficacy of everolimus-eluting stents compared to paclitaxel-eluting stents (from the spirit iii trial). *The American journal of cardiology*. 2011;107:833-840.

[70] Stone GW, Rizvi A, Newman W, Mastali K, Wang JC, Caputo R, Doostzadeh J, Cao S, Simonton CA, Sudhir K, Lansky AJ, Cutlip DE, Kereiakes DJ, Investigators SI. Everolimus-eluting versus paclitaxel-eluting stents in coronary artery disease. *N Engl J Med*. 2010;362:1663-1674.

[71] Alazzoni A, Al-Saleh A, Jolly SS. Everolimus-eluting versus paclitaxel-eluting stents in percutaneous coronary intervention: Meta-analysis of randomized trials. *Thrombosis*. 2012;2012:126369.

[72] Yamasaki M, Tsujino I, Lima-Filho MO, Ako J, Shimohama T, Hasegawa T, Sakurai R, Sudhir K, Stone GW, Waseda K, Honda Y, Fitzgerald PJ. Comparison of vascular response to the everolimus-eluting stent versus the paclitaxel-eluting stent: Intravascular ultrasound results from the spirit iii trial. *EuroIntervention*. 2012;8:724-731.

[73] de Waha A, Dibra A, Byrne RA, Ndrepepa G, Mehilli J, Fusaro M, Laugwitz KL, Massberg S, Schomig A, Kastrati A. Everolimus-eluting versus sirolimus-eluting stents: A meta-analysis of randomized trials. *Circ Cardiovasc Interv*. 2011;4:371-377.

[74] Kozuma K, Kimura T, Kadota K, Suwa S, Kimura K, Iwabuchi M, Kawai K, Miyazawa A, Kawamura M, Nakao K, Asano R, Yamamoto T, Suzuki N, Aoki J, Kyono H, Nakazawa G, Tanabe K, Morino Y, Igarashi K. Angiographic findings of everolimus-eluting as compared to sirolimus-eluting stents: Angiographic sub-study from the randomized evaluation of sirolimus-eluting versus everolimus-eluting stent trial (reset). *Cardiovascular intervention and therapeutics*. 2013;28:344-351.

[75] Kandzari DE, Leon MB, Popma JJ, Fitzgerald PJ, O'Shaughnessy C, Ball MW, Turco M, Applegate RJ, Gurbel PA, Midei MG, Badre SS, Mauri L, Thompson KP, LeNarz LA, Kuntz RE, Investigators EI. Comparison of zotarolimus-eluting and sirolimus-eluting stents in patients with native coronary artery disease: A randomized controlled trial. *J Am Coll Cardiol*. 2006;48:2440-2447.

[76] Miyazawa A, Ako J, Hongo Y, Hur SH, Tsujino I, Courtney BK, Hassan AH, Kandzari DE, Honda Y, Fitzgerald PJ, Investigators EI. Comparison of vascular response to

zotarolimus-eluting stent versus sirolimus-eluting stent: Intravascular ultrasound results from endeavor iii. *Am Heart J.* 2008;155:108-113.

[77] Leon MB, Mauri L, Popma JJ, Cutlip DE, Nikolsky E, O'Shaughnessy C, Overlie PA, McLaurin BT, Solomon SL, Douglas JS, Jr., Ball MW, Caputo RP, Jain A, Tolleson TR, Reen BM, 3rd, Kirtane AJ, Fitzgerald PJ, Thompson K, Kandzari DE, Investigators EI. A randomized comparison of the endeavor zotarolimus-eluting stent versus the taxus paclitaxel-eluting stent in de novo native coronary lesions 12-month outcomes from the endeavor iv trial. *J Am Coll Cardiol.* 2010;55:543-554.

[78] Waseda K, Miyazawa A, Ako J, Hasegawa T, Tsujino I, Sakurai R, Yock PG, Honda Y, Kandzari DE, Leon MB, Fitzgerald PJ, Investigators EIT. Intravascular ultrasound results from the endeavor iv trial: Randomized comparison between zotarolimus- and paclitaxel-eluting stents in patients with coronary artery disease. *JACC Cardiovasc Interv.* 2009;2:779-784.

[79] Eisenstein EL, Leon MB, Kandzari DE, Mauri L, Edwards R, Kong DF, Cowper PA, Anstrom KJ, Investigators EI. Long-term clinical and economic analysis of the endeavor zotarolimus-eluting stent versus the cypher sirolimus-eluting stent: 3-year results from the endeavor iii trial (randomized controlled trial of the medtronic endeavor drug [abt-578] eluting coronary stent system versus the cypher sirolimus-eluting coronary stent system in de novo native coronary artery lesions). *JACC Cardiovasc Interv.* 2009;2:1199-1207.

[80] Kandzari DE, Mauri L, Popma JJ, Turco MA, Gurbel PA, Fitzgerald PJ, Leon MB. Late-term clinical outcomes with zotarolimus- and sirolimus-eluting stents. 5-year follow-up of the endeavor iii (a randomized controlled trial of the medtronic endeavor drug [abt-578] eluting coronary stent system versus the cypher sirolimus-eluting coronary stent system in de novo native coronary artery lesions). *JACC Cardiovasc Interv.* 2011;4:543-550.

[81] Maeng M, Tilsted HH, Jensen LO, Krusell LR, Kaltoft A, Kelbaek H, Villadsen AB, Ravkilde J, Hansen KN, Christiansen EH, Aaroe J, Jensen JS, Kristensen SD, Botker HE, Thuesen L, Madsen M, Thayssen P, Sorensen HT, Lassen JF. Differential clinical outcomes after 1 year versus 5 years in a randomised comparison of zotarolimus-eluting and sirolimus-eluting coronary stents (the sort out iii study): A multicentre, open-label, randomised superiority trial. *Lancet.* 2014.

[82] Yeung AC, Leon MB, Jain A, Tolleson TR, Spriggs DJ, Mc Laurin BT, Popma JJ, Fitzgerald PJ, Cutlip DE, Massaro JM, Mauri L. Clinical evaluation of the resolute zotarolimus-eluting coronary stent system in the treatment of de novo lesions in native coronary arteries: The resolute us clinical trial. *J Am Coll Cardiol.* 2011;57:1778-1783.

[83] Waseda K, Ako J, Yamasaki M, Koizumi T, Sakurai R, Hongo Y, Koo BK, Ormiston J, Worthley SG, Whitbourn RJ, Walters DL, Meredith IT, Fitzgerald PJ, Honda Y. Impact of polymer formulations on neointimal proliferation after zotarolimus-eluting stent with different polymers: Insights from the resolute trial. *Circ Cardiovasc Interv.* 2011;4:248-255.

[84] Serruys PW, Silber S, Garg S, van Geuns RJ, Richardt G, Buszman PE, Kelbaek H, van Boven AJ, Hofma SH, Linke A, Klauss V, Wijns W, Macaya C, Garot P, DiMario C, Manoharan G, Kornowski R, Ischinger T, Bartorelli A, Ronden J, Bressers M, Gobbens P, Negoita M, van Leeuwen F, Windecker S. Comparison of zotarolimus-eluting and everolimus-eluting coronary stents. *N Engl J Med.* 2010;363:136-146.

[85] Silber S, Windecker S, Vranckx P, Serruys PW, investigators RAC. Unrestricted randomised use of two new generation drug-eluting coronary stents: 2-year patient-related versus stent-related outcomes from the resolute all comers trial. *Lancet.* 2011;377:1241-1247

[86] Taniwaki M, Stefanini GG, Silber S, Richardt G, Vranckx P, Serruys PW, Buszman PE, Kelbaek H, Windecker S, Investigators RA-C. 4-year clinical outcomes and predictors of repeat revascularization in patients treated with new-generation drug-eluting stents: A report from the resolute all-comers trial (a randomized comparison of a zotarolimus-eluting stent with an everolimus-eluting stent for percutaneous coronary intervention). *J Am Coll Cardiol.* 2014;63:1617-1625.

[87] Gutierrez-Chico JL, van Geuns RJ, Regar E, van der Giessen WJ, Kelbaek H, Saunamaki K, Escaned J, Gonzalo N, di Mario C, Borgia F, Nuesch E, Garcia-Garcia HM, Silber S, Windecker S, Serruys PW. Tissue coverage of a hydrophilic polymer-coated zotarolimus-eluting stent vs. A fluoropolymer-coated everolimus-eluting stent at 13-month follow-up: An optical coherence tomography substudy from the resolute all comers trial. *Eur Heart J.* 2011;32:2454-2463.

[88] Lee S YC, Oh I, et al. Changing morphologic patterns of restenosis with the 2nd generation drug-eluting stent: A shift towards focal restenosis. *J Am Coll Cardiol.*

[89] Ormiston JA, Serruys PW, Regar E, Dudek D, Thuesen L, Webster MW, Onuma Y, Garcia-Garcia HM, McGreevy R, Veldhof S. A bioabsorbable everolimus-eluting coronary stent system for patients with single de-novo coronary artery lesions (absorb): A prospective open-label trial. *Lancet.* 2008;371:899-907.

[90] Windecker S, Serruys PW, Wandel S, Buszman P, Trznadel S, Linke A, Lenk K, Ischinger T, Klauss V, Eberli F, Corti R, Wijns W, Morice MC, di Mario C, Davies S, van Geuns RJ, Eerdmans P, van Es GA, Meier B, Juni P. Biolimus-eluting stent with biodegradable polymer versus sirolimus-eluting stent with durable polymer for coronary revascularisation (leaders): A randomised non-inferiority trial. *Lancet.* 2008;372:1163-1173.

[91] Barlis P, Regar E, Serruys PW, Dimopoulos K, van der Giessen WJ, van Geuns RJ, Ferrante G, Wandel S, Windecker S, van Es GA, Eerdmans P, Juni P, di Mario C. An optical coherence tomography study of a biodegradable vs. Durable polymer-coated limus-eluting stent: A leaders trial sub-study. *European heart journal.* 2010;31:165-176.

[92] Stefanini GG, Kalesan B, Serruys PW, Heg D, Buszman P, Linke A, Ischinger T, Klauss V, Eberli F, Wijns W, Morice MC, Di Mario C, Corti R, Antoni D, Sohn HY, Eerdmans P, van Es GA, Meier B, Windecker S, Juni P. Long-term clinical outcomes of biodegradable polymer biolimus-eluting stents versus durable polymer sirolimus-eluting stents in patients with coronary artery disease (leaders): 4 year follow-up of a randomised non-inferiority trial. *Lancet.* 2011.

[93] Stefanini GG, Byrne RA, Serruys PW, de Waha A, Meier B, Massberg S, Juni P, Schomig A, Windecker S, Kastrati A. Biodegradable polymer drug-eluting stents reduce the risk of stent thrombosis at 4 years in patients undergoing percutaneous coronary intervention: A pooled analysis of individual patient data from the isar-test 3, isar-test 4, and leaders randomized trials. *Eur Heart J.* 2012;33:1214-1222.

[94] Serruys PW, Ormiston JA, Onuma Y, Regar E, Gonzalo N, Garcia-Garcia HM, Nieman K, Bruining N, Dorange C, Miquel-Hebert K, Veldhof S, Webster M, Thuesen L,

Dudek D. A bioabsorbable everolimus-eluting coronary stent system (absorb): 2-year outcomes and results from multiple imaging methods. *Lancet*. 2009;373:897-910.

[95] Nakatani S, Onuma Y, Ishibashi Y, Muramatsu T, Iqbal J, Zhang YJ, van Geuns RJ, Ormiston JA, Serruys PW. Early (before 6 months), late (6-12 months) and very late (after 12 months) angiographic scaffold restenosis in the absorb cohort b trial. *EuroIntervention*. 2014.

[96] Gomez-Lara J, Brugaletta S, Farooq V, Onuma Y, Diletti R, Windecker S, Thuesen L, McClean D, Koolen J, Whitbourn R, Dudek D, Smits PC, Chevalier B, Regar E, Veldhof S, Rapoza R, Ormiston JA, Garcia-Garcia HM, Serruys PW. Head-to-head comparison of the neointimal response between metallic and bioresorbable everolimus-eluting scaffolds using optical coherence tomography. *JACC Cardiovasc Interv*. 2011;4:1271-1280.

[97] Jaguszewski M, Obeid S, Luscher TF, Templin C. First three-dimensional optical frequency domain imaging evaluation of a bioabsorbable vascular scaffold implantation in an instent-restenosis 6 years after cypher stenting. *Eur Heart J*. 2014.

[98] Patel N, Banning AP. Bioabsorbable scaffolds for the treatment of obstructive coronary artery disease: The next revolution in coronary intervention? *Heart*. 2013;99:1236-1243.

[99] Gogas BD, Garcia-Garcia HM, Onuma Y, Muramatsu T, Farooq V, Bourantas CV, Serruys PW. Edge vascular response after percutaneous coronary intervention: An intracoronary ultrasound and optical coherence tomography appraisal: From radioactive platforms to first- and second-generation drug-eluting stents and bioresorbable scaffolds. *JACC Cardiovasc Interv*. 2013;6:211-221.

[100] Weissman NJ, Ellis SG, Grube E, Dawkins KD, Greenberg JD, Mann T, Cannon LA, Cambier PA, Fernandez S, Mintz GS, Mandinov L, Koglin J, Stone GW. Effect of the polymer-based, paclitaxel-eluting taxus express stent on vascular tissue responses: A volumetric intravascular ultrasound integrated analysis from the taxus iv, v, and vi trials. *Eur Heart J*. 2007;28:1574-1582.

[101] Weissman NJ, Koglin J, Cox DA, Hermiller J, O'Shaughnessy C, Mann JT, Turco M, Caputo R, Bergin P, Greenberg J, Kutcher M, Wong SC, Strickland W, Mooney M, Russell ME, Ellis SG, Stone GW. Polymer-based paclitaxel-eluting stents reduce in-stent neointimal tissue proliferation: A serial volumetric intravascular ultrasound analysis from the taxus-iv trial. *J Am Coll Cardiol*. 2005;45:1201-1205.

[102] Serruys PW, Degertekin M, Tanabe K, Russell ME, Guagliumi G, Webb J, Hamburger J, Rutsch W, Kaiser C, Whitbourn R, Camenzind E, Meredith I, Reeves F, Nienaber C, Benit E, Disco C, Koglin J, Colombo A. Vascular responses at proximal and distal edges of paclitaxel-eluting stents: Serial intravascular ultrasound analysis from the taxus ii trial. *Circulation*. 2004;109:627-633.

[103] Hoffmann R, Guagliumi G, Musumeci G, Reimers B, Petronio AS, Disco C, Amoroso G, Moses JW, Fitzgerald PJ, Schofer J, Leon MB, Breithardt G. Vascular response to sirolimus-eluting stents delivered with a nonaggressive implantation technique: Comparison of intravascular ultrasound results from the multicenter, randomized e-sirius, and sirius trials. *Catheter Cardiovasc Interv*. 2005;66:499-506.

[104] Weisz G, Leon MB, Holmes DR, Jr., Kereiakes DJ, Popma JJ, Teirstein PS, Cohen SA, Wang H, Cutlip DE, Moses JW. Five-year follow-up after sirolimus-eluting stent

implantation results of the sirius (sirolimus-eluting stent in de-novo native coronary lesions) trial. *J Am Coll Cardiol.* 2009;53:1488-1497.

[105] Shimohama T, Ako J, Yamasaki M, Otake H, Tsujino I, Hasegawa T, Nakatani D, Sakurai R, Chang H, Kusano H, Waseda K, Honda Y, Stone GW, Saito S, Fitzgerald PJ, Sudhir K. Spirit iii japan versus spirit iii USA: A comparative intravascular ultrasound analysis of the everolimus-eluting stent. *Am J Cardiol.* 2010;106:13-17.

[106] Applegate RJ, Yaqub M, Hermiller JB, Sood P, Yu S, Doostzadeh J, Williams JE, Farhat N, Caputo R, Lansky AJ, Cutlip DE, Sudhir K, Stone GW. Long-term (three-year) safety and efficacy of everolimus-eluting stents compared to paclitaxel-eluting stents (from the spirit iii trial). *Am J Cardiol.* 2011;107:833-840.

[107] Gogas BD, Bourantas CV, Garcia-Garcia HM, Onuma Y, Muramatsu T, Farooq V, Diletti R, van Geuns RJ, De Bruyne B, Chevalier B, Thuesen L, Smits PC, Dudek D, Koolen J, Windecker S, Whitbourn R, McClean D, Dorange C, Miquel-Hebert K, Veldhof S, Rapoza R, Ormiston JA, Serruys PW. The edge vascular response following implantation of the absorb everolimus-eluting bioresorbable vascular scaffold and the xience v metallic everolimus-eluting stent. First serial follow-up assessment at six months and two years: Insights from the first-in-man absorb cohort b and spirit ii trials. *EuroIntervention.* 2013;9:709-720.

[108] Bauters C, Hubert E, Prat A, Bougrimi K, Van Belle E, McFadden EP, Amouyel P, Lablanche JM, Bertrand M. Predictors of restenosis after coronary stent implantation. *J Am Coll Cardiol.* 1998;31:1291-1298.

[109] Kornowski R, Mintz GS, Kent KM, Pichard AD, Satler LF, Bucher TA, Hong MK, Popma JJ, Leon MB. Increased restenosis in diabetes mellitus after coronary interventions is due to exaggerated intimal hyperplasia. A serial intravascular ultrasound study. *Circulation.* 1997;95:1366-1369.

[110] Kaneda H, Ako J, Kataoka T, Takahashi T, Terashima M, Waseda K, Miyazawa A, Hassan A, Honda Y, Yock PG, Fitzgerald PJ. Heterogeneity of neointimal distribution of in-stent restenosis in patients with diabetes mellitus. *Am J Cardiol.* 2006;97:340-342.

[111] Kimura M, Mintz GS, Weissman NJ, Dawkins KD, Grube E, Ellis SG, Cannon LA, Masud Z, Mandinov L, Baim D, Stone GW. Meta-analysis of the effects of paclitaxel-eluting stents versus bare metal stents on volumetric intravascular ultrasound in patients with versus without diabetes mellitus. *Am J Cardiol.* 2008;101:1263-1268.

[112] Du R, Zhang RY, Zhu ZB, Zhang Q, Hu J, Yang ZK, Yan ZJ, Lv AK, Ding FH, Zhang JS, Shen WF. Impact of angiographic and intravascular ultrasound features on clinical outcome after sirolimus-eluting stent implantation for de-novo lesions in nondiabetic and type 2 diabetic patients. *Coron Artery Dis.* 2010;21:175-181.

[113] Kang SJ, Mintz GS, Park DW, Lee SW, Kim YH, Whan Lee C, Han KH, Kim JJ, Park SW, Park SJ. Mechanisms of in-stent restenosis after drug-eluting stent implantation: Intravascular ultrasound analysis. *Circ Cardiovasc Interv.* 2011;4:9-14.

[114] Kang SJ, Mintz GS, Park DW, Lee SW, Kim YH, Lee CW, Han KH, Kim JJ, Park SW, Park SJ. Tissue characterization of in-stent neointima using intravascular ultrasound radiofrequency data analysis. *Am J Cardiol.* 2010;106:1561-1565.

[115] Gonzalo N, Serruys PW, Okamura T, van Beusekom HM, Garcia-Garcia HM, van Soest G, van der Giessen W, Regar E. Optical coherence tomography patterns of stent restenosis. *Am Heart J.* 2009;158:284-293.

[116] Habara M, Terashima M, Nasu K, Kaneda H, Yokota D, Ito T, Kurita T, Teramoto T, Kimura M, Kinoshita Y, Tsuchikane E, Asakura Y, Suzuki T. Morphological differences of tissue characteristics between early, late, and very late restenosis lesions after first generation drug-eluting stent implantation: An optical coherence tomography study. *European heart journal cardiovascular Imaging*. 2013;14:276-284.

[117] Kang SJ, Mintz GS, Akasaka T, Park DW, Lee JY, Kim WJ, Lee SW, Kim YH, Whan Lee C, Park SW, Park SJ. Optical coherence tomographic analysis of in-stent neoatherosclerosis after drug-eluting stent implantation. *Circulation*. 2011;123:2954-2963.

[118] Ali ZA, Roleder T, Narula J, Mohanty BD, Baber U, Kovacic JC, Mintz GS, Otsuka F, Pan S, Virmani R, Sharma SK, Moreno P, Kini AS. Increased thin-cap neoatheroma and periprocedural myocardial infarction in drug-eluting stent restenosis: Multimodality intravascular imaging of drug-eluting and bare-metal stents. *Circ Cardiovasc Interv*. 2013;6:507-517.

[119] Teramoto T, Ikeno F, Otake H, Lyons JK, van Beusekom HM, Fearon WF, Yeung AC. Intriguing peri-strut low-intensity area detected by optical coherence tomography after coronary stent deployment. *Circ J*. 2010;74:1257-1259.

[120] Otake H, Shite J, Ikeno F, Shinke T, Teramoto T, Miyoshi N, Ako J, Honda Y, Fitzgerald PJ, Hirata K. Evaluation of the peri-strut low intensity area following sirolimus- and paclitaxel-eluting stents implantation: Insights from an optical coherence tomography study in humans. *Int J Cardiol*. 2012;157:38-42.

[121] Kilickesmez K, Dall'Ara G, Rama-Merchan JC, Ghione M, Mattesini A, Vinues CM, Konstantinidis N, Pighi M, Estevez-Loureiro R, Zivelonghi C, Lindsay AC, Secco GG, Foin N, De Silva R, Di Mario C. Optical coherence tomography characteristics of in-stent restenosis are different between first and second generation drug eluting stents. *IJC Heart & Vessels*. 2014.

[122] Lopez-Palop R, Pinar E, Lozano I, Saura D, Pico F, Valdes M. Utility of the fractional flow reserve in the evaluation of angiographically moderate in-stent restenosis. *European heart journal*. 2004;25:2040-2047.

[123] Dibra A, Kastrati A, Alfonso F, Seyfarth M, Perez-Vizcayno MJ, Mehilli J, Schomig A. Effectiveness of drug-eluting stents in patients with bare-metal in-stent restenosis: Meta-analysis of randomized trials. *J Am Coll Cardiol*. 2007;49:616-623.

[124] Alfonso F, Melgares R, Mainar V, Lezaun R, Vazquez N, Tascon J, Pomar F, Cequier A, Angel J, Perez-Vizcayno MJ, Sabate M, Banuelos C, Fernandez C, Garcia JM, Restensois Intra-stent: Ballon angioplasty versus elective Stenting I. Therapeutic implications of in-stent restenosis located at the stent edge. Insights from the restenosis intra-stent balloon angioplasty versus elective stenting (ribs) randomized trial. *Eur Heart J*. 2004;25:1829-1835.

[125] Alfonso F, Perez-Vizcayno MJ, Cardenas A, Garcia Del Blanco B, Seidelberger B, Iniguez A, Gomez-Recio M, Masotti M, Velazquez MT, Sanchis J, Garcia-Touchard A, Zueco J, Bethencourt A, Melgares R, Cequier A, Dominguez A, Mainar V, Lopez-Minguez JR, Moreu J, Marti V, Moreno R, Jimenez-Quevedo P, Gonzalo N, Fernandez C, Macaya C, Ribs V Study Investigators utaotWGoICotSSoC. A randomized comparison of drug-eluting balloon versus everolimus-eluting stent in patients with bare-metal stent-in-stent restenosis: The ribs v clinical trial (restenosis intra-stent of

bare metal stents: Paclitaxel-eluting balloon vs. Everolimus-eluting stent). *J Am Coll Cardiol.* 2014;63:1378-1386.

[126] Byrne RA, Neumann FJ, Mehilli J, Pinieck S, Wolff B, Tiroch K, Schulz S, Fusaro M, Ott I, Ibrahim T, Hausleiter J, Valina C, Pache J, Laugwitz KL, Massberg S, Kastrati A, investigators I-D. Paclitaxel-eluting balloons, paclitaxel-eluting stents, and balloon angioplasty in patients with restenosis after implantation of a drug-eluting stent (isar-desire 3): A randomised, open-label trial. *Lancet.* 2013;381:461-467.

[127] Mehilli J, Byrne RA, Tiroch K, Pinieck S, Schulz S, Kufner S, Massberg S, Laugwitz KL, Schomig A, Kastrati A, Investigators I-D. Randomized trial of paclitaxel- versus sirolimus-eluting stents for treatment of coronary restenosis in sirolimus-eluting stents: The isar-desire 2 (intracoronary stenting and angiographic results: Drug eluting stents for in-stent restenosis 2) study. *J Am Coll Cardiol.* 2010;55:2710-2716.

[128] Kufner S, Byrne RA, de Waha A, Schulz S, Joner M, Laugwitz KL, Kastrati A, Intracoronary S, Angiographic Results: Drug Eluting Stents for In-Stent Restenosis I. Sirolimus-eluting versus paclitaxel-eluting stents in diabetic and non-diabetic patients within sirolimus-eluting stent restenosis: Results from the isar-desire 2 trial. *Cardiovascular revascularization medicine: including molecular interventions.* 2014;15:69-75.

[129] Kitahara H, Kobayashi Y, Takebayashi H, Nakamura Y, Kuroda N, Miyazaki A, Haruta S, Komuro I. Angiographic patterns of restenosis after sirolimus-eluting stent implantation. *Circulation journal: official journal of the Japanese Circulation Society.* 2009;73:508-511.

[130] Bangalore S, Fusaro M, Amoroso N, Attubato MJ, Feit F, Slater J, Kumar S, Bhatt DL. Response to letter regarding article, "short- and long-term outcomes with drug-eluting and bare-metal coronary stents: A mixed-treatment comparison analysis of 117,762 patient-years of follow-up from randomized trials". *Circulation.* 2013;127:e447.

In: Coronary Artery Restenosis
Editor: Amir S. Lotfi
ISBN: 978-1-63321-346-3

Chapter 4

Coronary Restenosis: Clinical Outcomes

Hani Kozman, MD, FACC, FRCPC[1,•]
and Kan Liu, MD, PhD, FACC[2]
[1]Cardiac Catheterization Laboratory, Upstate Medical University, Syracuse, NY, US
[2]Non-invasive Laboratory, Upstate Medical University, Syracuse, NY, US

Abstract

Percutaneous coronary intervention is the primary mode of revascularization in patients with hemodynamically significant coronary artery stenosis. Despite advances in stent technology, restenosis remains a major issue with coronary intervention. In this chapter the clinical presentation and the impact of restenosis on clinical outcomes will be reviewed.

Introduction

The treatment of coronary artery disease focuses on improving morbidity and mortality. The field of interventional cardiology is a relative newcomer to the myriad of medical approaches to improve patient outcomes. The percutaneous treatment of coronary artery disease caused by arteriosclerosis was introduced by Grüntzig et al. in the late 1970s with the concept of balloon angioplasty (BA) [1]. Percutaneous coronary intervention (PCI) is now the primary mode of coronary revascularization in patients with significant coronary artery disease. Since the introduction of coronary artery stents, BA is rarely employed as a stand-alone management of significant coronary stenosis. The continued improvement in not only stent design but also the use stents as local drug-delivery agents has enabled treatment of more complex and difficult coronary lesions.

• Corresponding Author: Hani Kozman, MD Upstate University Hospital. University Health Care Center 5th Fl., 90 Presidential Plaza Syracuse, NY 13202. E-mail: kozmanh@upstate.edu.

Despite the technological improvements, coronary restenosis continues to be a major issue after coronary intervention. Even though the cause of restenosis varies based on the type of intervention (BA, bare metal stent (BMS), or drug eluting stent (DES)) its impact has important clinical consequences on the patient. Generally restenosis is not as dramatic as its acute counterpart, stent thrombosis, however it is associated with significant morbidity. The type of lesion treated and its contribution to the coronary circulation play a part in the incidence and symptomatology of restenosis respectively. Small vessels (< 3.0 mm diameter), long lesions, bifurcations, chronic total occlusions, vein grafts, aorto-ostial lesions are all angiographic characteristics found to be associated with restenosis occurrence [2]. Patient characteristics associated with restenosis include age, female sex, diabetes mellitus, and the presence of multivessel disease [3]. Procedural characteristics include final diameter stenosis, stent underexpansion, hypersensitivity, stent fracture, barotrauma outside the stented segment and type of stent used.

The relative contribution to the coronary circulation and degree of recurrent vessel occlusion would also predict the symptomatology of restenosis. Although chronic total occlusions have a higher rate of restenosis, symptomatology related to restenosis occurrence is often lacking [4]. On the other hand, restenosis in the situation of left main stenting has been associated with sudden cardiac death and has lead many practitioners to perform repeat diagnostic angiograms on these patients in order to help pre-empt a catastrophic event [5]. In this chapter we will discuss the symptomatology and clinical outcomes of stenting de novo and restenotic lesions in the DES era.

Definition

Binary angiographic restenosis is defined as > 50% luminal narrowing on follow-up angiography. The definition of clinical restenosis is the angiographic definition plus a history of angina pectoris, objective signs of ischemia at rest or during exercise test or abnormal invasive functional test (table 1). Also any recurrent lesion >70% in the absence of the above signs or symptoms would qualify as clinical restenosis [2].

In analyzing the clinical presentation of restenosis in the present era, we can infer that although the majority of patients are presenting with unstable or stable angina, a large number are asymptomatic at the time the restenosis is discovered and treated [6-8]. Multiple clinical trials have demonstrated that repeat revascularization tends to be driven by angiographic appearance than by symptoms [9-11]. There is little support for revascularization in asymptomatic individuals [12].

Table 1. Definition of Clinical Restenosis

Clinical restenosis - Abnormal invasive evaluation
o FFR ≤0.80
o IVUS CSA < 4mm^2 or < 6.0mm^2 for left main
o 70% recurrent stenosis and asymptomatic

FFR=Fractional Flow Reserve. IVUS=Intravascular Ultrasound. CSA=Cross-sectional Area.

Clinical Presentation

Clinical restenosis is suspected with recurrence of symptoms most often presenting as exertional or unstable angina. Walters et al. [13] in a group of 262 patients presenting with symptomatic restenosis either following BA or BMS had a very high rate of acute coronary syndrome (ACS) – 68% for BA and 46% for BMS. ACS was defined as either rest angina or acute myocardial infarction (AMI) with 4% of the BMS group and 8% of the BA group suffering a STEMI. Chen et al. [14] reviewed 10,472 PCIs at their center and identified 1186 cases of BMS in-stent restenosis (ISR) in 984 patients. 64.1% of patients with ISR presented with exertional angina, 26.4% were diagnosed as unstable angina, 7.3% were diagnosed as non-ST-segment elevation myocardial infarction, and 2.2% as ST-segment elevation myocardial infarction (STEMI). Rathore et al. [15] compared the clinical presentation of 487 patients with BMS ISR and 351 patients with sirolimus-eluting stent (SES) ISR. Approximately 18% of the patients presented with acute coronary syndrome in both groups with 2% presenting as a STEMI.

In the BA era the timing of restenosis tended to occur within 3-9 months after the procedure [16]. Similarly, the mean time to restenosis with BMS appears to be around 5-6 months post-procedure [13, 17]. Restenosis with DES appears to occur at a later time interval, beyond 1 year post-procedure [7]. The rate of angiographic in-stent restenosis with BMS has traditionally been in the range of 30% [16] while the clinical restenosis leading to repeat intervention is approximately 10-15% [3]. The utilization of DES has significantly decreased the need for repeat procedures and will be discussed in-depth later. Repeat events in the DES era appear to be as much related to target-lesion revascularization (TLR) as de novo stenoses [18].

Angiographic Patterns of Restenosis and Implications for Clinical Outcomes

The landmark 1999 observational study of Mehran et al. [19] demonstrated that the pattern of ISR in bare metal stents was most often diffuse in nature. The more extensive the restenosis, the higher the chance of major cardiac events including an almost exponential rise in TLR by coronary artery bypass grafting from focal to total occlusion. About 2.5-3% of patients died during the follow-up period of 12 months after treatment of the ISR. The pattern of restenosis with DES is more often focal most likely because of suppressed neointimal growth [7, 20, 21]. Over half of BMS restenosis is diffuse whereas it is focal over half the time with DES [19, 20, 21] (Figure 1). Despite being focal, DES restenosis is aggressive making it more difficult to treat. The incidence of repeat restenosis after re-intervention appears to be in the range of 20% [20, 22]. Stent fracture with an intra-stent gap, stent underexpansion and edge restenosis most likely play a more important role in DES versus BMS restenosis [23]. The long-term outcome for treatment of BMS restenosis with a DES is about equivalent to the treatment of a de novo stenosis with DES [21, 24]. The e-SELECT international registry [24] looking at a database of 15,400 patients receiving a cypher stent demonstrated an almost equivalent rate of death, myocardial infarction and TLR in patients with de novo lesions treated with SES versus those with previous BMS-ISR.

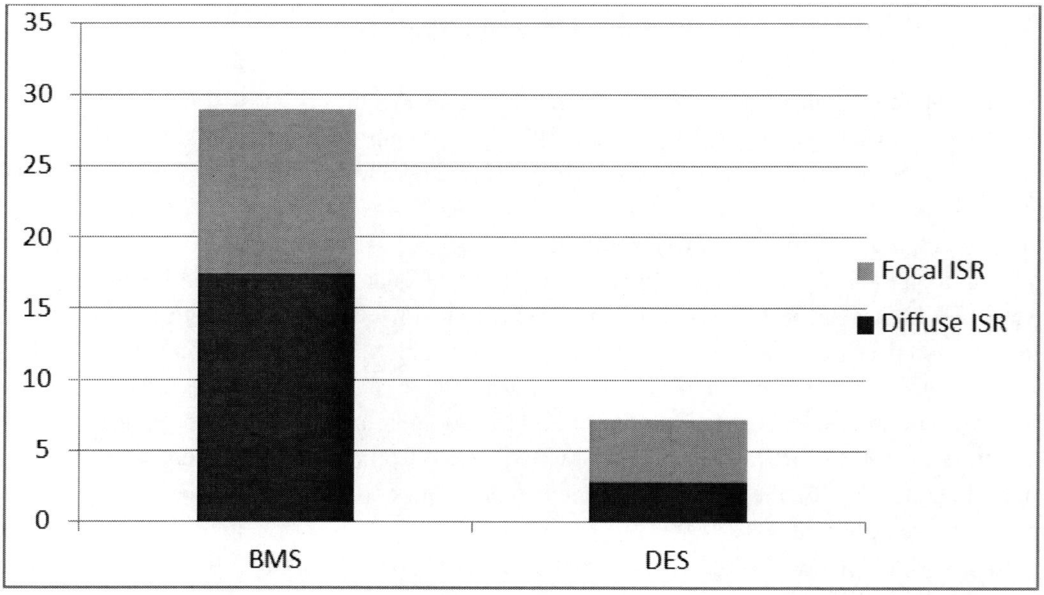

Figure 1. Approximate percentage rates of angiographic patterns of restenosis following treatment of de novo lesions in the reviewed stent trials.

The TLR rate for treatment of DES-ISR was significantly worse than either the BMS-ISR or the de novo group and the curves continued to diverge out to 3 years.

Restenosis in Major DES Trials

The first major randomized DES trial, SIRIUS [25], documented a TLR rate of 16.6% in the BMS group versus 4.1% in the SES group at 270 days. The increase in TLR did not translate into an increase in mortality however. That being said, less than 1% of patients in this study suffered stent thrombosis so the overwhelming majority of TLR would have been for restenosis.

The TAXUS-IV trial [26] demonstrated a 4.7% TLR in the paclitaxel-eluting stent (PES) group versus 12% in the BMS arm at 9 months. Follow-up angiography was performed on over half the patients. The pattern of restenosis was more often focal for PES as compared to the BMS group which was more often diffuse. The incidence of diffuse restenosis on follow-up angiography in the PES group was 2% compared to 17% in the BMS group. The SPIRIT III [27] trial comparing the 2nd generation everolimus-eluting stent with a cobalt-chromium platform, the XIENCE V, to the TAXUS stent demonstrated a decrease in major adverse cardiac events at both one and 2 years of follow-up. Late loss was markedly less in the everolimus-eluting stent (EES) group. Although the rate of in-stent and in-segment restenosis was about half in the EES group, this did not reach statistical significance. No comment was made about the angiographic pattern of restenosis. The RESOLUTE All Comers trial [28] comparing Zotarolimus-eluting stent with a cobalt-chromium platform, the RESOLUTE stent, versus the XIENCE V stent in more of a real-world setting demonstrated essentially no difference in target-vessel failure. Sixty-six percent of patients in this study had an off-label criterion for stent placement. A small number of patients (<20%) had planned angiographic follow-up at 13 months.

Table 2. Restenosis in DES Trials

	TLR rate	Duration of Follow-up
SIRIUS	BMS – 16.6% versus SES – 4.1% (p<0.001)	9 months
TAXUS-IV	BMS – 12% versus PES – 4.7% (p<0.001)	9 months
SPIRIT III	PES – 6.9% versus EES – 4.3% (p=0.07)	2 years
RESOLUTE All Comers	ZES – 3.9% versus EES – 3.4% (non-inferiority)	1 year
E-SELECT	DES-ISR – 6.9% versus BMS-ISR 3.1% (p=0.003)	1 year

In-segment and in-stent binary restenosis was equal for the 2 stents at about 6% for zotarolimus-eluting stent (ZES) and 4% for EES. The patients with definite or probable stent thrombosis appeared to contribute to at least 20% of the major adverse cardiac events indicating that restenosis in the real-world with DES plays a much more negligible role in contributing to morbidity and mortality than it had with BMS previously.

Conclusion

Coronary restenosis is not a benign clinical entity with the incidence of presentation varying with the type of treatment. The rate of restenosis has decreased with technological improvements. As advances in technology continues to improve the morbidity associated with coronary restenosis it needs to be recognized that each advancement has its unique benefit and limitation and the clinician needs to be cognizant of the time-course of restenosis and its presentation.

References

[1] Grüntzig A. R., Senning A., Siegenthaler W. E. Nonoperative Dilatation of Coronary-Artery Stenosis — Percutaneous Transluminal Coronary Angioplasty. *New Eng. J. Med.*, 1979; 301:61-68.

[2] Dangas G. D., Claessen B. E., Caixeta A., et al. In-stent restenosis in the drug-eluting stent era. *J. Am. Coll. Cardiol.*, 2010; 56:1897-907.

[3] Cutlip D. E., Chauhan M. S., Baim D. S., et al. Clinical restenosis after coronary stenting: Perspectives from Multicenter Trials. *J. Am. Coll. Cardiol.*, 2002; 40:2082-9.

[4] Buller C. E., Dzavik V., Carere R. G., et al. Primary stenting versus balloon angioplasty in occluded coronary arteries: the Total Occlusion Study of Canada (TOSCA). *Circulation,* 1999;100:236-42.

[5] Tan W. A., Park S.-J., Plokker T., et al. Long-term Outcomes after unprotected left main trunk percutaneous revascularization in 279 patients. *Circulation*, 2001; 104: 1609-14.

[6] Adlam D., Evans N., Malhotra A., et al. Repeat percutaneous revascularization: indications and outcomes in a real world cohort. *Catheter Cardiovasc. Interv.*, 2012; 80:539-45.

[7] Maleunda G., Ben-Dor I., Gaglia M. A., et al. Clinical outcomes and treatment after drug-eluting stent failure. *Circ. Cardiovasc. Interv.*, 2012;5:12-19.

[8] Patel M. R., Dehmer G. J., Hirshfeld J. W., et al.

[9] Hernández R. A., Macaya C., Iñiguez A., et al. Midterm outcome of patients with asymptomatic restenosis after coronary baloon angioplasty. *J. Am. Coll. Cardiol.*, 1992; 19: 1402-1409.

[10] Ruygrok P. N., Webster M. W. I., de Valk V., etal. Clinical and angiographic factors associated with asymptomatic restenosis after percutaneous coronary intervention. *Circulation,* 2001;104:2289-2294.

[11] Popma J. J., van der Berg E. K., Dehmer G. J. Long term outcome of patients with asymptomatic restenosis after percutaneous transluminal coronary angioplasty. *Am. J. Cardiol.*, 1988;62:1298-1299.

[12] ACCF/SCAI/AATS/AHA/ASNC/HFSA/SCCT 2012 Appropriate use criteria for coronary revascularization focused update. *J. Am. Coll. Cardiol.*, 2012; 59:857-81.

[13] Walters D. L., Harding S. A., Walsh C. R., et al. Acute coronary syndrome is a common clinical presentation of in-stent restenosis. *Am. J. Cardiol.*, 2002;89:491-4.

[14] Chen M. S., John J. M., Chew D. P., et al. Bare metal stent restenosis us not a benign clinical entity. *Am. Heart J.*, 2006;151:1260-4.

[15] Rathore S., Kinoshita Y., Terashima M., et al. A comparison of clinical presentation, angiographic patterns and outcomes of in-stent restenosis between bare metal stents and drug eluting stents. *Eurointervention,* 2010;5(7):841-6.

[16] Nobuyoshi M., Kimura T., Nosaka H., et al. Restenosis after successful percutaneous transluminal coronary angioplasty: serial angiographic follow-up of 229 patients. *J. Am. Coll. Cardiol.*, 1988; 12:616-23.

[17] Bossi I., Klersy C., Black A. J., et al. In-stent restenosis: long-term outcome and predictors of subsequent target lesion revascularization after repeat balloon angioplasty. *J. Am. Coll. Cardiol.,* 200;35:1569-76.

[18] Al Muradi H., Mehra A., Okolo J., et al. Clinical presentation and predictors of target vessel revascularization after drug-eluting stent implantation. *Cardiovasc. Revasc. Med.*, 2012; 13:311-15.

[19] Mehran R., Dangas D., Abizaid A. S., et al. Angiographic patterns of in-stent restenosis, classification and implications for long-term outcome. *Circulation*, 1999; 100:1872-1878.

[20] Latib A., Mussardo M., Ielasi A., et al. Long-term outcomes after the percutaneous treatment of drug-eluting stent restnosis. *J. Am. Coll. Cardiol. Cardiovasc. Intv.,* 2011;4:155-64.

[21] Kastrati A., Mehilli J., von Beckerath N., et al. Sirolimus-eluting stent or paclitaxel-eluting stent vs balloon angioplasty for prevention of recurrences in patients with coronary in-stent restenosis. *JAMA,* 2005;293:165-71.

[22] Lemos P. A., van Mieghem C. A., Arampatzis C. A., et al. Post-sirolimus-eluting stent restenosis treated with repeat percutaneous intervention: late angiographic and clinical outcomes. *Circulation,* 2004;109:2500-2.

[23] Cutlip D. E., Windecker S., Mehran R., et al. Clinical endpoints in coronary stent trials: a case for standardized definitions. *Circulation*, 2007; 115:2344-51.

[24] Abizaid A., Costa J. R., Banning A., et al. The sirolimus-eluting sypher select coronary stent fot the treatment of bare-metal and drug-eluting stent restenosis. *J. Am. Coll. Cardiol. Intv.*, 2012;5:64-71.

[25] Moses J. W., Leon M. B., Popma J. J., et al. Sirolimus-eluting stents versus standard stents in patients with stenosis in a native coronary artery. *N. Engl. J. Med.,* 2003; 349: 1315-23.

[26] Stone G. W., Ellis S. G., Cox D. A., et al. A Polymer-based, paclitaxel-eluting stent in patients with coronary artery disease. *N. Engl. J. Med.,* 2004; 350:221-31.

[27] Stone G. W., Midei M., Newman W., et al. Randomized Comparison of everolimus-eluting and paclitaxel-eluting stents. *Circulation,* 2009; 119:680-6.

[28] Serruys P. W., Silber S., Garg S., et al. Comparison of zotarolimus-eluting and everolimus-eluting coronary stents. *N. Engl. J. Med.*, 2010;363:136-46.

In: Coronary Artery Restenosis
Editor: Amir S. Lotfi

ISBN: 978-1-63321-346-3

Chapter 5

Late Phase In-Stent Restenosis after Coronary Stent Implantation

Shigenori Ito, MD, PhD [•]
Division of Cardiology, Nagoya City East Medical Center, Nagoya, Aichi-ken, Japan

Abstract

In the field of coronary artery stenting, the issue of restenosis has been largely resolved since the development of drug-eluting stents (DES). In-stent restenosis (ISR) is generally considered to be a stable process, with an early peak in intimal hyperplasia followed by a quiescent period beginning 1 year after stent implantation. However, recently, long-term problems (over 1 year) have been reported in both bare-metal stents (BMS) and DES. This phenomenon seems to be different from early ISR within one year in terms of its mechanism, prevention, and treatment. In this article, we discuss the cause of this ISR from the standpoint of intracoronary imaging such as intravascular ultrasound and optical coherence tomography and histopathology, referencing several interesting cases we experienced. The relationship between late stent restenosis and stent thrombosis is also addressed. Furthermore, although there is no definite treatment strategy for the late phase restenosis occurring after drug-eluting stent implantation, we provide an overview of the publications concerning the best treatment for this relatively rare phenomenon which should not be overlooked.

Keywords: Bare-Metal stents, drug-eluting stents, in-stent restenosis, optical coherence tomography, intravascular ultrasound, pathology, late catch up

Introduction

In the field of coronary artery stenting, the development of drug-eluting stents (DES) significantly reduced the rate of restenosis. In-stent restenosis (ISR) is generally considered to

[•] Corresponding Author: Shigenori Ito, Division of Cardiology, Nagoya City East Medical Center, Nagoya, Aichi-ken Japan. Phone: 81-52-721-7171, Fax: 81-52-721-1308, E-mail: sito@higashi-hosp.jp.

be a stable process, with an early peak in intimal hyperplasia followed by a quiescent period beginning 1 year after stent implantation.

However, recently, problems after an extended term (greater than 1 year) in both bare-metal stents (BMS) and DES have been reported. Very late stent thrombosis (greater than 1 year) is a challenging problem in patients who underwent DES implantation. It may occur at a low incidence of 0.2-0.6% yearly, however, the consequence of stent thrombosis can be catastrophic. Late ISR is also a problem in both DES and BMS implantation. This phenomenon seems to be different from early ISR within one year in terms of its mechanism, prevention, and treatment.

In this review chapter, we discuss this topic from the standpoint of intracoronary imaging and histopathology, referencing several interesting cases we have experienced. This Chapter presents an overview of publications concerning the optimal treatment for late phase restenosis after DES implantation.

Clinical Course of ISR after BMS Implantation

In spite of the efficacy and stability of coronary BMS in the early and medium-term phase, the long-term safety of implanted stents remains controversial. Choussal et al. [1] reported the clinical stability of the stented target site at 8-10 years after coronary stenting. In contrast, Kimura et al. [2] reported that 7-11 years of angiographic follow-up demonstrated late luminal re-narrowing beyond 4 years, which did not necessarily require target lesion percutaneous coronary intervention (PCI). They also reported that the long-term luminal response after coronary stenting was triphasic: an early restenotic phase (until 6 months), an intermediate-term regression phase (from 6 months to 3 years), and a late re-narrowing phase (beyond 4 years). A late re-narrowing represents late ISR.

Late In-Stent Restenosis after BMS Implantation

A previous study [3] and our first case (Figures 1-7) [4] clearly demonstrated that new atherosclerotic progression is observed in late ISR, especially in extended late phase ISR (over 5 years) after BMS implantation.

In our case [4], pathologically the retrieved tissue appeared to be double-layered facing the healed neointimal layer inside the implanted stents, suggesting that accumulation of the tissue might have occurred in 2 stages. In fact, the ISR occurred with a time lag of over 10 years after the last angiography at another hospital that showed moderate intimal hyperplasia with 50% angiographic stenosis.

The detection of macrophages by CD 68 staining and pleomorphic smooth muscle cells (SMC) by anti-SMC alpha-actin staining might suggest that activation of the intimal hyperplasia may have restarted or continued once the intimal hyperplasia had remained stabilized for over 10 years following BMS implantation. Pathologic studies have demonstrated that the mechanism of very late ISR is quite different from that of early ISR. It is likely that neoatherosclerosis is a major cause of ISR in patients with late ISR after BMS implantation.

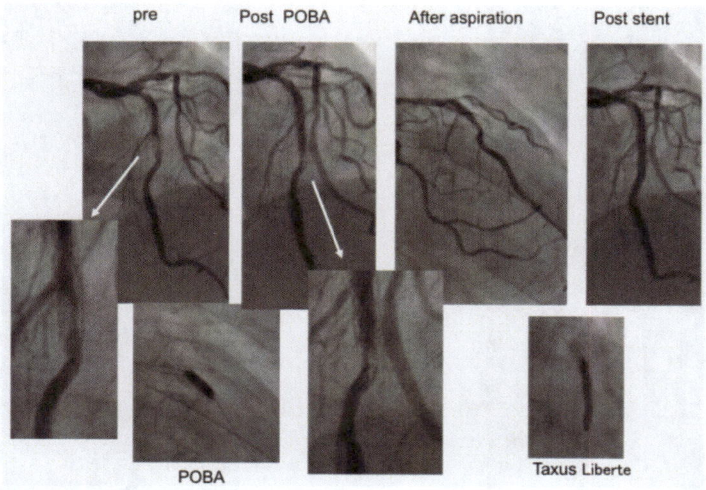

Adapted from J. Invasive Cardiol., 2011;23:E86-91.

Figure 1. Coronary angiograms during index percutaneous coronary intervention. Balloon angioplasty was performed for in-stent restenosis in the mid-left anterior descending coronary artery. After balloon dilatation, a filling defect was seen just distal to the stent with resultant improvement of in-stent stenosis. After aspiration, the defect was not angiographically visible. A 2.5 x 20 mm Taxus Liberte stent was deployed to cover the in-stent restenotic lesion and the result was good.

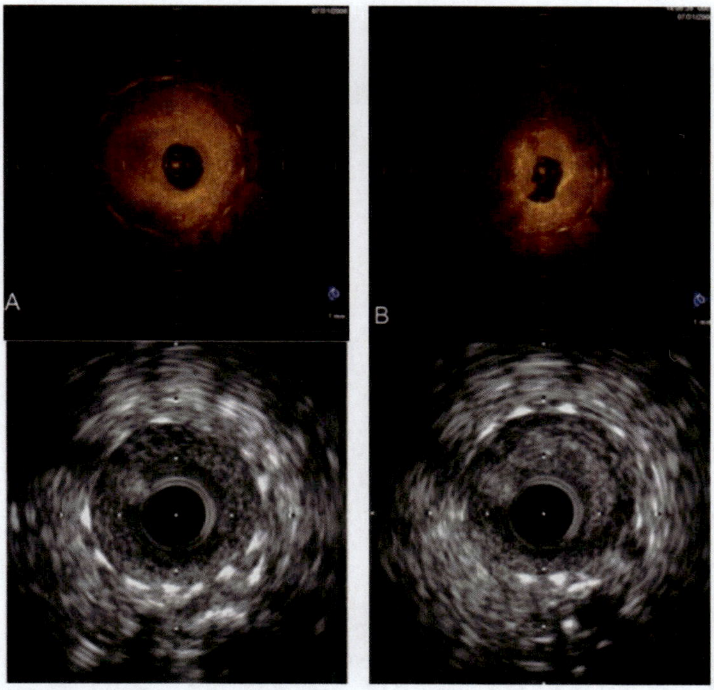

Adapted from J. Invasive Cardiol., 2011;23:E86-91.

Figure 2. Optical coherence tomography (OCT) and intravascular ultrasound (IVUS) findings of in-stent restenosis before balloon angioplasty. OCT showed homogeneous high intensity in the distal segment. IVUS revealed a homogeneous and __ slightly hyperechoic material. High intensity accompanied by attenuation was observed in the proximal segment by OCT. Peri-stent area was hypoechoic by IVUS; however, there was no clear difference between (A) and (B) compared to OCT.

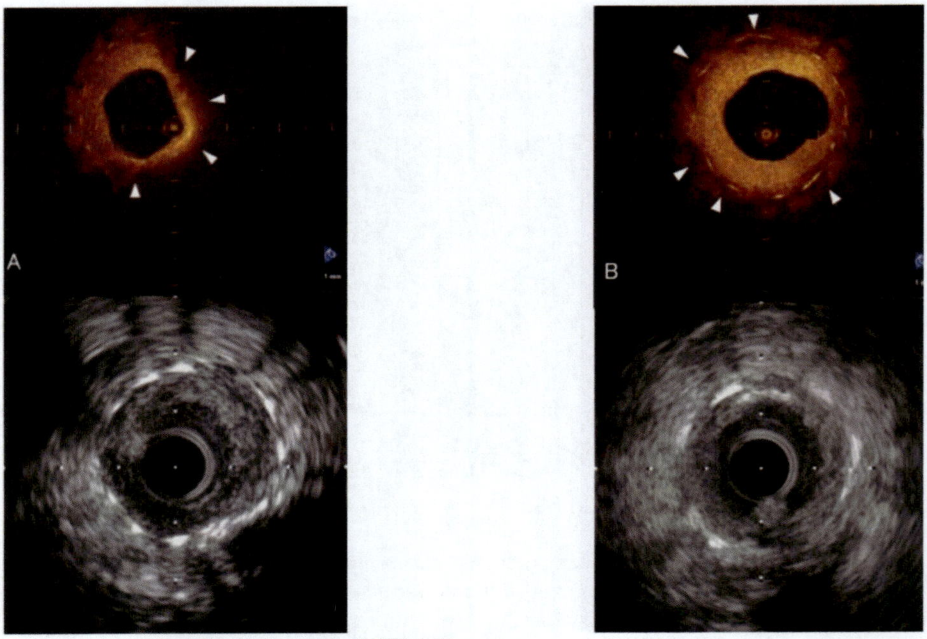

Adapted from J. Invasive Cardiol., 2011;23:E86-91.

Figure 3. Thin cap fibroatheroma without significant stenosis proximal to the in-stent restenotic lesion. Low signals surrounding some stent struts. Intravascular ultrasound could not identify the thin-cap fibroatheroma or low signals surrounding the stent struts.

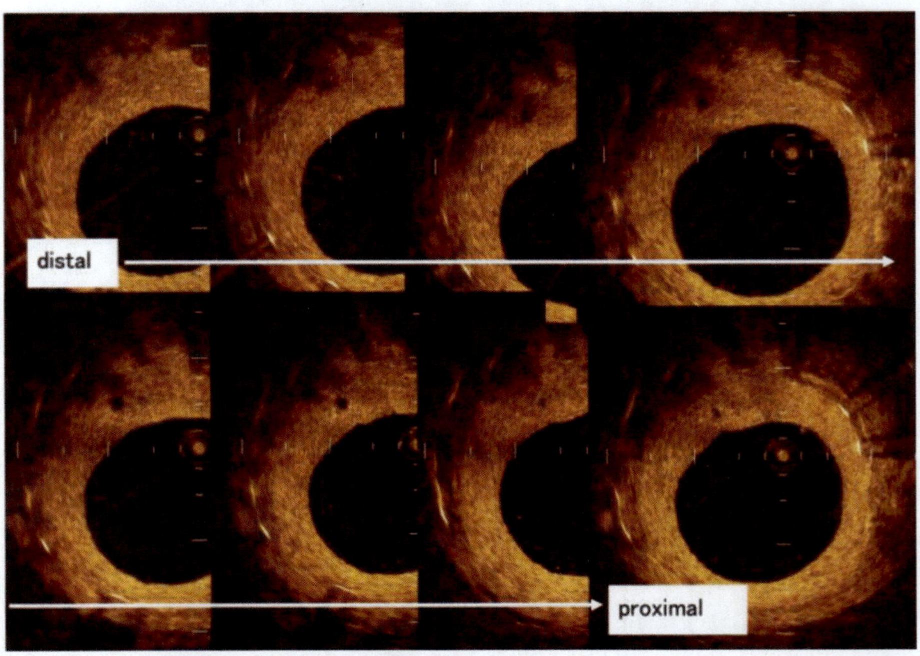

Adapted from J. Invasive Cardiol., 2011;23:E86-91.

Figure 4. Frame by frame OCT images showing a microvessel. There was a tubular structure (diameter = 100 □m) expanding the peri-stent to the intima suggesting neovascularization observed 3 mm distal to the proximal edge.

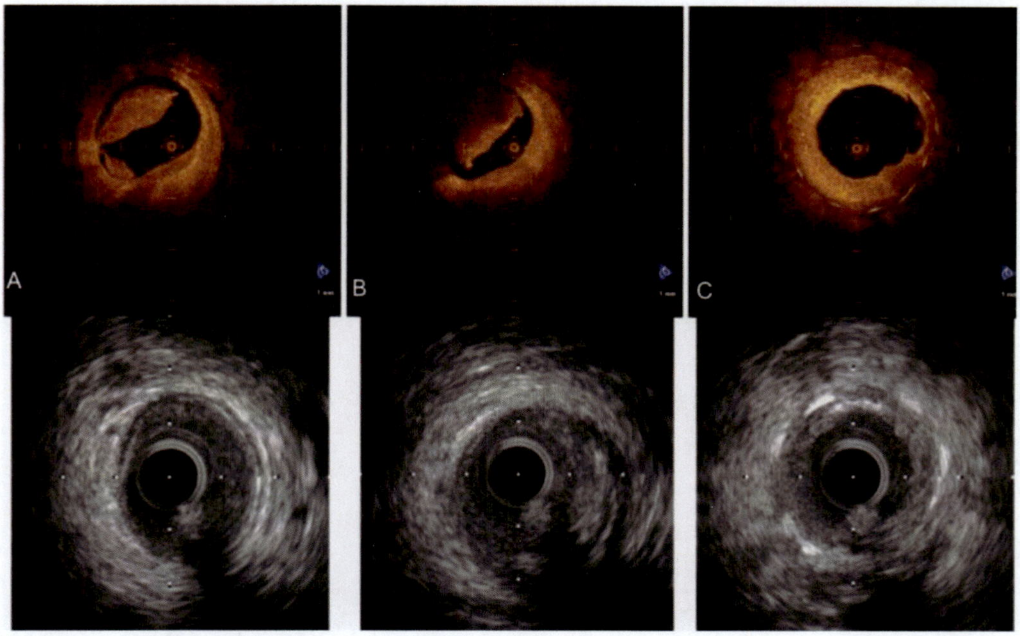

Adapted from J. Invasive Cardiol., 2011;23:E86-91.

Figure 5. Optical coherence tomographic findings of in-stent restenosis after balloon angioplasty. Distal part of in-stent restenosis. The distal half of the material had a high-intensity homogenous signal. Proximal part of in-stent restenosis. The proximal half of the retrieved material showed superficial high-intensity with attenuation, suggesting that they were composed of different components. Resultant tissues showed heterogeneous plaque containing partial low signals.

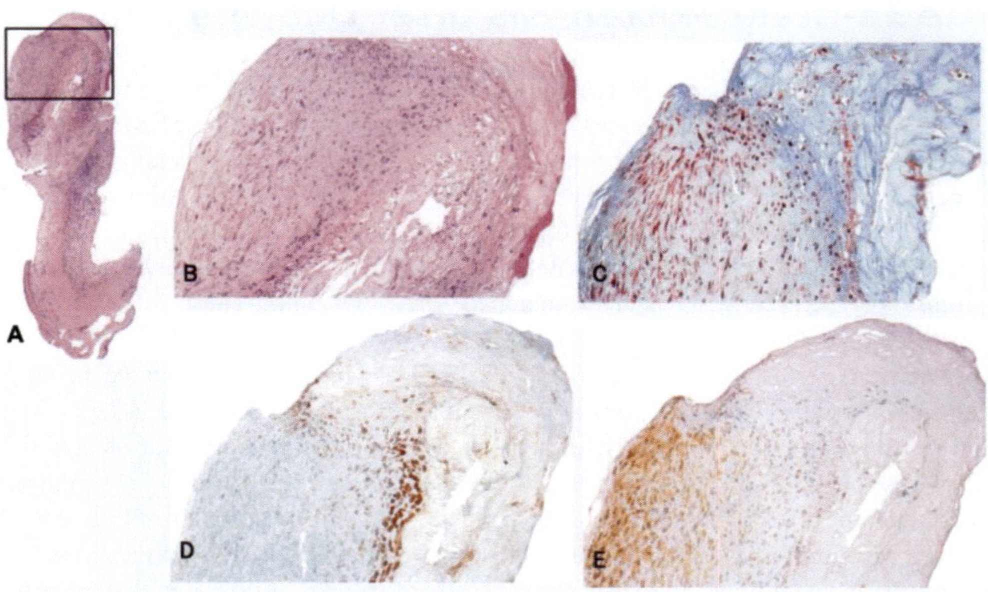

Adapted from J. Invasive Cardiol., 2011;23:E86-91.

Figure 6. A) Hematoxylin-eosin stain The entire body of this material seemed to be composed of two layers. Box in A is magnified in Figures B-E. B) Hematoxylin-eosin stain: C) Masson's trichrome stain: D) Immunoreactivity to CD 68:E) Immunoreactivity to SMC α-actin.

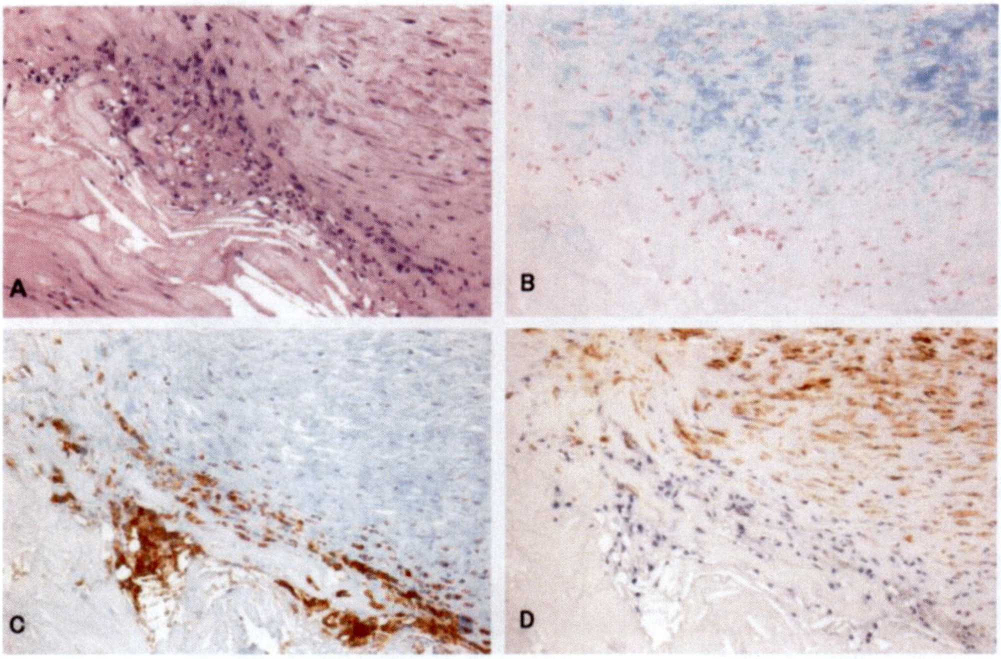

Adapted from J. Invasive Cardiol., 2011;23:E86-91.

Figure 7. Microscopic findings (Higher magnification). A) Hematoxylin-eosin stain: B) Alcian blue stain C) Immunoreactivity to CD 68: D) Immunoreactivity to SMC α-actin. Fibrous collagenous plaque is adjacent to the lesion where polymorphic SMCs proliferate with rich proteoglycans in the background.

Late In-Stent Restenosis after DES Implantation

The phenomenon of late ISR is rather infrequent, occurring in only 2.6% of treated lesions [5], but exhibits a steady annual rate after sirolimus-eluting stent (SES) implantation. The mechanisms of the late catch-up phenomenon are incompletely understood after DES implantation. Long-term inflammation has been reported after SES implantation by pathological observation in humans [6]. Since the sirolimus is eluted from the stent completely within about 120 days, this inflammation might be due to polymer toxicity or hypersensitivity. Recently, 3 studies reported that the other cause of late ISR is neoatherosclerosis that formed in the stent [7-9]. As another cause of SES late ISR, we encountered an interesting case [10] in which fibrin deposition was observed in an SES implanted 39 months previously. It is also conceivable that fibrin retrieved in this case had been formed during a previous rupture of neoatherosclerosis that formed in the stent [7, 8]. In our third case (Figures 10-11) we speculated that the inflammation and delayed healing with coronary endothelial dysfunction [11, 12] might have been related to the fibrin thrombus formation. Also, thin-cap fibroatheroma (TCFA) was recognized in the short segment of the restenotic tissue suggesting the existence of neoatherosclerosis. Sawada et al. [13] recently reported that some subclinical intra-stent thrombi might eventually result in DES ISR and partial area of DES restenosis neointima might be configured by thrombi.

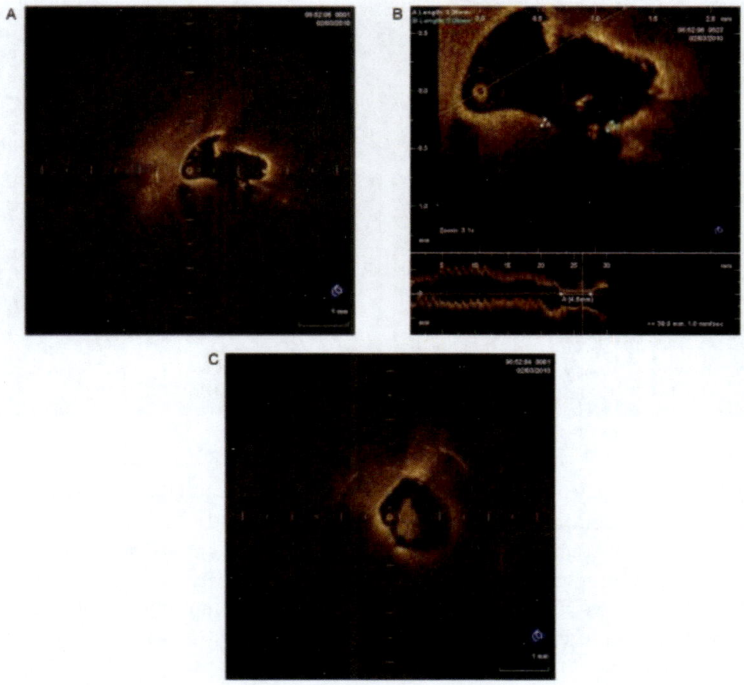

Adapted form J. C. Cases, 2012;5:e1-e3.

Figure 8. Optical coherence tomography findings. A: Ruptured thin cup fibroatheroma with homogeneous low intensity signals. B: Measurements of thin fibrous cap (A: 60μm, B: 90 μm). C: White thrombus can been detected on the thin fibrous cap near the ruptured site.

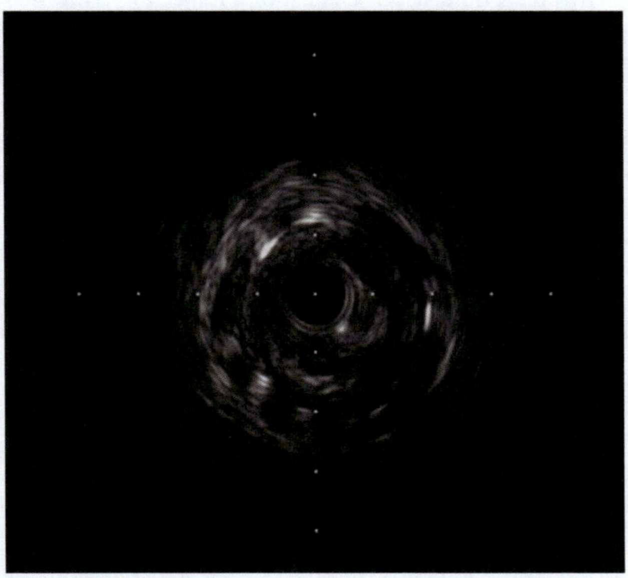

Adapted form J. C. Cases, 2012;5:e1-e3.

Figure 9. Intravascular ultrasound finding. Heterogeneous and mainly echolucent plaque can be seen nearly at the identical. site of ruptured site detected by optical coherence tomography. There was also homogeneous echolucent appearance observed outside the stent struts. Obvious stent malapposition was not detected.

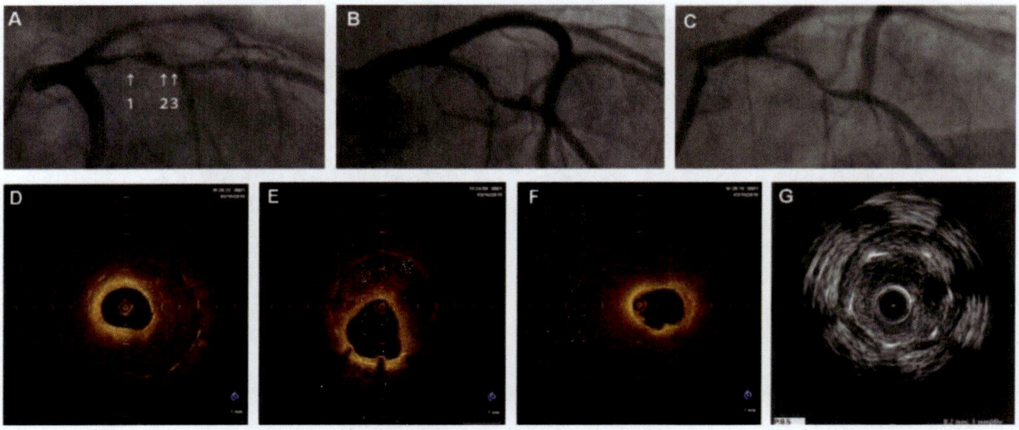

Adapted from J. C. Cases, 2012;5:e83-e86.

Figure 10. A) Follow-up coronary angiography at 39 months (RAO caudal view). Arrows 1, 2, and 3 indicate corresponding cross sections of the OCT findings in Figures D-F. Follow-up coronary angiography at 39 months (AP cranial view). Control coronary angiography before PCI two months after the diagnostic coronary angiography (AP cranial view). There was no progression of stenosis in the proximal LAD during the two months. OCT findings before PCI in the proximal stenosis (Arrow 1 in Figure 1A). OCT findings before PCI in the distal stenosis (Arrow 3 in Figure 1A). OCT findings before PCI in the distal stenosis (Arrow 2 in Figure 1A). IVUS findings before PCI. Abbreviations: RAO right anterior oblique view; AP anterioposterior; PCI percutaneous coronary intervention; OCT optical coherence tomography; IVUS intravascular tomography; LAD left anterior descending coronary artery.

This possibility leads to the hypothesis that the CYP2C19*2 polymorphism is associated with DES restenosis as well as intra-stent thrombus through a poor response to clopidogrel. Although the patient had taken both aspirin and ticlopidine, drug resistance should also be considered. Fujii et al. [14] also demonstrated the contribution of organized thrombi to in-stent restenosis after SES implantation by OCT findings 12 months after implantation. At the ISR site, OCT revealed a low-backscattering irregular mass protruding into the lumen. This finding also may suggest an organized thrombus that was the main component of restenotic tissue after SES implantation. The mechanism of late ISR after DES implantation is multifactorial.

In-Stent Restenosis and Inflammation

Shiode et al. [15] reported that at 6 months to 3 years, the stenosis of BMS-treated lesions had regressed, while that of DES-treated lesions had progressed, suggesting a phenomenon of late catch-up [15]. Their data suggest that later relapse and persistence of inflammation might cause this late catch-up phenomenon of DES. As the local concentration of the drugs coated on the stent surface decreases, inflammatory relapse is likely to occur along with impaired and incomplete wound healing. Another possibility is that the inflammation is a result of late toxicity or hypersensitivity to the polymer coating on the stent surface [6]. The inflammatory response to residues of non-erodible polymers, which are used in SES, plays an important role and may cause nonspecific monocyte/macrophage adherence and activation or hypersensitivity-related reaction [16].

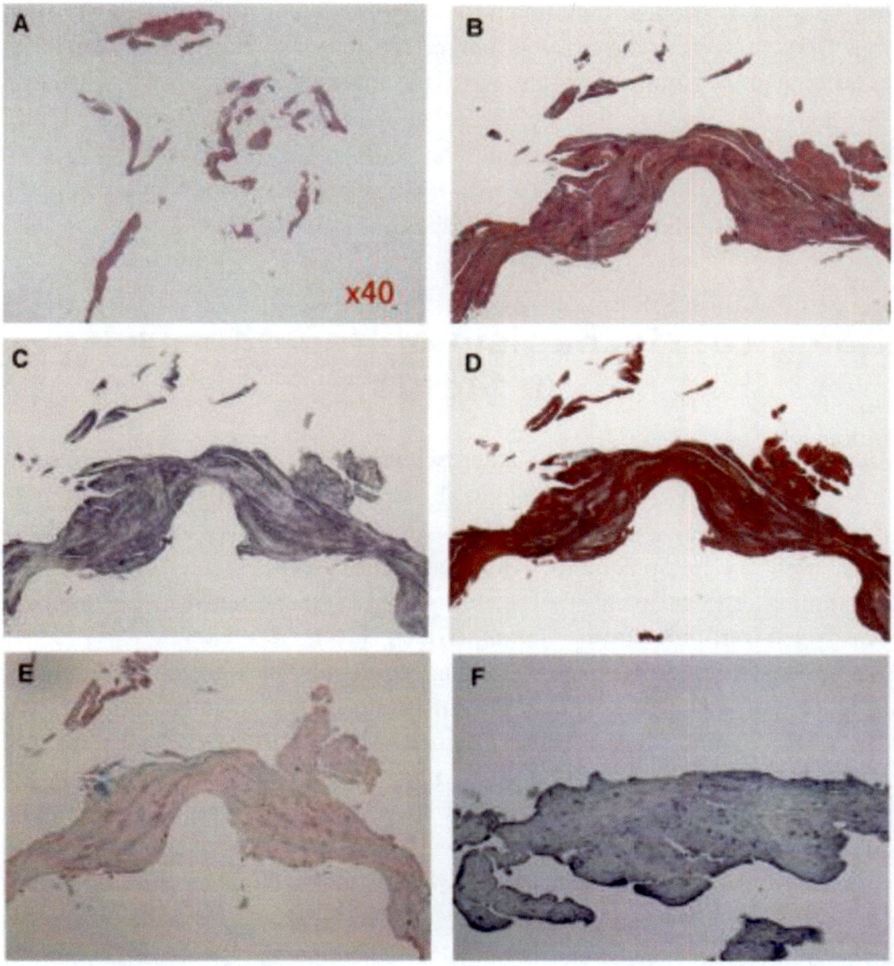

Adapted from J. C. Cases, 2012;5:e83-e86.

Figure 11. Materials retrieved on the Filtrap™. After the procedure, the net of the Filtrap™ was cut and fixed in formalin. The main samples captured on the net were stained with hematoxylin-eosin staining, special staining, and immunohistological staining. Microscopic findings of main retrieved samples. Hematoxylin-eosin stain: x200. The retrieved samples consisted of hypocellular deposits and were mainly composed of fibrin deposits with a few inflammatory cells (neutrophils). C) Phosphotungstic acid hematoxylin staining (PTAH): x200. Fibrin deposits were confirmed by PTAH staining as blue. Masson's trichrome staining: x200. Fibrin deposits were also confirmed by this special staining as red. Alcian blue staining: x200. Proteoglycans were only slightly detected. Immunoreactivity to SMC α actin: x200. Smooth muscle cells were not detected in this material.

Yoneda et al. [17] hypothesized that the mechanism of in-stent restenosis after DES stenting might be different from that after BMS stenting as well as atherosclerosis. They used tissues obtained by directional coronary atherectomy (DES: 7 specimens, BMS: 17 specimens, and de-novo: 15 specimens) which were immunostained for T lymphocytes (CD45), macrophages (CD68), smooth muscle cells (alpha-smooth muscle actin), endothelial cells (Von Willebrand factor), and activated platelets (P-selectin). The accumulation of T lymphocytes tended to increase and that of macrophages increased significantly in the DES lesions compared with BMS lesions. No significant differences were observed for the other parameters evaluated. Thus, the pathological features of restenotic tissues after DES implantation showed a stronger inflammatory response compared with those after BMS implantation. DES suppresses the acute inflammatory response considerably because of the strong anti-inflammatory action of the drugs coated in the stent surface [18, 19]. However, impaired or delayed wound healing by DES stenting potentially causes inflammation to relapse and persist thereafter. Their findings that DES restenotic lesions showed stronger inflammatory cell accumulation compared with BMS restenotic lesions, might support DES-induced delayed wound healing or subsequent persistent inflammation.

Pathological Mechanism of Neoatherosclerosis in Stents

The pathological mechanism of new atherosclerotic plaque formation at extended long-period follow-up is not well known. Takano et al. [8] demonstrated that expanded intraintima neovascularization may play a key role in atherosclerotic progression and surrounding tissue instability, as well as intraplaque neovascularization of non-stented segments. In our pathological findings shown in the first case, there was sparse neovascularization because material was retrieved only from the superficial layer [4]. However, OCT detected microvessels near the stent struts. The trigger that causes microvessels to develop into plaque should be elucidated, and persistent chronic inflammation may somehow be related to it. Inoue et al. [20] reported that autopsied samples after implantation of Palmaz-Schatz coronary stents (19 patients autopsied after noncardiac death 2-7 years post-stenting) demonstrated that stainless steel stents evoked a remarkable foreign-body inflammatory reaction to the metal. In this study, they concluded that persistent peri-strut chronic inflammatory cells might accelerate new indolent atherosclerotic changes and plaque vulnerability. We could not obtain material from the peri-stent area, however, there were low signals surrounding some stent struts, potentially indicating the presence of inflammation even 11 years after BMS deployment [4]. Autopsy studies have suggested that coronary thrombosis may occur in the absence of cardiac symptoms, resulting in progression of atherosclerosis [21]. Burke et al. [22] supported the hypothesis of plaque rupture as a mechanism of increased luminal narrowing. In their study, there was a low but significantly increased rate of cell proliferation in the SMC-rich regions of healed rupture sites, providing evidence of further plaque expansion. The matrix within the healed fibrous cap consists of a proteoglycan-rich mass or a collagen-rich scar, depending on the healing phase. The pathological findings in this case seems to have similarity to that reported by Burke et al. [22]. Regarding the pathological mechanism of in-stent restenosis after 11 years, we speculate that persistent peri-stent chronic inflammation [20] might have yielded neovascularization, accelerating new indolent atherosclerotic change [23] and consequent plaque vulnerability, which may have caused plaque ruptures or plaque erosions. After that, as healing process, proteoglycan–rich mass associated with SMC narrowed the lumen like in the non-stented vessels.

Iijima et al. [24] investigated the clinical relevancy of late phase ISR after DES implantation. A total of 923 patients treated with first-generation DES to detect independent predictors of late catch–up (LCU), defined as secondary revascularization one year after index stenting. Retreatment for very late stent thrombosis was considered to be part of the

LCU phenomenon. LCU phenomenon was seen in 33 patients (3.6%), consisting of very late stent thrombosis in 5 patients (0.6%) and very late ISR in 28 patients (3.0%). In the multivariate analysis, hemodialysis [odds ratio (OR) 6.07, p=0.003], number of stents (OR 1.58, p=0.02), and coronary bifurcation lesions (OR 2.06, p=0.048) were identified as independent predictors of the LCU phenomenon.

Difference in Neoatherosclerosis between BMS and DES

Nakazawa et al. investigated the pathology of neoatherosclerosis in human coronary stent implantations in 299 autopsy cases with a total of 406 lesions (197 BMS, 209 DES (103 SESs and 106 paclitaxel-eluting stents)) [7]. The incidence of neoatherosclerosis was significantly higher in the DES lesions than BMS lesions (31% vs. 16%; p<0.001). The median stent duration with neoatherosclerosis was shorter in DES than BMS (DES, 420 days [interquartile range: 361 to 683 days]; BMS, 2,160 days [interquartile range; 1,800 to 2,880 days], p<0.001). Unstable lesions characterized as TCFA or plaque rupture were more frequent in BMS (7.4%) than in DES (3.1%, p=0.17), with relatively shorter implant duration for DES (1.5±0.4 years) compared to BMS (6.1±1.5 years). Thus, they concluded that neoatherosclerosis is a frequent finding in DES and occurs earlier than in BMS [7]. The development of neoatherosclerosis may be yet another rare contributing factor to late stent thrombosis. That is, this phenomenon manifest as stable stenosis irrespective of its degree followed by stent thrombosis due to plaque rupture in the stent.

Optical Coherence Tomography and Plaque Characteristics in ISR

Optical coherence tomography (OCT) has been the most powerful tool to delineate restenotic tissue imaging and to classify the tissue components. On the other hand, intravascular ultrasound (IVUS) has some limitations in visualizing its complex tissue structure as can be documented by histopathology. In 2009 Gonzalo et al. [25] evaluated the morphologic characteristics of ISR by OCT. They classified the ISR tissue in terms of restenotic tissue structure (homogeneous, heterogeneous, and layered), restenotic tissue backscatter (high, low), presence or absence of microvessels, lumen shape (regular, irregular), and presence of intraluminal material in 24 patients with 25 ISR tissue samples (DES 84% BMS 16%). Tissue structure was layered in 52%, homogeneous in 28%, and heterogeneous in 20%. The predominant backscatter was high in 72% of the samples. Stents implanted ≤12 months previously more frequently had restenotic tissue with a layered appearance (84.6% vs. 16.7%, p=0.003). Homogeneous and heterogeneous appearances were more frequent in stents implanted greater than 12 months. Their classification has been well recognized and adopted in the following reports about the OCT findings of ISR. Goto K et al. [26] analyzed neointimal characteristics by OCT in 59 ISR patients and reported there were differences in the neointima according to stent type and restenotic phase, and that this may lead to a better understanding of the different mechanisms of ISR. The OCT signal patterns of tissues at the minimal lumen area were categorized into three patterns: (1) homogeneous high-signal band, (2) heterogeneous mixed-signal band, and (3) lipid-laden intima. The predominant OCT pattern was a homogeneous high-signal band in the BMS early phase (19/21 [91%]), lipid-laden intima in the BMS late phase (12/16 [76%]), and a heterogeneous mixed-signal band in the DES late phase (9/13 [69%]). Heterogeneous mixed-signal band was seen more frequently in the DES early phase compared with BMS early phase (44% vs. 9%, $p<0.05$) suggesting a different mechanism in DES early phase.

Intracoronary Imaging of Late Phase ISR after BMS Implantation

As a relatively rare cause of early ISR after BMS implantation, although probably common in very late ISR, neoatherosclerosis has been reported in the extended long-term follow-up periods in two pathological [7, 20] and one OCT study [8]. We also successfully obtained both IVUS and OCT images of such a ruptured plaque in an acute coronary syndrome case [27] with late ISR 8 years after BMS implantation. Reflecting the difference in their mechanisms, the image characteristics of ISR after BMS may be different between the early phase and extended late phase (usually over 5 years) [28]. Early stage ISR is characterized by both IVUS and OCT as homogenous high intensity signals [26]. On the other hand, extended late phase ISR shows various signal patterns in plaque composition [28]. The proportion of cross-sections with heterogeneous intima in the entire stent was significantly higher in the very late ISR (over 5 years) group compared to the early ISR (within the first year) group (60.5±28.5% versus 5.8±11.5%, $p<0.0001$), with heterogeneous intima being more frequently observed at the minimum lumen area site in the very late ISR group (90.7% versus 17.9%). This might imply that several types of tissue are formed during an extended follow-up period. The OCT findings in the very late ISR are similar to the morphology observed with typical native atherosclerotic lesions. That is, the signal-poor area with a diffuse lumen border was similar to the OCT image of lipid laden plaque in the atherosclerotic lesion. Our second case [27] (Figures 8-9) clearly shows the disruption of the fibrous cap associated with white thrombus by OCT. Deep attenuation under a thin fibrous cap might be expressed as echolucent plaque by IVUS, because the location of the plaque is almost identical between IVUS and OCT images in the same cross section level. OCT was very useful, like it is for de novo vulnerable plaques, to evaluate vulnerable plaque that had formed in a previously implanted stent. On the other hand, tissue outside the stent struts could be visualized by IVUS with good penetration. Combined use of OCT and IVUS was useful to understand the characteristics of a ruptured vulnerable plaque that had formed in a previously implanted BMS even after stabilization of neointimal hyperplasia. If such plaque rupture repeats silently in patients with coronary stents, tissue in the stent accumulates gradually leading to severe stenosis like in this case.

Intracoronary Imaging of Late Phase ISR after DES Implantation

Kang et al. [9] reported findings from OCT of in-stent neoatherosclerosis as a cause of DES failure in 50 patients (30 stable, 20 unstable angina) with 50 DES ISR lesions and intimal hyperplasia >50% of stent area. Compared with DES <20 months after implantation, DES ≥ 20 months after implantation had a higher incidence of TCFA-containing neointima (69% versus 33%, p=0.012) and red thrombi (27% versus 0%, p=0.007). Furthermore, their study showed that patients with late DES-ISR were more likely to have an unstable clinical manifestation compared to those with early DES-ISR. We encountered the third case with typical presentation 6 years after SES implantation. As a second cause of ISR after SES, fibrin thrombus and fibrinoid are important. To date, there are no OCT criteria for organized thrombus and fibrinoid corresponding with the histological validation [29]. However, in our very late ISR after SES [10], we speculated that homogeneous low signals with a superficial high signal fibrous cap by OCT, where stent struts were identified, by OCT and low echoic plaque by IVUS might suggest fibrin thrombus. Special staining and immunohistological study showed that there was no massive deposition of proteoglycans or smooth muscle cells. Because all restenotic tissue could not be retrieved by Filtrap™ (Nipro Corporation) in this case, it is impossible to definitively determine the OCT and IVUS features of a fibrin thrombus. It is sometimes difficult to discern fibrin from neoatherosclerosis. Massive fibrin accumulation is seen on OCT as a dark area without a clear border, which resembles necrotic core [30].

Relationships between ISR, Neoatherosclerosis, and Stent Thrombosis

Kang et al. [9] recently showed that, on OCT, in-stent neoatherosclerosis and intimal ruptures were frequent in DES-treated patients with ISR. Miyazaki also [31] showed that there was lipid-laden-like neointima involved in several cases of late ISR. Moreover, 34% of patients (4/11) with lipid-laden-like neointima with disruption presented clinically with unstable angina. All 4 patients with unstable angina in the late ISR group were also found to have lipid-laden-like neointima with disruption and intracoronary thrombus. This result indicates that progression of lipid-laden-like neointima may promote the disruption and the subsequent late thrombosis, and that these processes may be overlapping in part in cases of late restenosis or late thrombosis. Also, a previous pathological study demonstrated that ISR was an additional risk factor for late stent thrombosis [32].

Prevention of Very Late ISR

It is well known that a high cholesterol level is related to the coronary events from the Framingham study and for the secondary prevention of cardiovascular events, lowering the LDL cholesterol level to 70 mg/dl is recommended. However, it is still unknown whether neoatherosclerosis occurring in BMS or DES is also related to the LDL level. To the best of our knowledge, there is no data showing greater progression of atherosclerosis in the non-stented coronary segments in patients with very late ISR. Although histological studies reported residual stent struts cause inflammation around the struts and work as a trigger of neoatherosclerosis, particular medical treatment for this phenomenon is not realistic right now. The study by Yoneda et al. [17] only referred to additive medical treatment with statins, angiotensin receptor blockers, or others, which potentially promote re-endothelialization, stabilize inflammation, and subsequently induce normal wound healing have potential after DES implantation [18, 19]. Instead, recent investigations have focused on the development and improvement of bioresorbable vascular scaffolds [33-36], which resorbs leaving no permanent scaffold.

Previous studies have showed that approximately 15-30% of patients after DES implantation, who had high residual platelet reactivity after dual anti-platelet therapy (DAPT), were associated with higher cardiovascular complications and restenosis [37-39]. Although several original or meta-analyses [40-42] showed the additive effect of cilostazol to DAPT regarding the prevention of cardiovascular events and restenosis, this is still controversial. According to a meta analysis by Chen et al. [43], cilostazol in addition to usual DAPT reduced the cardiac events after DES implantation. Five clinical trials were involved in the study. Triplet anti-platelet therapy (TAT) was associated with a 36% reduction in major adverse cardiac events (MACE; odds ratio (OR) = 0.64; 95% confidence interval (CI) = 0.51-0.81, P <0.01), a 40% reduction (OR = 0.60, 95% CI = 0.44-0.80; P < 0.01) in target vessel revascularization (TVR), a 44% reduction (OR = 0.56, 95% CI = 0.34-0.91; P = 0.02) in target lesion revascularization (TLR), a 47%/44% reduction in in-segment/in-stent restenosis (P < 0.01), and lower in-segment/in-stent late loss (P <0.01). However, the risk of gastrointestinal adverse events were significantly higher in the TAT group (OR = 2.46, 95% CI = 1.25-4.86; P <0.01). TAT seems promising based on these study results, however, the long-term effect for over 1 year ISR was not evaluated in this study.

Interventional Strategy for Very Late ISR

An interventional strategy for ISR is still controversial, and depends on the timing, index stent implanted (BMS or DES), and pattern of ISR (focal, diffuse, proliferative, or occluded according to the Mehran classification [44]). In the cases with early ISR after BMS or DES, in which intimal hyperplasia is a predominant factor, we usually use DES to prevent proliferation of smooth muscle cells. Scoring balloons such as Cutting balloon (Boston Scientific Corporation, Natick, MA, USA), Angiosculpt (Biotronik, Fremont, CA, USA), Scoreflex (Orbus Neich Medical Corporation, Shenzhen, China), or Lacrosse NSE (Goodman, Nagoya, Japan) also might be effective for focal ISR with acceptable long-term results. This simple method can avoid overlapping stent struts that have the potential risk of inflammation and stent thrombosis. Paclitaxel–coated balloon (PCB) angioplasty is not inferior to paclitaxel–eluting stents for BMS restenosis [45]. Strut thickness and polymer-mediated inflammatory reactions may act as stimuli for recurrent neointimal growth. Several studies have been conducted on ISR after DES implantation [33, 46, 47]. It should be determined whether the same or another DES is more beneficial in preventing recurrence of

ISR. Recently, the PEPCAD-DES (PEPCAD DES–Treatment of DES-In-Stent Restenosis With SeQuent® Please Paclitaxel Eluting PTCA Catheter) study revealed the superiority of PCB angioplasty compared with plain balloon angioplasty for DES restenosis [48]. On the other hand, because the mechanism of very late ISR is different from early ISR, a treatment decision is further complicated due to lack of evidence. If the inflammation caused by the polymer is considered to be the cause of ISR BMS or cutting balloon angioplasty would be recommended at the expense of superiority in suppressing smooth muscle cell proliferation with DES. DES implantation might induce additional inflammation during further follow-up. In the patients and/or lesions with potential high ISR rate such as diffuse, proliferative, occluded IRS lesions, diabetes, or hemodialysis, DES could be the choice to prevent early ISR. At the present time, no definite data is available and case based decisions would be important to yield better clinical outcomes after additional PCI for very late ISR.

Cheverier et al. [49] compared the efficacy of the Cypher Select (Cordis Corporation, Bridgewater, NJ, USA) sirolimus-eluting stent (SES) versus balloon angioplasty (BA) in ISR of Taxus or Taxus Liberte paclitaxel-eluting stents (PES; Boston Scientific, Natick, MA, USA) or Cypher/Cypher Select SES. There was no difference in the primary end-point, LLL at 12 months, between the SES and BA groups. However, follow-up MLD and immediate and net gain favored SES. Yu et al. [50] systematically reviewed the efficacy and safety of drug (paclitaxel)-eluting balloon (DEB) in the treatment of coronary artery disease (CAD). Five studies involving 349 patients were included as control POBA in 3 trials and DES in 2 trials; DEB improved angiographic measures with no significant effect on clinical outcomes in the overall CAD population. There was clear superiority of DEB in 289 patients with ISR in TLR (OR 0.17, 95% CI 0.07 to 0.38, $p<0.0001$, I(2)=0%), MACE (OR 0.22, 95% CI 0.10 to 0.51, $p=0.0005$, I(2)=13%), LLL (in-stent: MD -0.51, 95% CI -0.73 to -0.28, $p<0.00001$, I(2)=60%; in-segment: MD -0.51, 95% CI -0.77 to -0.24, $p=0.0002$, I(2)=72%;), minimal lumen diameter (in-stent: MD 0.49, 95% CI 0.05 to 0.93, $p=0.03$, I(2)=85%; in-segment: MD 0.49, 95% CI 0.13 to 0.86, $p=0.008$, I(2)=79%), and binary restenosis (in-stent: OR 0.15, 95% CI 0.05 to 0.47, $p=0.001$, I(2)=37%; in-segment: OR 0.11, 95% CI 0.05 to 0.27, $p<0.00001$, I(2)=17%). Currently, further data from randomized clinical trials with clinical endpoints are required to assess the long term benefits of this technology.

Yamashita et al. [51] investigated the efficacy and safety of a second-generation DES (Everolimus-eluting stent; EES) for ISR after first-generation DES implantation in a single center non-randomized study. The subjects were 145 consecutive patients who underwent re-stenting, including 93 given a first-generation DES (Cypher 27 Taxus 66 patients) and 52 given an EES. The two groups were followed up for 37.8 ± 16.7 months and 13.8 ± 2.1 months, respectively. Follow-up angiography showed that late luminal loss (0.26 ± 0.31 mm vs. 0.58 ± 0.67 mm; $P= 0.01$), the binary restenosis rate (2.6% vs. 16.7%; $P = 0.03$), and the target lesion revascularization (TLR) rate (1.9% vs. 11.8%; log-rank=0.04) were smaller in the second-generation group than in the first-generation group. There was no definite stent thrombosis in either group. During follow-up, there were no significant between-group differences in MACE without TLR, myocardial infarction, death, and death and myocardial infarction. Multivariate analysis demonstrated that using a first-generation DES was the only independent predictor of TLR after 1 year (odds ratio, 2.78; 95% confidence interval, 1.22-5.43; $P = 0.03$). Thus, when ISR occurs after DES implantation, treatment with a second-generation DES reduces LLL, binary restenosis, and TLR after 1 year compared with a first-generation DES. Treatment of patients with DES ISR remains a challenge.

Alfonso et al. [52] reported the results of the RIBS III (Restenosis Intra-Stent: Balloon Angioplasty Versus Drug-Eluting Stent), prospective, multicenter study that included 363 consecutive patients with DES ISR from 12 Spanish sites. The use of a different DES was the recommended strategy (274 patients for different DES, 89 patients for the other strategies). The main angiographic endpoint was minimal lumen diameter at 9-month follow-up. The main clinical outcome measure was a composite of cardiac death, myocardial infarction, and TLR. The different-DES strategy was used in 274 patients (75%) and alternative therapeutic modalities (no switch) were used in 89 patients (25%). Baseline characteristics were similar in the 2 groups, although lesion length was longer in the switch group. Time to ISR (days) tended to be shorter in the switch group (279 (180-576) vs. 324 (245-597)). However, both groups had patients with over 1 year late restenosis, which seems to be longer than the BMS cases. The strength of this study was that a second–generation DES was used in 335 of the patients treated for DES ISR. At late angiographic follow-up (77% of eligible patients, median: 278 days) the minimal lumen diameter was larger (1.86 ± 0.7 mm vs. 1.40 ± 0.8 mm, $p = 0.003$) and recurrent restenosis rate lower (22% vs. 40%, $p = 0.008$) in the different-DES group. At the last clinical follow-up (99% of patients, median: 771 days), the combined clinical endpoint occurred less frequently (23% vs. 35%, $p = 0.039$) in the different-DES group. After adjustment using propensity score analyses, restenosis rate (relative risk: 0.41, 95% confidence interval [CI]: 0.21 to 0.80, $p = 0.01$), minimal lumen diameter (difference: 0.41 mm, 95% CI: 0.19 to 0.62, $p = 0.001$), and the event-free survival (hazard ratio: 0.56, 95% CI: 0.33 to 0.96, $p = 0.038$) remained significantly improved in the switch group.

Drug-coated balloons (DCB) might be the most realistic and promising option. Several studies [48, 53-55] have shown the superiority of DCB to plain old balloons for in-stent restenosis. Hehrlein, et al. [56] studied patients with ISR to investigate the safety and efficacy of a novel drug-coated balloon (DCB) incorporating paclitaxel into a microcrystalline structure by applying the inert excipient butyryltri-n-hexyl citrate (BTHC) in a prospective first-in-man trial. Eighty-one patients were enrolled at 9 European sites, 43 (53.1%) presenting with bare metal stent (BMS)-ISR and 38 (46.9%) with DES-ISR. At 6 months, overall in-stent late lumen loss (LLL) (primary endpoint) was 0.07 ± 0.31 mm showing differences in BMS-ISR and DES-ISR treatment (-0.05 ± 0.28 mm vs. 0.19 ± 0.29 mm, respectively, $P= 0.001$). Overall MACE rates at 6 and 12 months (secondary endpoint) were 6.5% and 11.8%, respectively. At the 12-month follow-up, one myocardial infarction, and no cardiac death or stent thrombosis had occurred. Application of a novel PCB using BTHC as an excipient in patients with ISR is safe and results in very low LLL, revascularization, and MACE rates at follow-up. This effect was only limited to the short term ISR and further studies are warranted to determine the efficacy of late phase ISR. On the other hand, serial clinical and angiographic follow-up data that support PCB for the treatment of BMS-ISR and DES-ISR have been reported. In Japan, Habara et al. [57] revealed that PCB reduced neointimal hyperplasia more effectively in BMS-ISR than in DES-ISR during follow-up. In their study, the duration of ISR after stent implantation was not clearly described, however, those with DES ISR within 6 months were excluded. LLL was lower in the PCB group than in the balloon angioplasty group (0.11 ± 0.33 mm vs. 0.49 ± 0.50 mm, $P <0.001$). In PCB-treated lesions, recurrent restenosis occurred in 1.1% of patients with BMS-ISR and in 9.1% of patients with DES-ISR ($P = 0.04$). LLL was lower in patients with BMS-ISR than in patients with DES-ISR (0.05 ± 0.28 mm vs. 0.18 ± 0.38 mm, $P = 0.03$). There was no death, myocardial infarction, or stent thrombosis in either group. Although the mechanisms of DES-

ISR are similar to BMS-ISR in some particular aspects, such as stent underexpansion, stent fracture, and stent malapposition, DES-ISR has another unique mechanism that includes drug-specific factors such as localized hypersensitivity, nonuniform drug deposition, polymers, and drug resistance. According to Habara et al. [57], BMS-ISR and DES-ISR had different biological responses after PCB.

Bioabsorbable vascular scaffolding (BVS) might be a potential candidate for DES-ISR therapy. However, the thick struts of the present version of BVS could be a negative factor in this clinical situation depending on the vessel size. Further investigations on this new technology are warranted.

PCI for recurrent ISR presents a challenging problem with limited data for treatment. Recently, Kubo et al. reported the optimal treatment of recurrent restenosis lesions after DES implantation for study [58].

148 recurrent ISR lesions (142 patients) among 1,101 ISR lesions treated by DES implantation were intervened. They were treated with balloon angioplasty (76 lesions, 72 patients) and DES implantation (i.e. third stent implantation) (72 lesions, 70 patients). Index stent was BMS in 61.1% and DES in 38.9% in the DES group and BMS in 68.4% and DES in 31.6% in the balloon angioplasty group. Index DES included sirolimus–eluting stents (SES) and paclitaxel-eluting stents (PES). Second PCI used SES in 86.1% and PES in 13.9% in the DES group and SES in 85.5% and PES in 14.5% in the balloon angioplasty group. The mean number of days from index PCI to second PCI was 903±1,070 in the DES group and 780±1,038 in the balloon angioplasty group.

Also, the mean number of days from second PCI to third PCI was 597±442 in the DES group and 400±387 in the balloon angioplasty group. Thus, subjects in this study included those with very late ISR. DES implantation had better outcomes than balloon angioplasty, mainly because of a higher TLR rate in the balloon angioplasty group regardless of whether the recurrent ISR pattern was focal or non-focal. Although LLL was similar between the two groups (0.80±0.78 mm in DES group vs. 0.87±0.79 mm in balloon angioplasty group, $P = 0.60$), the angiographic restenosis rate after PCI for recurrent ISR after DES implantation was significantly lower in DES implantation (25.0%) than in balloon angioplasty (64.4%, $p<0.001$). IVUS-guided PCI was associated with a lower TLR rate after PCI for recurrent ISR lesions, particularly after DES implantation. These results suggest that the IVUS-guided larger acute gain works in the DES group but is less effective in balloon angioplasty. The authors recommended a third stent implantation with a DES should be selected in residual stenosis lesions only after balloon dilatation [58].

Conclusion

Late ISR is a relatively rare phenomenon compared with early ISR after coronary stent implantation and its clinical consequence can be severe if the underlying mechanism is not appreciated.

Its mechanism is not simple (related to inflammation and neoatherosclerosis) and is different from that of early ISR. Prevention and treatment for late ISR is not established however, BVS and DCB have great potential.

References

[1] Choussat R., Klersy C., Black A. J., et al. Long-term (> or =8 years) outcome after Palmaz-Schatz stent implantation. *Am. J. Cardiol.*, 2001;88:10-6.

[2] Kimura T., Abe K., Shizuta S., et al. Long-term clinical and angiographic follow-up after coronary stent placement in native coronary arteries. *Circulation*, 2002;105: 2986-91.

[3] Hasegawa K., Tamai H., Kyo E., et al. Histopathological findings of new in-stent lesions developed beyond five years. *Catheter Cardiovasc. Interv.*, 2006;68:554-8.

[4] Ito S., Yoshida T., Suzuki S. A case of extended late-phase in-stent restenosis after implantation of a bare-metal stent: intravascular ultrasound, optical coherence tomography and immunohistochemical findings. *J. Invasive Cardiol.*, 2011;23:E86-91.

[5] Cosgrave J., Corbett S. J., Melzi G., et al. Late restenosis following sirolimus-eluting stent implantation. *Am. J. Cardiol.*, 2007;100:41-4.

[6] Virmani R., Guagliumi G., Farb A., et al. Localized hypersensitivity and late coronary thrombosis secondary to a sirolimus-eluting stent: should we be cautious? *Circulation,* 2004;109:701-5.

[7] Nakazawa G., Otsuka F., Nakano M., Vorpahl M., Virmaani R. The pathology of neoatherosclerosis in human coronary implants. *J. Am. Coll. Cardiol.*, 2011; 57: 1314-22.

[8] Takano M., Yamamoto M., Inami S., et al. Appearance of lipid-laden intima and neovascularization after implantation of bare-metal stents. *J. Am. Coll. Cardiol.*, 2010; 55: 26-32.

[9] Kang S. J., Mintz G. S., Akasaka T., et al. Optical coherence tomographic analysis of in-stent neoatherosclerosis after drug-eluting stent implantation. *Circulation,* 2011; 123:2954-63.

[10] Ito S., Nakasuka K., Miyata K., et al. Late in-stent restenosis after sirolimus-eluting stent implantation is related to thrmobus foramtion-Insight from a case with IVUS, OCT, and histological findings. *J. C. Cases*, 2012;5:e83-e6.

[11] Ito S., Nakasuka K., Morimoto K., et al. Angiographic and clinical characteristics of patients with acetylcholine-induced coronary vasospasm on follow-up coronary angiography following drug-eluting stent implantation. *J. Invasive Cardiol.*, 2011; 23:57-64.

[12] Kim J. W., Seo H. S., Park J. H., et al. A prospective randomized, 6-month comparison of the coronary vasomotor response asociated with a zotarolimus- versus a sirolimus-eluting stent. *J. Am. Coll. Cardiol.*, 2009;53:1653-9.

[13] Sawada T., Shinke T., Shite J., et al. Inpact of cytochrome P450 2C19*2 polymorphism on intra-stent thrombus after drug-eluting stent implantation in Japanese patients receiving clopidogrel. *Circ.,* J 2010;75:99-105.

[14] Fujii K., Masutani M., Ohyanagi M. Contribution of organized thrombus to in-stent restenosis after sirolimus-eluting stent implantation: optical coherence tomography findings. *Eur. Heart J.,* 2008;29:1385.

[15] Shiode N., Shirota Y., Katou Y., tsunoda F., Fujiwara M., Miura M. Late progression after progression sirolimu-eluting stent implantation:comparison with bare metal stent implantation. *J. Am. Coll. Cardiol.,* 2009;53 (Supple):A12.

[16] Byme R. A., Joner M., Kastrati A. Polymer coatings and delayed arterial healing following drug-eluting stent implantation. *Minerva Cardioangiol.*, 2009;57:567-84.

[17] Yoneda S., Abe S., Kanaya T., et al. Late-phase inflammatory response as a feature of in-stent restenosis after drug-eluting stent implantation. *Coron. Artery Dis.*, 2013; 24: 368-73.

[18] Inoue T., Node K. Molecular basis of restenosis and novel issues of drug-eluting stents. *Circ. J.*, 2009;73:615-21.

[19] Inoue T., Croce K., Morooka T., Sakuma M., Node K., Simon D. I. Vascular inflammation and repair:implication for re-endothelialization, restenosis, and stent thrombosis. *J. Am. Coll. Cardiol. Interv.*, 2011;4:1057-66.

[20] Inoue K., Abe K., Ando K., et al. Pathological amalyses of long-term intracoronary Palmaz-Schatz stenting Is its efficacy permanent? *Cardiovascular pathology*, 2004; 13:109-15.

[21] Mann J., Davies M. J. Mechanisms of progression in native coronary artery disease: role of healed plaque disruption. *Heart*, 1999;82:265-8.

[22] Burke A. P., Kolodgie F. D., Farb A., et al. Healed plaque ruptures and sudden coronary death: evidence that subclinical rupture has a role in plaque progression. *Circulation*, 2001;103:934-40.

[23] Kolodgie F. D., Gold H. K., Burke A. P., et al. Intraplaque hemorrhage and progression of coronary atheroma. *N. Engl. J. Med.*, 2003;349:2316-25.

[24] Iijima R., Araki T., Nagashima Y., et al. Incidence and predictors of the late catch-up phenomenon after drug-eluting stent implantation. *Int. J. Cardiol.*, 2013.

[25] Gonzaro N., Serruys P. W., Okamura T., et al. Optical coherence tomography pattern of stent restenosis. *Am. Heart J.*, 2009;158:284-93.

[26] Goto K., Takebayashi H., Kihara Y., et al. Appearance of neointima according to stent type and restenotic phase: analysis by optical coherence tomography. *EuroIntervention*, 2013.

[27] Ito S., Nakasuka K., Miyata K., et al. Ruptured plaque in a bare-metal stent 8 years after implantation-Comparison of IVUS and OCT findings. *J. C. Cases*, 2012;5:e1-e3.

[28] Habara M., Terashima M., Nasu K., et al. Difference of tissue characteristics between early and very late restenosis lesions after bare-metal stent implantation: an optical coherence tomography study. *Circ. Cardiovasc. Interv.*, 2011;4:232-8.

[29] Takano M., Xie Y., Murakami D., et al. Various optical coherence tomographic findings in restenotic lesions after sirolimus-eluting stent implantation. *Int. J. Cardiol.*, 2009;134:263-5.

[30] Nakano M., Otsuka F., Virmani R. Letter by Nakano et al. regarding article, "optical coherence tomographic analysis of in-stent neoatherosclerosis after drug-eluting stent implantation". *Circulation*, 2011;124:e954; author reply e5.

[31] Miyazaki S., Hiasa Y., Takahashi T., et al. In vivo optical coherence tomography of very late drug-eluting stent thrombosis compared with late in-stent restenosis. *Circ. J.*, 2012;76:390-8.

[32] Joner M., Finn A. V., Farb A., et al. Pathology of drug-eluting stents in humans: delayed healing and late thrombotic risk. *J. Am. Coll. Cardiol.*, 2006;48:193-202.

[33] Song H. G., Park D. W., Kim Y. H., et al. Randomized trial of optimal treatment strategies for in-stent restenosis after drug-eluting stent implantation. *J. Am. Coll. Cardiol.*, 2012;59:1093-100.

[34] Stefanini G. G., Byrne R. A., Serruys P. W., et al. Biodegradable polymer drug-eluting stents reduce the risk of stent thrombosis at 4 years in patients undergoing percutaneous coronary intervention: a pooled analysis of individual patient data from the ISAR-TEST 3, ISAR-TEST 4, and LEADERS randomized trials. *Eur. Heart J.*, 2012;33:1214-22.

[35] Onuma Y., Muramatsu T., Kharlamov A., Serruys P. W. Freeing the vessel from metallic cage: what can we achieve with bioresorbable vascular scaffolds? *Cardiovasc. Interv. Ther.*, 2012.

[36] Nishio S., Kosuga K., Igaki K., et al. Long-Term (>10 Years) clinical outcomes of first-in-human biodegradable poly-l-lactic acid coronary stents: Igaki-Tamai stents. *Circulation,* 2012;125:2343-53.

[37] Marcucci R., Gori A. M., Paniccia R., et al. Cardiovascular death and nonfatal myocardial infarction in acute coronary syndrome patients receiving coronary stenting are predicted by residual platelet reactivity to ADP detected by a point-of-care assay: a 12-month follow-up. *Circulation,* 2009;119:237-42.

[38] Matetzky S., Shenkman B., Guetta V., et al. Clopidogrel resistance is associated with increased risk of recurrent atherothrombotic events in patients with acute myocardial infarction. *Circulation*, 2004;109:3171-5.

[39] Patti G., Nusca A., Mangiacapra F., Gatto L., D'Ambrosio A., Di Sciascio G. Point-of-care measurement of clopidogrel responsiveness predicts clinical outcome in patients undergoing percutaneous coronary intervention results of the ARMYDA-PRO (Antiplatelet therapy for Reduction of MYocardial Damage during Angioplasty-Platelet Reactivity Predicts Outcome) study. *J. Am. Coll. Cardiol.*, 2008;52:1128-33.

[40] Biondi-Zoccai G. G., Lotrionte M., Anselmino M., et al. Systematic review and meta-analysis of randomized clinical trials appraising the impact of cilostazol after percutaneous coronary intervention. *Am. Heart J.*, 2008;155:1081-9.

[41] Jennings D. L., Kalus J. S. Addition of cilostazol to aspirin and a thienopyridine for prevention of restenosis after coronary artery stenting: a meta-analysis. *J. Clin. Pharmacol.*, 2010;50:415-21.

[42] Singh I., Shafiq N., Pandhi P., et al. Triple antiplatelet therapy vs. dual antiplatelet therapy in patients undergoing percutaneous coronary intervention: an evidence-based approach to answering a clinical query. *Br. J. Clin. Pharmacol.*, 2009;68:4-13.

[43] Chen Z., Qian J., Chen Y., Ma J., Ge J. Addition of cilostazol to conventional dual antiplatelet therapy reduces the risk of cardiac events and restenosis after drug-eluting stent implantation: a meta-analysis. *J. Clin. Pharmacol.*, 2013;53:532-9.

[44] Mehran R., Dangas G., Abizaid A. S., et al. Angiographic patterns of in-stent restenosis: classification and implications for long-term outcome. *Circulation,* 1999;100:1872-8.

[45] Unverdorben M., Vallbracht C., Cremers B., et al. Paclitaxel-coated balloon catheter versus paclitaxel-coated stent for the treatment of coronary in-stent restenosis. *Circulation,* 2009;119:2986-94.

[46] Maluenda G., Ben-Dor I., Gaglia M. A., Jr., et al. Clinical outcomes and treatment after drug-eluting stent failure: the absence of traditional risk factors for in-stent restenosis. *Circ. Cardiovasc. Interv.*, 2012;5:12-9.

[47] Ko Y. G., Kim J. S., Kim B. K., et al. Efficacy of drug-eluting stents for treating in-stent restenosis of drug-eluting stents (from the Korean DES ISR multicenter registry study [KISS]). *Am. J. Cardiol.*, 2012;109:607-13.

[48] Rittger H., Brachmann J., Sinha A. M., et al. A randomized, multicenter, single-blinded trial comparing paclitaxel-coated balloon angioplasty with plain balloon angioplasty in drug-eluting stent restenosis: the PEPCAD-DES study. *J. Am. Coll. Cardiol.,* 2012;59: 1377-82.

[49] Chevalier B., Moulichon R., Teiger E., et al. One-year results of the CRISTAL Trial, a randomized comparison of cypher sirolimus-eluting coronary stents versus balloon angioplasty for restenosis of drug-eluting stents. *J. Interv. Cardiol.*, 2012;25:586-95.

[50] Yu C. M., Kwong J. S., Sanderson J. E. Drug-eluting balloons for coronary artery disease: A meta-analysis of randomized controlled trials. *Int. J. Cardiol.*, 2012.

[51] Yamashita K., Ochiai M., Yakushiji T., et al. Repeat drug-eluting stent implantation for in-stent restenosis: first- or second-generation stent. *J. Invasive Cardiol.*, 2012;24: 574-8.

[52] Alfonso F., Perez-Vizcayno M. J., Dutary J., et al. Implantation of a drug-eluting stent with a different drug (switch strategy) in patients with drug-eluting stent restenosis. Results from a prospective multicenter study (RIBS III [Restenosis Intra-Stent: Balloon Angioplasty Versus Drug-Eluting Stent]). *JACC Cardiovasc. Interv.*, 2012;5:728-37.

[53] Steinberg D. H., Gaglia M. A., Jr., Pinto Slottow T. L., et al. Outcome differences with the use of drug-eluting stents for the treatment of in-stent restenosis of bare-metal stents versus drug-eluting stents. *Am. J. Cardiol.*, 2009;103:491-5.

[54] Wohrle J., Zadura M., Mobius-Winkler S., et al. SeQuentPlease World Wide Registry: clinical results of SeQuent please paclitaxel-coated balloon angioplasty in a large-scale, prospective registry study. *J. Am. Coll. Cardiol.*, 2012;60:1733-8.

[55] Scheller B., Clever Y. P., Kelsch B., et al. Long-term follow-up after treatment of coronary in-stent restenosis with a paclitaxel-coated balloon catheter. *JACC Cardiovasc. Interv.*, 2012;5:323-30.

[56] Hehrlein C., Dietz U., Kubica J., et al. Twelve-month results of a paclitaxel releasing balloon in patients presenting with in-stent restenosis First-in-Man (PEPPER) trial. *Cardiovasc. Revasc. Med.*, 2012;13:260-4.

[57] Habara S., Iwabuchi M., Inoue N., et al. A multicenter randomized comparison of paclitaxel-coated balloon catheter with conventional balloon angioplasty in patients with bare-metal stent restenosis and drug-eluting stent restenosis. *Am. Heart J.,* 2013;166:527-33.

[58] Kubo S., Kadota K., Otsuru S., et al. Optimal treatment of recurrent restenosis lesions after drug-eluting stent implantation for in-stent restenosis lesions. *EuroIntervention*, 2013;9:788-96.

In: Coronary Artery Restenosis
Editor: Amir S. Lotfi

ISBN: 978-1-63321-346-3

Chapter 6

Stent Sizing Without Intravascular Imaging: Impact on Restenosis

Yohan Chacko[1,2], J. Kimberly Haladyn[1] and Richard Lim[1,2*]

[1]The University of Queensland, Brisbane, Australia

[2]Department of Cardiology, Princess Alexandra Hospital, Brisbane, Australia

Abstract

Intravascular ultrasound (IVUS) use is promoted to guide optimal stent implantation. However, cost and time constraints limit the uptake of routine intravascular imaging in many interventional centres. In laboratories where intravascular imaging is available but not routine, the synergistic practice of angiographic assessment combined with reference to balloon compliance charts is a popular method of optimising stent deployment especially in non-complex cases.

This chapter gives an overview of stent sizing without the use of intravascular imaging and its effect on clinical restenosis. Lessons learnt from the balloon angioplasty era and trials using IVUS to optimize stent placement are reviewed, guiding the interventional cardiologist on appropriate balloon to artery ratios, achieving largest minimal lumen diameter and to be alert for diffuse atherosclerosis of the reference vessel. For further guidance, data on strengths and pitfalls of manufacturers' balloon compliance chart use in optimal stent sizing are presented alongside real world data of aggressive angiographic guided stent expansion and restenosis.

In summary, in non-complex stenting, aggressive stent expansion without intravascular guidance is common and there is no signal that such aggressive stent expansion predisposes to restenosis even in small coronary arteries. Recent studies confirm the clinical validity of the synergistic strategy of visual angiographic assessment coupled with reference to manufacturers' compliance charts as a guide – a popular approach that previously lacked an evidence base.

* Corresponding Author: Associate Professor Richard Lim, Email: r.lim@uq.edu.au, Telephone: +61-7-3176 7143, Fax: +61-7-3176 7630.

Introduction

There is ample evidence to support the use of intravascular ultrasound (IVUS) and more recently optical coherence tomography (OCT) to guide optimal stent expansion [1-7]. Early studies showed that stent deployment guided only by angiography often resulted in suboptimal apposition of struts despite appearing angiographically adequate. Clinical outcome data, although not robust, have suggested a reduction in major adverse cardiac events in the patients receiving IVUS-guided stent deployment [6, 8]. In particular, when drug-eluting stents are used, stent thrombosis risk – early or late, and even restenosis may be heightened by poor strut apposition [9]. Interventional cardiologists have therefore learnt to aggressively post-dilate stents to improve strut apposition and patient outcomes.

Stenting has come of age and operators have also become confident about the need to optimise stent sizing. At the same time, there is an emerging breed of younger interventional cardiologists who rely heavily on intravascular imaging as a routine. However, cost and time constraints conspire to reduce the uptake of routine intravascular imaging in many busy publicly-funded centres. In such laboratories where intravascular imaging is available but not routine, angiographically-guided expansion of stents above nominal size to maximise luminal diameter is commonly practised especially in non-complex cases. This approach relies not only on reasonably accurate angiographic assessment but also reference to manufacturers' balloon compliance charts to guide stent sizing. Outcome data however are limited to support this popular real-world practice [10-12].

Thus the interventional cardiologist must balance optimal stent apposition against the risk of vessel trauma and restenosis when expanding stents without IVUS guidance. Deciding on how aggressive to be during final stent optimisation is a routine challenge. This chapter summarises research addressing stent sizing and its effect on clinical restenosis.

Lessons in Balloon Sizing from the Balloon Angioplasty Era

Balloon dilatation fractures the intimal plaque and partially disrupts the media and adventitia leading to acute enlargement of vessel lumen and overall outer vessel diameter [13]. There is however elastic recoil of the vessel and fibrotic contraction of the vessel wall known as negative remodeling. This commonly explains the immediate 30% residual stenosis following balloon deflation. Further, the physiological response to balloon-induced injury includes platelet and fibrin deposition as well as infiltration of smooth muscle cells and fibroblasts. This results in neointimal hyperplasia. Restenosis rates in the balloon angioplasty era were 30-60% at 6 months, unsurprisingly [14].

Coronary stents were originally developed to act as a scaffold in the bailout situation and also to mitigate the elastic recoil and negative remodeling. After the initial acute gain, every stented lesion then undergoes some degree of late loss due to neointimal hyperplasia. Just as stents were being commercialised, there was recognition that larger lumen diameters immediately after intervention translated into larger diameters at follow up on 6 month repeat angiography [15]. This instigated the 'bigger is better' dogma – one that was intuitively acceptable.

This philosophy however did not escape controversy, initially being tempered by observational and randomised data reporting higher rates of dissection, Q wave infarction and emergency bypass surgery when balloons were oversized. Nichols et al. described a 37% rate of dissection with a balloon to artery ratio of >1.3 : 1 [16]. Roubin et al. randomised patients to receive either a larger or smaller balloon than reference vessel [17]. A balloon to artery ratio >1.1 : 1 caused increased rates of emergency bypass surgery (7.1% vs 3.6%) and peri-procedural Q wave myocardial infarction. These studies also showed that undersizing the balloon with a balloon to artery ratio less than 0.9 : 1 predisposed to late loss or restenosis. How balloon to artery ratio was measured was not fully defined.

So the search continued for the procedural and device factors that help to achieve the perfect balance of size, expansion and optimum patient outcomes.

Lessons on Stent Sizing and Drivers of Restenosis from Intravascular Ultrasound Trials

Studies assessing the use of IVUS for coronary stenting provided early valuable information on stent sizing. They emphasised the importance of optimal stent apposition, obtaining maximal lumen area and symmetric stent expansion.

One recurring theme was that larger intra-stent minimal lumen area (MLA), as a percentage of reference vessel lumen area, correlated with less restenosis. Therefore an under-expanded stent, with resultant small intra-stent MLA, is a procedural driver for restenosis.

Criteria for optimal stent expansion varied between trials (Table 1) and were not easy to meet in the trials even with use of IVUS. When inplanting stents without the use of IVUS, MLA or cross-sectional area (CSA) cannot be measured. Instead, minimum lumen diameter (MLD) is the objective measure and can be deduced either by visual inspection or quantitative coronary angiography. In the mid 1990's, trials reported that using angiography alone, up to 80% of stents were sub-optimally expanded [18, 19], judged against IVUS criteria mandating that the lumen CSA be >70% of the dilatation balloon CSA. Then came trials testing IVUS-guided optimisation for stent sizing. One such trial reported that IVUS optimisation by post-dilatation could significantly improve CSA and in turn MLD (3.12 mm to 3.61 mm) [18].

Based on angiographic imaging, the risk of restenosis correlates inversely with post-intervention intra-stent lumen diameter also termed final MLD. Moussa et al. [4] examined numerous proposed IVUS criteria for optimal stent sizing to test which best predicted freedom from restenosis. They compared:

1. Intra-stent minimal lumen cross-sectional area (ISMLCSA) ≥ 9 mm^2
2. ISMLCSA ≥ 9 mm^2 and ≥ 80% of average reference lumen cross sectional area (CSA) [measured outlining lumen-intima interface]
3. ISMLCSA ≥ 90% of average reference lumen CSA
4. ISMLCSA ≥ 90% of distal reference lumen CSA
5. ISMLCSA ≥ 55% of average reference *vessel* CSA [measured outlining vessel media- adventitia interface]

These were tested on 425 patients who underwent IVUS-guided stenting. The balloon to artery ratio required to achieve the above IVUS criteria was typically ≥ 1.2 : 1. This is outside the safe limit of 1.1 : 1 derived from data in the balloon angioplasty era [16, 17].

Only ISMLCSA ≥ 9 mm^2 and ISMLCSA ≥ 55% of average reference vessel CSA were significantly associated with freedom from restenosis. However, ISMLCSA ≥ 9 mm^2 was only achieved in 29% of patients and predominantly in large vessels. Assuming a circular vessel shape, CSA of 9mm^2 requires a lumen diameter of 3.39 mm, which could be considered unlikely to be safely achieved in vessels much smaller than 3 mm. So when vessel size was taken into account, ISMLCSA ≥ 9 mm^2 as an absolute metric was no longer an independent predictor of freedom from restenosis, but ISMLCSA ≥ 55% of average reference vessel CSA was still predictive as a relative index.

Notably, ISMLCSA ≥ 55% of average reference vessel CSA was more predictive of freedom from restenosis than ISMLCSA ≥ 90% of average reference lumen CSA. This highlights the importance for operators assessing lesions angiographically to be alert to the possibility of diffuse atherosclerosis along the length of the vessel giving a false impression of reference vessel size on the 'lumen-ogram.' It also emphasizes the importance, if stenting were to be performed without intravascular imaging, to visually examine the *entire* vessel to gauge its true size perhaps with the aid of liberal intracoronary boluses of nitroglycerin.

Variation in intra-stent lumen diameter is common. Symmetrical stent expansion by improving MLD is thought to protect against restenosis. The MUSIC investigators [20] defined symmetric stent expansion as a ratio of minimum lumen diameter: maximum lumen diameter of ≥0·7. Newer non-compliant balloons should assist in achieving this.

De Feyter et al. [21] combined data from 3 large IVUS registries (MUSIC, WEST-II and ESSEX) and 2 RCTs in an attempt to identify the most strongly predictive factors for angiographic restenosis (>50%) at 6 months. They found that in-stent area and stent length were the most predictive factors and developed a reference chart to predict restenosis risk using only these 2 parameters.

Despite multiple reports including some randomised controlled trials showing improved lumen diameter and target lesion revascularisation rates at 6 months, IVUS use is still not routine. The limitations of applying these trial results to contemporary practice include [22]:

- No established uniform IVUS criteria for stent optimization
- Lack of experience/expertise in interpreting IVUS images online by operator
- Post-dilatation not being standard practice after stent implantation in the era of these trials; if post-dilatation was carried out, balloon diameter was chosen on the basis of complex numerical formulae based on IVUS measurements
- Non-compliant balloons not commonly available in these trials
- Increased time and cost of procedure
- Limited data with drug-eluting stents

The only randomised clinical trial of IVUS guided versus angiography-guided stenting in the current era of drug-eluting stents and non-compliant balloons is the AVIO trial [23]. This trial of 284 patients looked only at complex lesions which included long lesions > 28 mm, chronic total occlusions, bifurcations, small vessels ≤ 2.5 mm and those requiring ≥ 4 stents. IVUS guided compared with angiography-guided stent implantation increased the final MLD

(2.55 mm vs 2.39 mm) but there was no significant difference in clinical endpoints at one or 24 months. The AVIO authors noted that in their top enrolling centre which had extensive IVUS experience, there was no difference in final MLD between IVUS guided and angiography-guided stenting. They suggested that experienced operators thoroughly familiar with the angiographic correlates of IVUS could develop the "IVUS eye" *i.e.* the ability to perform aggressive post-dilatation with only angiographic guidance.

It is a defensible view that clinical endpoint data for IVUS-guided stenting, being only modest and conflicting in parts, do not support a definite mandate for the routine use of IVUS to guide all coronary stenting. The Society for Cardiovascular Angiography and Interventions (SCAI) guidelines [24] give only a Class II B recommendation for the use of IVUS to guide coronary stenting, with the exception of left main disease. If IVUS or intravascular imaging is not mandatory for routine non-complex stenting, how are we doing in the current era of latest-generation stents, refined pharmacotherapy and aggressive post-dilatation practices empowered by lessons from IVUS and common use of non-compliant balloons?

Table 1. Summary of IVUS Guided vs Angiography-Guided PCI Trials

	Balloon Sizing	IVUS Criteria	Results	
			Angiographic	IVUS
CLOUT 1997 155 pts; Observational study; only post-procedural endpoints	(MLD+MVD) *0.5 in the proximal and distal segment	If PTCA balloon size was already equal to BS obtained according to the formula, no further dilatation performed (27% lesions)	MLA 2.21±0.47 Acute gain 0.20	MLA 4.52±1.14, p<0.001 Acute gain 0.26, p<0.001
MUSIC 1998 161 pts; Observational study	IVUS used for evaluation of appropriate stent apposition.	1. Complete apposition against the vessel wall of the entire stent. 2. a) MLA≥90% of the average reference lumen area or ≥100% of lumen area of the reference segment with the lowest lumen area. b) MLA >9.0 mm^2. c) MLA ≥80% of the average reference lumen area or ≥90% of lumen area of the reference segment with the lowest lumen area. 3. Symmetric stent expansion	MLD 2.90±0.36; Acute gain 1.79±0.39	MLD 3.10±0.40
RESIST 1998 155 pts; Multicentre, randomised, single-blinded study		Stent CSA>80% of the mean proximal and distal reference vessel CSA *Only 77% of pts with adequate angiographic result*	MLD 2.46±0.46 Acute gain 1.45±0.53 MLA 7.16±2.48 6 month Restenosis 28.8%	MLD 2.57±0.41 Acute gain 1.62±0.43, p=0.04 MLA

Table 1. (Continued)

	Balloon Sizing	IVUS Criteria	Results	
		satisfied *IVUS criteria*	MLA 4.47±2.59	7.95±2.21, p=0.04 6 month Restenosis 22.5%, p=0.25 MLA 5.36±2.81, p=0.03
SIPS 2000 269 pts; Randomised prospective; 6 mths angiographic and 2 years clinical FU	(MLD+MVD) *0.5 in the prox and distal segment	MUSIC criteria	MLD 2.38±0.67; Acute gain 1.67±0.76 2yr clinically driven TLR 43%	MLD 2.49±0.66, p=0.12; Acute gain 1.85±0.72; p=0.02 2yr clinically driven TLR 21%, p=0.02
CRUISE 2000 525 pts, Multicentre, prospective observational, IVUS substudy	No detailed IVUS criteria	Post procedure IVUS analysis in the core lab	MLD 2.59±0.43 MLA 7.06±2.13 TLR 9 months 15.3%	MLD, 2.96±0.55, p<0.001 MLA 7.78±1.72 TLR 9 months 8.5%, p< 0.05
AVID 2000 800 pts, Multicentre, randomized study		1. MLA ≥90% of distal minimal vessel lumen CSA; 2. Stent fully apposed; 3. Dissections covered by stent *Criteria accomplished only in 48% patients*	MLD 2.89±0.51 MLA 6.90±2.43 12 month TLR 10.1%	MLD 2.95±0.49, p=0.15 MLA 7.55±2.82, p=0.001 12 month TLR 4.3%, p=0.01
OPTICUS 2001 550 pts; multicentre, randomised		MUSIC criteria for optimal stent implantation achieved in only 56% of patients	MLD 2.91±0.41 Acute gain 1.91±0.66 6 month Binary restenosis 22.8% Late loss 1.00±0.58	MLD 3.02±0.49; p=0.01 Acute gain 2.07±0.50; p<0.0001 MLA 8.10±2.30 6 month binary restenosis Binary restenosis 24.5%, p=0.68 Late loss 1.07±0.62; p=0.20
TULIP 2002 150 pts, Multicentre, randomized study		1) complete stent apposition; 2) MLD≥80% of the mean of prox and distal reference diameters; 3) MLA≥ distal reference lumen area. Criteria accomplished	MLD 2.80±0.31 Acute gain 1.81±0.45 6 month Binary restenosis 46% 6 month Late loss 1.33±0.55 6 month TLR 10%	MLD 3.01±0.40, p=0.008 Acute gain 2.04±0.62, p=0.045 MLA 6.00±3.30 6 month Binary restenosis 23%, p=0.008

	Balloon Sizing	IVUS Criteria	Results	
		in 89% of patients		6 month Late loss 1.20±0.51, p=NS 6 month TLR 3%, p=0.037
BEST 2003 254 pts, Multicentre, randomized study	Balloon diameter closest to the vessel diameter (EEM mean diameter)	IVUS criteria for crossover to stent: >30% stenosis or MLA< 6 mm^2	MLD 2.55±0.49 MLA 6.60±2.05 6-mo FU: no significant angiographic and MACE differences	MLD 2.75±0.49, p=0.013 MLA 7.28±2.22, p=0.02
AVIO 2013 284 pts, Multicentre, randomised, DES only in complex lesions only		1. Avg media to media diameter of prox & distal segment & MLD. Corresponding balloon size CSA. 2. 10% less diameter allowed at stent edges. Criteria achieved in 48% of patients	MLD 2.51± 0.46 24months FU Cumulative MACE 23.2% Death 1.4% TLR 11.9%	MLD 2.7±0.46, p=0.0002 24months FU Cumulative MACE 16.9% p=NS Death 0% p=NS TLR 9.2% p=NS

CLOUT [25], MUSIC [20], RESIST[3], SIPS[8], CRUISE[26], AVID[1], OPTICUS[27], TULIP[6], BEST [28], AVIO[23]

Table Adapted from Rogacka et al. [22]

IVUS intravascular ultrasound; MLD minimal lumen diameter (mm), MVD minimal vessel diameter (mm), MLA intra stent minimal lumen area (mm^2); CSA Cross sectional area(mm^2), TLR target lesion revascularisation; MACE Major Adverse Cardiac Event, FU follow-up; EEM external elastic membrane

Concerns with Stent Over-Expansion

Stent over-expansion without IVUS guidance raises concerns that stent deformation, compromised strut integrity and exaggerated arterial wall stress may predispose to restenosis and lead to poorer short- and long-term outcomes, especially in small vessels or when the stent used is much smaller than vessel size. We have earlier described the concerns seen with oversized balloons in the balloon angioplasty era. Rationally, these concerns have carried over to the era of stenting [29]. One contemporary registry of complications during PCI has reported rates of major dissection at 2%, abrupt closure 0.3% and death 0.7% [30]. Improved device technology, angiographic imaging and operator experience can reduce the risk of complications related to aggressive expansion of stents.

An important consideration in stent expansion is the composition and compliance characteristics of the dilatation balloon. Inflating a compliant or semi-compliant balloon at the lesion to pressures above nominal can often over-distend the adjacent "normal" segment where there is less resistance to balloon expansion – the "dog-bone" effect. Tissue trauma may accentuate neointimal hyperplasia. Worse, edge dissection may require further stents which in turn will increase the restenotic risk. With DES, neointimal hyperplasia may be amplified at the adjacent traumatised segments, leading to restenosis [13, 31]. The more predictable and uniform expansion with non-compliant balloons can mitigate these issues by concentrating dilatation force at the lesion point to maximise acute gain and minimise any dog-bone effect.

The risk of dissection or abrupt closure during coronary stenting is magnified by well-described factors defining lesion complexity including proximal tortuousity [32]. These lesions often require predilatation or other lesion preparation then aggressive post-dilatation of the stent. Clearly the more aggressive the stent expansion, the higher the risk of short-term complication. In the long term however, the risk of restenosis is probably influenced more by the patient and lesion factors that define the baseline complexity, rather than any procedural drivers particularly if intravascular imaging is used. Conversely, when focusing on non-complex lesions, procedural drivers of restenosis become relatively more important. Thus, if intravascular imaging is deemed unnecessary in straightforward stenting, the onus falls on the operator guided only by angiography, to achieve the best outcomes based on a sound understanding of how to safely optimise stent and lumen size.

Reliability of Manufacturers' Balloon Compliance Charts

Manufacturers' balloon compliance charts tabulate the balloon size at various inflation pressures and also include the rated burst pressure. Up to this pressure, the probability of balloon rupture is <0.1%. Inflating the balloon to above rated burst pressure increases the risk of balloon or vessel rupture and potential air embolisation.

Manufacturers' compliance charts are also available for all stent delivery systems to estimate the maximum diameter a stent may reach at various inflation pressures. These charts are derived from *in vitro* testing in a water bath or related phantom at 37 Celsius [33]. Their accuracy based on *in vitro* measurements has been disputed by *in vivo* studies using quantitative coronary angiography (QCA) and IVUS [33-36], suggesting they over-estimate intra-stent lumen diameter by 14-25% and hence cannot be relied upon in clinical practice.

The intra-stent lumen diameter is conventionally known as final MLD. However, variation in lumen diameter along the length of a stent is well-described [36-39] (Figure 1). QCA lacks consensus terminology to address this variation. Current literature in the main refer only to the absolute *smallest* diameter along the length of a stent to compare against compliance chart sizes [33-35]. It seems more intuitive that the balloon compliance chart measurement should more closely correlate with the *largest* lumen diameter achieved across the stent length.

The authors studied 50 randomly selected cases undergoing single-vessel, non-complex stenting to assess the accuracy of balloon compliance chart-derived lumen diameter against QCA [40]. An emphasis was placed on small vessels, with 30 cases with final lumen diameter < 3 mm included.

Figure 2 shows that compliance chart *Derived final MLD* and *QCA maximum intra-stent lumen diameter (ISLD)* correlate near the line of equality, suggesting the two measurements have good agreement.

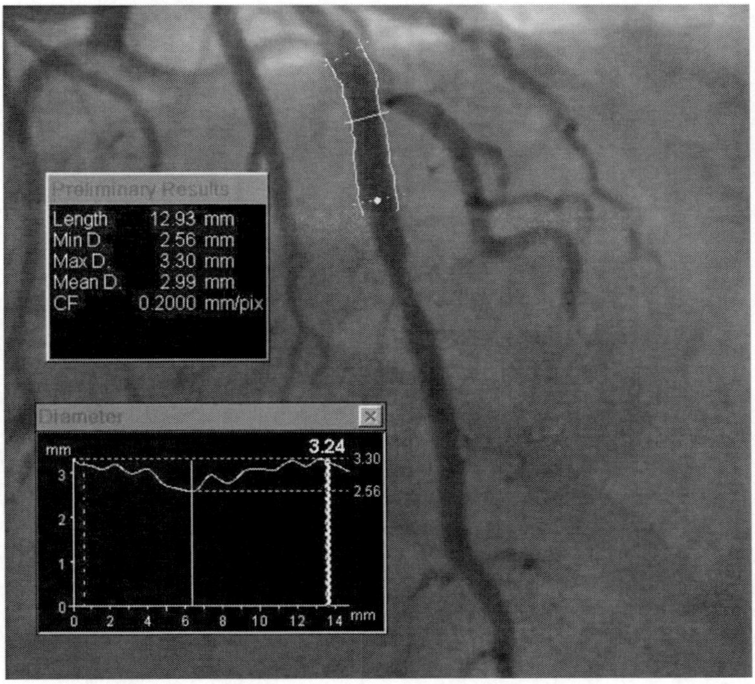

Figure 1. Quantitative Coronary Angiography measuring maximum, mean and minimum intra stent diameter.

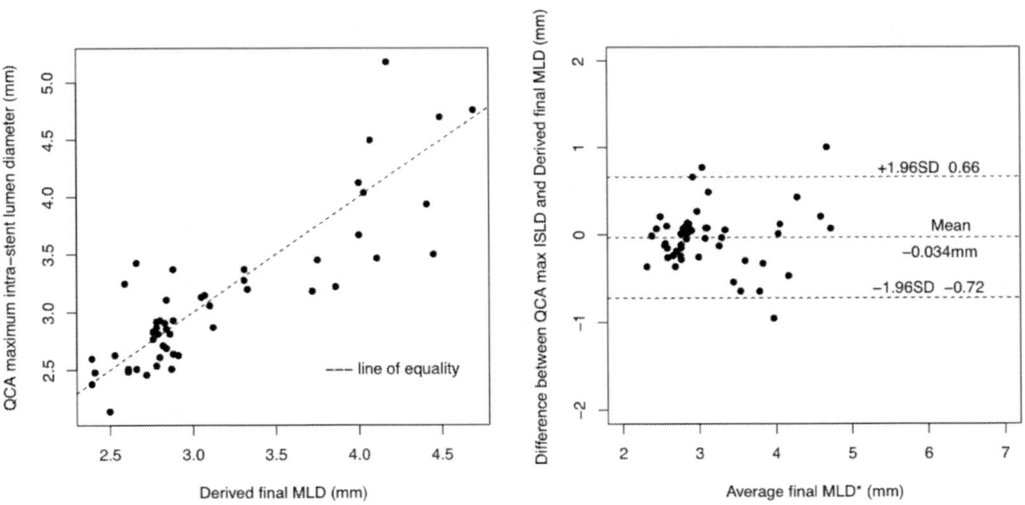

*Average final MLD = (QCA max ISLD + Derived final MLD)/2

Figure 2. Derived final MLD vs QCA maximum intra-stent lumen diameter (left) and Bland-Altman Analysis (right) [*n*=50]. Figures 2-4 reproduced from [Compliance charts to guide non-complex small artery stenting: validation by quantitative coronary angiography, Chacko Y, Haladyn JK, Smith D, Lim R, Heart Asia. 2013;5(1):76-9] with permission from BMJ Publishing Group Ltd.

The Bland-Altman plot (Figure 2) shows the 95% limits of agreement, which suggests no consistent difference of one method of measurement over the other. The scatter however is greater at larger stent sizes – an observation with lesser clinical impact.

Patients with stent size < 3 mm (Figure 3) are of particular interest because they are at greater risk of restenosis [42,43].

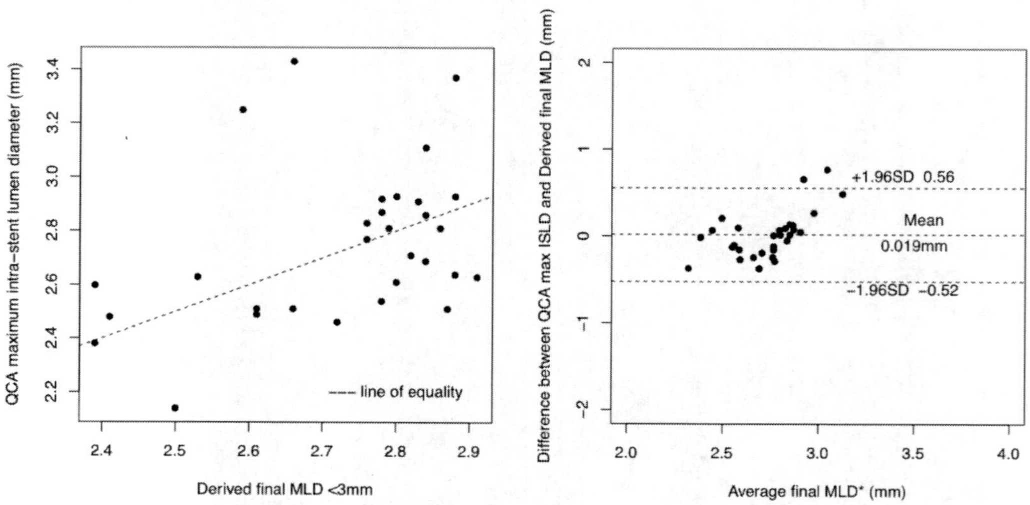

*Average final MLD = (QCA max ISLD + Derived final MLD)/2
The Bland-Altman plot shows narrow 95% limits of agreement between -0.52 to +0.56mm.

Figure 3. Derived final MLD < 3mm vs QCA maximum intra-stent lumen diameter (left) and Bland-Altman Analysis (right) [n=30]. In contrast, when comparing the QCA-measured absolute *minimum* intra-stent lumen diameter and lumen diameter derived from compliance chart (Derived final MLD), the measurements did not correlate (Figure 4). Balloon compliance chart-derived measurements were consistently greater than the minimum intra-stent lumen diameters measured by QCA (Table 2).

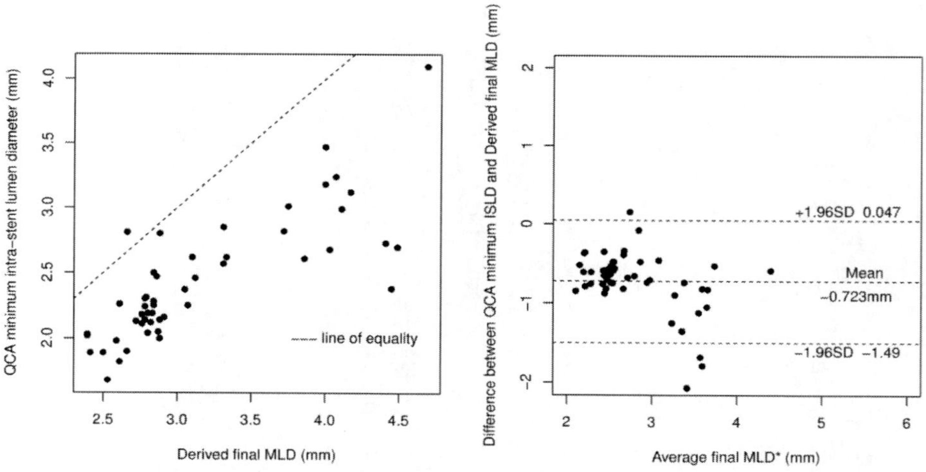

*Average final MLD = (QCA minimum ISLD + Derived final MLD)/2.

Figure 4. Derived final MLD vs QCA *minimum* intra-stent lumen diameter (left) and Bland-Altman Analysis (right) [n=50].

Table 2. Derived final MLD vs QCA maximum and minimum intra-stent lumen diameter

	Compliance Chart Derived final lumen diameter	vs QCA *maximum* intra-stent lumen diameter	vs QCA *minimum* intra-stent lumen diameter
Overall (*n*=50)	Mean difference (95% CI) (mm)	-0.034, (-0.13 to +0.06); *p*=0.49	-0.723 (-0,83 to -0.61); *p*=0.0001
	Bland-Altman 95% LOA (mm)	-0.72 to +0.66	-1.49 to +0.05
Derived Final MLD <3 mm (*n*=30)	Mean difference (95% CI) (mm)	0.019 (-0.08 to 0.12); *p*=0.71	-0.563 (-0.65 to -0.48); *p*=0.0001
	Bland-Altman 95% LOA (mm)	-0.52 to +0.56	-1.01 to -0.12

95% CI = 95% confidence intervals; 95% LOA = 95% limits of agreement from Bland-Altman analysis.

Sizing Stents Without IVUS

The compliance chart is meant only as a guide; as a sizing tool, it cannot be as dynamic or accurate as on-line QCA, IVUS or OCT. In non-complex cases, stents are commonly sized initially by visual assessment of the lesion and vessel size relative to the guide catheter. On-line quantitative coronary angiography can also be used to size vessels especially if there is uncertainty about the visual assessment. Limitations as for visual inspection are that only the vessel lumen is measured and imaging is only 2-dimensional. Although QCA is no longer considered the gold standard, QCA and IVUS measures of lumen dimensions correlate reasonably well for most clinical purposes [41].

Once stent length and nominal size have been selected, stent size is optimised by visual inspection, with reference to the balloon compliance chart as needed. Post- dilatation is common practice to optimise strut apposition and lumen diameter. A stent to vessel ratio of at least 1.1 : 1 is desirable. Drug-eluting stents also benefit from post-dilatation [10]. Haldis et al. (9) described a 'step up, step down' angiographic image after stenting as an objective way to ensure good stent expansion and saw no adverse outcomes. In the early stenting era, Moussa et al. [4] showed that post-dilatation balloon to artery ratios required to meet IVUS stent optimisation criteria were at least 1.2 : 1 with IVUS guidance. Compliance charts can also be referred to for post-dilatation balloon sizing. A real world experience of aggressive stent expansion without intravascular imaging is described in the next section.

Aggressive Stent Expansion without Intravascular Imaging: Incidence and Impact on Restenosis

At a high-volume, publicly funded tertiary referral centre, the authors analysed 243 patients who had ischaemia-driven repeat angiography up to 48 months after the index single-vessel, non-complex PCI in 277 *de novo* coronary stenoses [42]. During the index PCI, stents were sized by angiographic inspection plus reference to manufacturers' balloon compliance charts, as previously described [40]. High-pressure post-dilatation was carried out at the operator's discretion.

Of the 277 lesions, 194 (70%) were treated with bare-metal stents (BMS) and 83 (30%) with drug-eluting stents (DES). Table 3 lists the nominal stent sizes used. In 274 (99%) lesions, the stent was deployed at above nominal size according to the balloon compliance chart. There were 4 (1.4%) cases of coronary artery dissection. One occurred on pre-dilatation of the lesion. Three related to stents over-expanded by < 20% only. No intra-procedural death occurred.

Table 3. Stent Sizes

Nominal Stent Size (mm)	Frequency (%)	Mean Final Stent Size (mm)
2.25	12 (4.3)	2.86
2.50	35 (12.6)	2.93
2.75	17 (6.1)	3.18
3.00	104 (37.5)	3.34
3.50	78 (28.2)	3.90
4.00	26 (9.4)	4.35
4.50	3 (1.1)	4.79
5.00	2 (0.07)	5.26

Stent size mismatch - as a surrogate for degree of stent (over)expansion - was the difference between final stent size and nominal stent size. There was no significant positive correlation between stent size mismatch and percent restenosis for the entire group (R^2 = -0.01, P=0.09) (Figure 5).

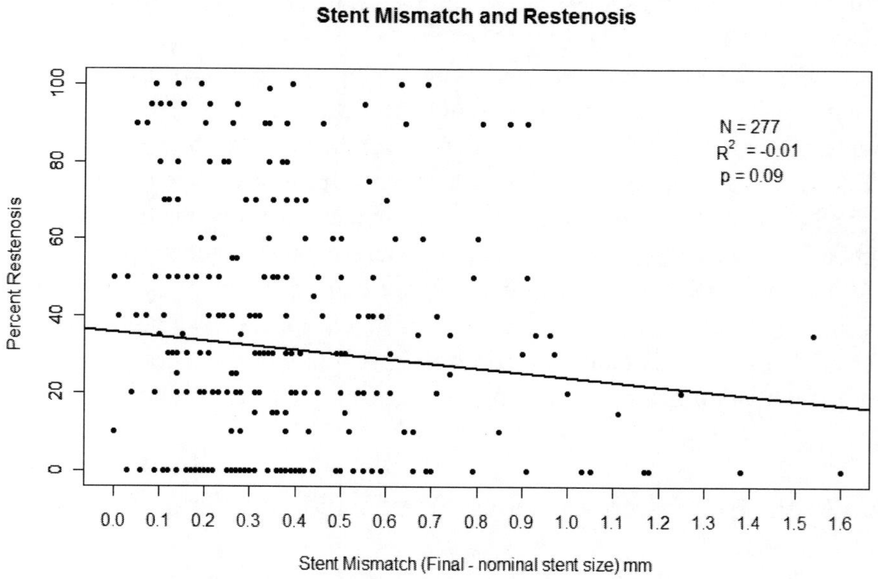

Figure 5. Stent mismatch vs. restenosis for all lesions. Figures 5-7 reproduced from [Overaggresive stent expansion without intravascular imaging: impact on restenosis, Chacko Y, Chan R, Haladyn JK, Lim R, *Heart Asia* 2014; 6 (1):32-35] with permission from BMJ Publishing Group Ltd.

Further analysis stratified by final stent size (Figure 6) was undertaken as small vessels < 3.0 mm are known to be at increased risk of restenosis. Stent size mismatch did not predispose to restenosis in lesions with final stent size < 3.0 mm; indeed there was an inverse relationship.

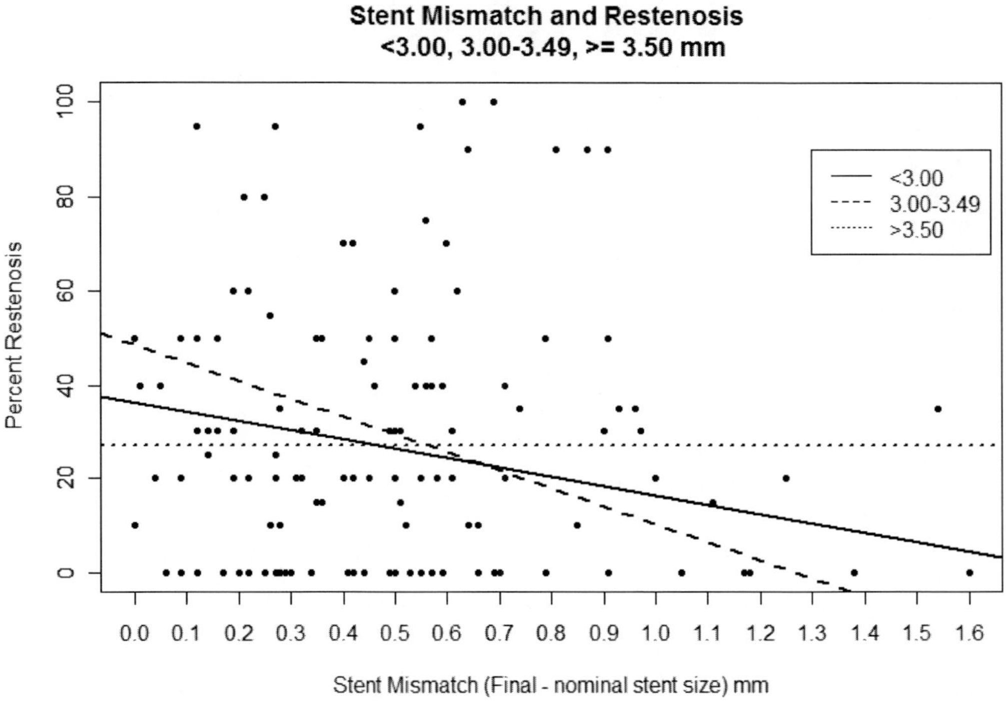

Figure 6. Stent mismatch vs. restenosis stratified by final stent size.

No correlation was seen between restenosis and over-expansion by >20% or >25% above nominal size. Rather there was an inverse relationship between stent over-expansion >20% and restenosis (Figure 7). Stents over-expanded by >20% were smaller (2.87 v 3.19 mm), longer (24 v 19 mm) and more often drug-eluting (53% v 27%,). Stents were expanded to sizes above the balloon rated burst pressure in 52% of lesions. This group did not have a higher rate of restenosis or target lesion revascularisation (TLR).

In this real-world population, the degree of mismatch (over-expansion) was significantly greater in patients *without* binary restenosis (0.41 vs 0.34 mm; P=0.049). There was no significant relationship between the degree of mismatch and TLR.

Conclusion

This chapter discusses how, in non-complex stenting, aggressive stent expansion without intravascular guidance is common and there is no signal that such aggressive stent expansion predisposes to restenosis even in small coronary arteries. Recent studies [40, 42] have confirmed the clinical validity of the synergistic strategy of visual angiographic assessment coupled with reference to manufacturers' compliance charts as a guide – a popular approach that previously lacked an evidence base.

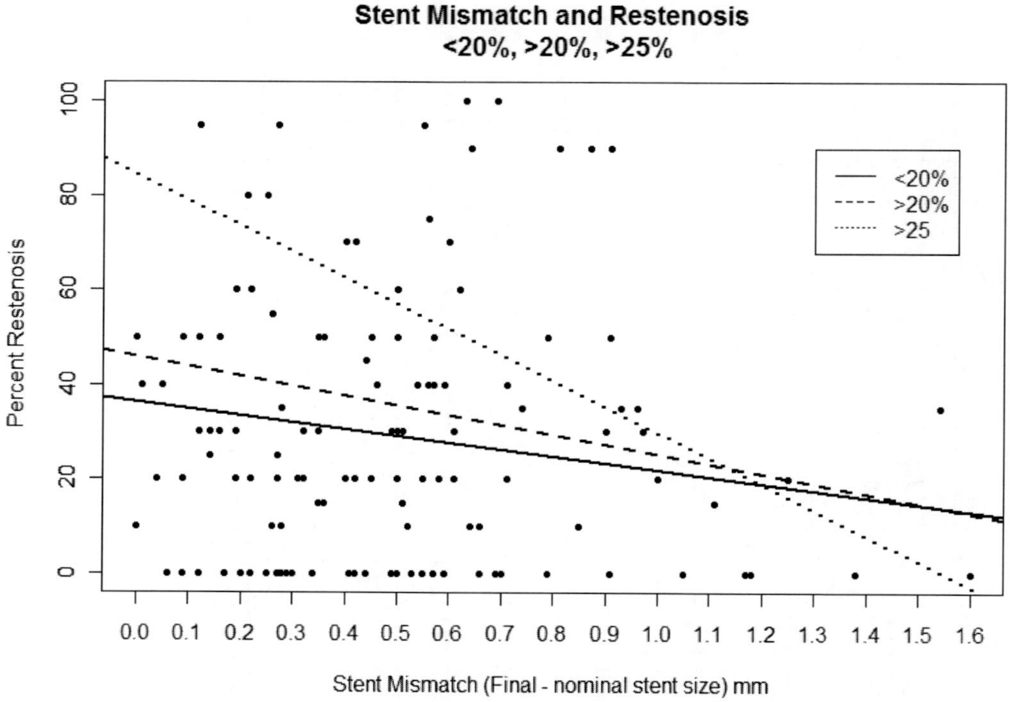

Figure 7. Stent mismatch vs restenosis stratified by percent over-expansion above nominal stent size.

References

[1] Russo RJ, Silva PD, Teirstein PS, Attubato MJ, Davidson CJ, DeFranco AC, et al. A randomized controlled trial of angiography versus intravascular ultrasound-directed bare-metal coronary stent placement (the AVID Trial). *Circ. Cardiovasc. Interv.* 2009 Apr;2(2):113-23.

[2] Choi JW, Goodreau LM, Davidson CJ. Resource utilization and clinical outcomes of coronary stenting: a comparison of intravascular ultrasound and angiographical guided stent implantation. *Am. Heart J.* 2001 Jul;142(1):112-8.

[3] Schiele F, Meneveau N, Vuillemenot A, Zhang DD, Gupta S, Mercier M, et al. Impact of intravascular ultrasound guidance in stent deployment on 6-month restenosis rate: a multicenter, randomized study comparing two strategies--with and without intravascular ultrasound guidance. RESIST Study Group. REStenosis after Ivus guided STenting. *J. Am. Coll. Cardiol.* 1998 Aug;32(2):320-8.

[4] Moussa I, Moses J, Di Mario C, Albiero R, De Gregorio J, Adamian M, et al. Does the specific intravascular ultrasound criterion used to optimize stent expansion have an impact on the probability of stent restenosis? *Am. J. Cardiol.* 1999 Apr 1;83(7):1012-7.

[5] Brodie BR. Adjunctive balloon postdilatation after stent deployment: is it still necessary with drug-eluting stents? *J. Interv. Cardiol.* 2006 Feb;19(1):43-50.

[6] Oemrawsingh PV, Mintz GS, Schalij MJ, Zwinderman AH, Jukema JW, van der Wall EE. Intravascular ultrasound guidance improves angiographic and clinical outcome of stent implantation for long coronary artery stenoses: final results of a randomized comparison with angiographic guidance (TULIP Study). *Circulation.* 2003 Jan 7;107(1):62-7.

[7] Brodie BR, Cooper C, Jones M, Fitzgerald P, Cummins F. Is adjunctive balloon postdilatation necessary after coronary stent deployment? Final results from the POSTIT trial. *Catheter Cardiovasc. Interv.* 2003 Jun;59(2):184-92.

[8] Frey AW, Hodgson JM, Muller C, Bestehorn HP, Roskamm H. Ultrasound-guided strategy for provisional stenting with focal balloon combination catheter: results from the randomized Strategy for Intracoronary Ultrasound-guided PTCA and Stenting (SIPS) trial. *Circulation.* 2000 Nov 14;102(20):2497-502.

[9] Cook S, Wenaweser P, Togni M, Billinger M, Morger C, Seiler C, et al. Incomplete stent apposition and very late stent thrombosis after drug-eluting stent implantation. *Circulation.* 2007 May 8;115(18):2426-34.

[10] Gao Z, Yang YJ, Xu B, Chen JL, Qiao SB, Yao M, et al. Is adjunctive balloon postdilatation necessary with drug-eluting stents? One center experience in Chinese patients. *Chin. Med. J.* (Engl). 2008 Mar 20;121(6):513-7.

[11] Haldis TA, Fenster B, Gavlick K, Singh KD, Iliadis E, Blankenship JC. The angiographic step-up and step-down: a surrogate for optimal stent expansion by intravascular ultrasound. *J. Invasive Cardiol.* 2007 Mar;19(3):101-5.

[12] Johansson B, Allared M, Borgencrantz B, Brorson L, Geijer H, Kellerth T, et al. Standardized angiographically guided over-dilatation of stents using high pressure technique optimize results without increasing risks. *J. Invasive Cardiol.* 2002 May;14(5):221-6.

[13] Baim DS. Percutaneous Balloon Angioplasty and General Coronary Intervention In: Baim DS, editor. Cardiac Catherterization, Angiography and Intervention. 7th ed: Lippincott Williams & Wilkins; 2006. p. 433-66.

[14] Alegria J, Holmes, DR Jr. History of Coronary Balloon Angioplasty and Current Indications. In: Topol E, Teirstein, PS, editor. *Textbook of Interventional Cardiology.* 6th ed: Elsevier; 2012. p. 203-8.

[15] Kuntz RE, Safian RD, Carrozza JP, Fishman RF, Mansour M, Baim DS. The importance of acute luminal diameter in determining restenosis after coronary atherectomy or stenting. *Circulation.* 1992 Dec;86(6):1827-35.

[16] Nichols AB, Smith R, Berke AD, Shlofmitz RA, Powers ER. Importance of balloon size in coronary angioplasty. *J. Am. Coll Cardiol.* 1989 Apr;13(5):1094-100.

[17] Roubin GS, Douglas JS, Jr., King SB, 3rd, Lin SF, Hutchison N, Thomas RG, et al. Influence of balloon size on initial success, acute complications, and restenosis after percutaneous transluminal coronary angioplasty. A prospective randomized study. *Circulation.* 1988 Sep;78(3):557-65.

[18] Nakamura S, Colombo A, Gaglione A, Almagor Y, Goldberg SL, Maiello L, et al. Intracoronary ultrasound observations during stent implantation. *Circulation.* 1994 May;89(5):2026-34.

[19] Colombo A, Hall P, Nakamura S, Almagor Y, Maiello L, Martini G, et al. Intracoronary stenting without anticoagulation accomplished with intravascular ultrasound guidance. *Circulation.* 1995 Mar 15;91(6):1676-88.

[20] de Jaegere P, Mudra H, Figulla H, Almagor Y, Doucet S, Penn I, et al. Intravascular ultrasound-guided optimized stent deployment. Immediate and 6 months clinical and angiographic results from the Multicenter Ultrasound Stenting in Coronaries Study (MUSIC Study). *Eur. Heart J.* 1998 Aug;19(8):1214-23.

[21] de Feyter PJ, Kay P, Disco C, Serruys PW. Reference chart derived from post-stent-implantation intravascular ultrasound predictors of 6-month expected restenosis on quantitative coronary angiography. *Circulation.* 1999 Oct 26;100(17):1777-83.

[22] Rogacka R, Latib A, Colombo A. IVUS-Guided Stent Implantation to Improve Outcome: A Promise Waiting to be Fulfilled. Curr Cardiol Rev. 2009 May;5(2):78-86.

[23] Chieffo A, Latib A, Caussin C, Presbitero P, Galli S, Menozzi A, et al. A prospective, randomized trial of intravascular-ultrasound guided compared to angiography guided stent implantation in complex coronary lesions: the AVIO trial. *Am. Heart J.* 2013 Jan;165(1):65-72.

[24] Lotfi A, Jeremias A, Fearon WF, Feldman MD, Mehran R, Messenger JC, et al. Expert consensus statement on the use of fractional flow reserve, intravascular ultrasound, and optical coherence tomography: A consensus statement of the society of cardiovascular angiography and interventions. *Catheter Cardiovasc. Interv.* 2013 Oct 6.

[25] Stone GW, Hodgson JM, St Goar FG, Frey A, Mudra H, Sheehan H, et al. Improved procedural results of coronary angioplasty with intravascular ultrasound-guided balloon sizing: the CLOUT Pilot Trial. Clinical Outcomes With Ultrasound Trial (CLOUT) Investigators. *Circulation.* 1997 Apr 15;95(8):2044-52.

[26] Fitzgerald PJ, Oshima A, Hayase M, Metz JA, Bailey SR, Baim DS, et al. Final results of the Can Routine Ultrasound Influence Stent Expansion (CRUISE) study. *Circulation.* 2000 Aug 1;102(5):523-30.

[27] Mudra H, di Mario C, de Jaegere P, Figulla HR, Macaya C, Zahn R, et al. Randomized comparison of coronary stent implantation under ultrasound or angiographic guidance to reduce stent restenosis (OPTICUS Study). *Circulation.* 2001 Sep 18;104(12):1343-9.

[28] Schiele F, Meneveau N, Gilard M, Boschat J, Commeau P, Ming LP, et al. Intravascular ultrasound-guided balloon angioplasty compared with stent: immediate and 6-month results of the multicenter, randomized Balloon Equivalent to Stent Study (BEST). *Circulation.* 2003 Feb 4;107(4):545-51.

[29] Weintraub WS. The pathophysiology and burden of restenosis. *Am. J. Cardiol.* 2007 Sep 3;100(5A):3K-9K.

[30] Venkitachalam L, Kip KE, Selzer F, Wilensky RL, Slater J, Mulukutla SR, et al. Twenty-year evolution of percutaneous coronary intervention and its impact on clinical outcomes: a report from the National Heart, Lung, and Blood Institute-sponsored, multicenter 1985-1986 PTCA and 1997-2006 Dynamic Registries. *Circ. Cardiovasc. Interv.* 2009 Feb;2(1):6-13.

[31] Croce K, Costa, MA, Simon, DI. Restenosis. In: Topol E, Teirstein, PS, editor. Textbook of Interventional Cardiology. 6th ed: *Elsevier*; 2012. p. 421-31.

[32] Eng M, Moses, JW, Teirstein, PS. Complications of Percutaneous Coronary Intervention. In: Topol E, Teirstein, PS, editor. *Textbook of Interventional Cardiology.* 6*th* ed: Elsevier; 2012. p. 357-71.

[33] Hehrlein C, DeVries JJ, Wood TA, Haller SD, Arab A, Kloostra AC, et al. Overestimation of stent delivery balloon diameters by manufacturers' compliance tables: a quantitative coronary analysis of Duet and NIR stent implantation. *Catheter Cardiovasc. Interv.* 2001 Aug;53(4):474-8; discussion 9.

[34] de Ribamar Costa J, Jr., Mintz GS, Carlier SG, Costa RA, Fujii K, Sano K, et al. Intravascular ultrasonic assessment of stent diameters derived from manufacturer's compliance charts. *Am. J. Cardiol.* 2005 Jul 1;96(1):74-8.

[35] de Ribamar Costa J, Jr., Mintz GS, Carlier SG, Fujii K, Sano K, Kimura M, et al. Intravascular ultrasound assessment of drug-eluting stent expansion. *Am. Heart J.* 2007 Feb;153(2):297-303.

[36] More RS, Brack MJ, Gershlick AH. Angioplasty balloon compliance: can in vivo size be predicted from in vitro pressure profile measurements? *Clin. Cardiol.* 1996 May;19(5):393-7.

[37] Hjemdahl-Monsen CE, Ambrose JA, Borrico S, Cohen M, Sherman W, Alexopoulos D, et al. Angiographic patterns of balloon inflation during percutaneous transluminal coronary angioplasty: role of pressure-diameter curves in studying distensibility and elasticity of the stenotic lesion and the mechanism of dilation. *J. Am. Coll. Cardiol.* 1990 Sep;16(3):569-75.

[38] Hermans WR, Rensing BJ, Strauss BH, Serruys PW. Methodological problems related to the quantitative assessment of stretch, elastic recoil, and balloon-artery ratio. *Cathet. Cardiovasc. Diagn.* 1992 Mar;25(3):174-85.

[39] Gerber RT, Latib A, Ielasi A, Cosgrave J, Qasim A, Airoldi F, et al. Defining a new standard for IVUS optimized drug eluting stent implantation: the PRAVIO study. *Catheter Cardiovasc. Interv.* 2009 Aug 1;74(2):348-56.

[40] Chacko Y, Haladyn JK, Smith D, Lim R. Compliance charts to guide non-complex small artery stenting: validation by quantitative coronary angiography. *Heart Asia.* 2013;5(1):76-9.

[41] Berry C, L'Allier PL, Gregoire J, Lesperance J, Levesque S, Ibrahim R, et al. Comparison of intravascular ultrasound and quantitative coronary angiography for the assessment of coronary artery disease progression. *Circulation.* 2007 Apr 10;115(14):1851-7.

[42] Chacko Y, Chan R, Haladyn JK, Lim R, Overaggresive stent expansion without intravascular imaging: impact on restenosis. *Heart Asia* 2014; 6 (1):32-35.

Part II. Diagnosis of Restenosis – Need Something Here on Angiographic Definition and Their Diagnosis

In: Coronary Artery Restenosis
Editor: Amir S. Lotfi

ISBN: 978-1-63321-346-3

Chapter 7

Physiological Assessment of Coronary Restenosis

Mauro Echavarría-Pinto, MD,[1] Tim P. van de Hoef, MD[1,2] and Javier Escaned, MD, PhD[1,*]
[1]Cardiovascular Institute, Hospital Clínico San Carlos and Centro Nacional de Investigaciones Cardiovasculares Carlos III (CNIC), Madrid, Spain;
[2]AMC Heart Centre, Academic Medical Centre, University of Amsterdam, Amsterdam, The Netherlands

Abstract

The limitation of coronary angiography to assess the functional significance of coronary restenosis has been well recognized. Therefore, the decision to proceed with repeat intervention is usually based on angiographic findings rather than using physiological measurements. With the potential of procedural complications, both short and long term, it is essential to have objective evidence of myocardial ischemia prior proceeding with repeat intervention. In this chapter the potential of physiological assessment of coronary artery restenosis is discussed.

Introduction

Over the last decades an important body of evidence has been gathered on the relevance of physiological assessment of ischemic heart disease [1, 2]. Randomized and non-randomized trials have consistently shown that most of the benefit of mechanical strategies targeting myocardial flow restoration - i.e., surgical or percutaneous coronary revascularisation-- is confined to the treatment of those coronary stenosis associated with

* Corresponding Author: Dr. Javier Escaned MD PhD, Cardiovascular Institute, Hospital Clínico San Carlos and Centro Nacional de Investigaciones Cardiovasculares Carlos III (CNIC), Madrid, Spain. Email: escaned@secardiologia.es.

objective signs of significant myocardial ischemia in downstream area [3, 4]. In this regard, intracoronary physiology techniques have become powerful diagnostic and adjuvant tools to establish the hemodynamic relevance of epicardial stenoses, and have been pivotal in promoting ischemia-driven coronary revascularization [5]. These notions are of utmost importance when investigating coronary restenosis (ISR), as the risk and benefit ratio of further interventions in this particular scenario is already influenced by the presence of the latter entity. In the following paragraphs, we firstly describe the hemodynamic consequences of coronary stenosis; then briefly discuss the concept of fractional flow reserve (FFR), and finally we outline the contributions of intracoronary physiology to the ISR field.

Physiological Consequences of An epicardial Stenosis

The anatomical impediment to flow imposed by an epicardial stenosis (including ISR) is determined by the stenosis geometry and the magnitude of trans-stenotic flow; which is governed by the amount of functional myocardium supplied by the epicardial vessel [5]. Physiologically, epicardial stenosis generate pressure drops; that are the sum of pressure losses due to viscous friction (when blood passes through the stenosis) and to flow separation (due to transformation of normal flow first to high velocity flow in the stenosis and then to turbulent non-laminar flow that eddies at the exit throat) [6, 7]. It has been established that this complex interaction can be expressed in the form of aquadratic equation as follows: $\Delta P = fQ + sQ^2$; where ΔP is the trans-stenotic pressure drop, $Q$is flow, and the constants f and s (which are functions of stenoses geometry) represent for pressure losses due to the viscous friction and to passive expansion (flow separation), respectively [8]. Ultimately, if the total trans-stenotic pressure drop is significant, distal perfusion pressure will be limited, and therefore flow to distal myocardium.

Fractional Flow Reserve as the Most Widely Used Index to Assess the Ischemic Potential of an Epicardial Stenosis

Several indices for the assessment of stenoses severity based on intracoronary measurements of pressure, flow, or both, have been proposed [9-12]. Many of them have clinically important limitations. In this regard, FFR has become accepted as the technique of choice because of its accuracy and relatively easiness to perform and interpret [1, 9]. In order to understand the theoretical framework of FFR, it is important to recognize some key aspects of the coronary pressure-flow relationship (*figure 1*). First of all, at rest, the relationship between pressure and flow in the coronary arteries is non-lineal and its characteristics vary with the metabolic status of the heart. Second, during coronary hyperemia (which occurs as a response to intense metabolic myocardial demand or to the administration of vasodilator agents) resistance is minimised and the relation between coronary pressure and flow is assumed to be linear [9] (full detail is beyond the scope of this chapter and the interested reader is referred to specialized literature [5]). This linear relation is the cornerstone for obtaining information on coronary flow from coronary pressure measurements. FFR calculation requires two pressures: the aortic pressure (P_a) and the pressure distal to an interrogated stenosis (P_d). Since the pressure flow relationship is assumed linear a thyperemia, the ratio of pressures P_d/P_a is proportional to the ratio of flows.

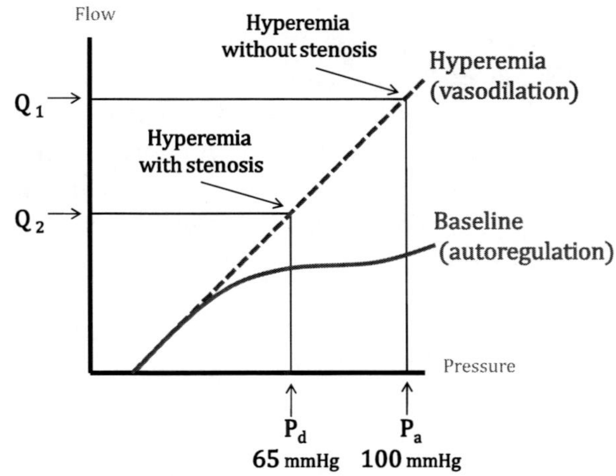

$$\frac{Q_2}{Q_1} \cong \frac{P_d}{P_a} = \frac{65}{100} = FFR = 0.65$$

Figure 1. Conceptual plot of the relationship between intracoronary pressure and flow at baseline and hyperemia in the presence and absence of a significant stenosis. Please note how at baseline (blue line) the relationship between pressure and flow is non-lineal and its characteristics vary with the metabolic status of the heart. Then, at coronary hyperemia (red line) resistance is minimised and the relation between coronary pressure and flow becomes linear. In the absence of epicardial stenosis (red line at Q_1), the driving pressure (P_a) determines a normal (100%) maximal myocardial blood flow (Q_1). In the presence of a stenosis responsible for a hyperaemic pressure gradient of 35 mm Hg (red line at Q_2), the driving pressure will no longer be 100 mm Hg but instead will be 65 mm Hg (P_d). FFR is derived from this pressures ratio (P_d/P_a) and is defined as the ratio of maximal flow in a stenotic artery to the flow in the same artery in the theoretic absence of the stenosis. In this example, an FFR of 0.65impliesthat the stenosis causes a 35% impairment in blood supply.

Consequently, pressure can be used as a surrogate of flow. FFR is simply derived from this pressures ratio (P_d/P_a) and is defined as the ratio of maximal flow in a stenotic artery to the flow in the same artery in the theoretic absence of the stenosis. For example, an FFR of 0.65means that the myocardium in the area of distribution of the interrogated vessel receives only 65% of the expected flow in the absence of that stenosis; or, conversely, that the stenosis causes a 35% impairment in blood supply. Since coronary pressure is transmitted without significant losses throughout the bifurcations of the coronary tree, the highest possible value of FFR is 1.0, being the latter the normal one in every patient and every vessel. FFR has a narrow ischemic threshold of 0.75-0.80, below which the potential for significant inducible ischemia is very high, and above which it is very unlikely [13]. Moreover, FFR informs about the expected gain in myocardial flow should the epicardial stenosis be relieved. This theoretical background is strongly supported by many observational studies as well as by three clinical decision-making, landmark randomised trials [14]. First, the DEFER trial (Deferral of Percutaneous Coronary Intervention) demonstrated that the annual rate of myocardial infarction and death due to epicardial stenoses with associated FFR values in the non-ischemic range ($\geq$0.75) was very low (<1%) and not decreased by stenting [15]. Second, the FAME trial (Fractional Flow Reserve versus Angiography for Guiding PCI in Patients with Multivessel Coronary Artery Disease) showed that a tailored revascularization approach based in FFR (using 0.80 as revascularization threshold) resulted in better clinical outcomes and reduced costs, as compared to angiographic guidance [3]. Finally, the FAME II trial (Fractional Flow Reserve–Guided PCI versus Medical Therapy in Stable Coronary Disease) established that in patients with stable coronary artery disease and functionally significant stenoses (using also the 0.80 threshold), FFR-guided PCI plus optimal medical treatment decreased the need for urgent revascularization, as compared with lone-optimal medical treatment [4]. Altogether, this theoretical framework and the clinical evidence—including outcomes— clearly supports FFR as the index of choice for the invasive assessment of epicardial disease [1]. In the following section we now discuss available information on the physiological assessment of ISR.

Functional Treatment of Coronary Restenosis

Deciding whether to further treat or not a particular ISR is a significant clinical problem, and its management remains a technical challenge [16]. This holds true, even in the drug eluting stent era, due to increasing numbers of patients undergoing PCI and the use of stents in more complex clinical and anatomic scenarios, resulting in an increase in absolute number of cases at a time with reduced relative rates of restenosis. Whilst in patients with typical anginal symptoms, proven ischemia and severe ISR, there is little discussion that an intervention is of probable benefit; it is not uncommon to find patients with recurrent angina and variable degrees of neointimal proliferation in control angiography. This leaves unanswered the pivotal question whether this hyperplasia or ISR is responsible for the symptoms and/or ischemia, and if the risk and benefit ratio of further interventions is satisfactory; since a repeat intervention in this context has a higher risk of triggering a restenotic response than in de novo coronary stenoses. Moreover, the latter decision is additionally complicated by the heterogeneous amount of functional myocardial mass being jeopardized. As the ratio of percutaneous coronary interventions (PCI) due to acute coronary syndromes over stable symptoms keeps increasing, the proportion of contemporary ISR arising from vessels supplying infarcted territories can be expected to be growing [17]. In this scenario, the functional myocardial mass supplied by the given ISR is reduced; and so will be its ischemic potential—because less flow will suffice the metabolic demands of the reduced mass [18]. In clinical practice, this implies that even severe ISR might not lead to ischemia if proven distal functional mass is significantly reduced (figure 2). In addition to these physiological considerations, several angiographic aspects may cause difficultly in the visual assessment of stenosis severity in stented and non-stented segments. Marked radiopacity of some stent designs may interfere with QCA systems and with visual assessment; and the functional relevance of diffuse neointimal proliferation, particularly in long stents, can be also more difficult to assess than that of focal stenoses. Altogether, this highlights why visual interpretation of coronary angiograms is insufficient to depict the ischemic potential of epicardial stenoses and therefore making ISR one of the most challenging scenarios.

Several non-randomised trials have investigated the clinical value of FFR to guide ISR treatment. In the bare metal stent-era, Lopez-Palop et al., studied 65 ISR of moderate severity (40 to 70% diameter stenosis (DS) by visual assessment) using FFR for further intervention guidance, with<0.75 as the threshold for treatment [19]. This study provided two key conclusions.

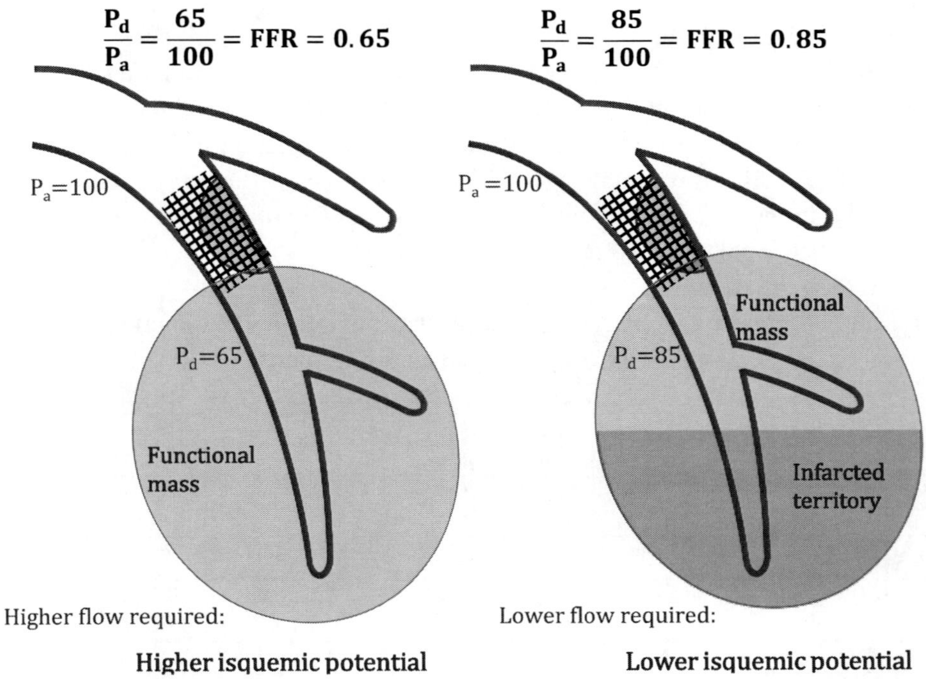

Figure 2. This figure illustrates the influence of the functional myocardial mass on the ischemic potential of an epicardial stenosis, including a ISR. In panel A, hyperaemic flow to a large normal amount of functional mass is comprised by a severe ISR. Since a large amount flow is required to cover its metabolic demands, the ischemic potential is high (FFR=0.65). Assuming that the geometry of the ISR remains identical, contrariwise, in panel B, the amount of functional myocardial mass was reduced by a chronic infarction. In this scenario, less flow will suffice the metabolic demands of the reduced functional mass and thus hyperaemic gradient will decrease as well (FFR=0.85). This figure also illustrates how the mere morphology of an ISR does not necessarily reflect its functional importance.

First, that quantitative coronary angiography (QCA) is inappropriate for assessing the physiological significance of moderate ISR, since only half of stenosis with a lumen reduction>50% were hemodynamically significant; and second, that deferral based on FFR is probably safe, as no single death or myocardial infarction related to deferred-ISR developed during the one year follow-up; and only one (2%) required further target lesion revascularization (TLR). In the same line and era, Kobori et al., investigated 155 ISR from which 113 (72.9%) were deferred based on FFR $\geq$ 0.75. At 25 ± 11 months, only 4 patients (3.5%) developed cardiac events:TVR in 1 and positive SPECTs in 3 patients [20]. Moreover, discordance between anatomical severity (defined as DS $\geq$ 50%) and functional significance (defined as FFR<0.75) was also very high (45% of the cases) under lining also the limitations of angiography to predict the functional significance of ISR. Consistent findings were additionally provided byKruger et al., that investigated 42 patients with bare metal-ISR and compared its angiographical severity (DS) with that of 57 intermediate de novo epicardial stenoses [21]. While DS was comparable in both groups (de novo, 52 ± 11%; ISR, 52 ± 9%; p=NS), FFR was lower in the ISR group (0.77 ± 0.15 vs. 0.82 ± 0.12, $p < 0.05$) and more often < 0.75 (48% vs. 26%, $p < 0.05$). Of note, none of the 22 deferred-ISR suffered an adverse event in the 6-month period of follow-up. Finally, in the drug eluting stent era, Nam et al. investigated 50 ISR lesions from 49 patients [22]. Based on FFR<0.80, 30 (60%) received additional treatment [17 (56.6%) balloon angioplasty and 13 (43.3%) repeated DES-PCI] and the remainder 20 (40%) were deferred (FFR≥0.80). This work adds to the growing evidence supporting the poor association between functional ischemia as defined by FFR and angiographic-ISR as defined by DS (%) [since a only a moderate correlation between the latters was observed (r=-0.61, p<0.01)] and further suggests that an FFR-guided strategy in patients with DES-ISR is favourable, as at 12 months of follow-up, only 2 cases (10%) of TVR developed in the deferred arm; while 7 events [one (2.3%) acute myocardial infarction and 6 (20.0%)TVR] were observed in the FFR<0.80 arm.

Table 1. Safety of percutaneous coronary intervention deferral based on fractional flow reserve for in-stent coronary restenosis

	Year of publication	*n*	*Stent*	*FFR cut-off*	*deferred-ISR*	*Follow up*	*Events*	*Event rate*
Lopez-Palop et al	2004	65	NA	<0.75	41	12 months	1 TLR	2%
Kruger et al	2005	42	BMS	<0.75	22	6 months	-	-
Kobori et al	2005	155	BMS	<0.75	113	25 months	1 TVR, 3 (+) SPECTS	3.5%
Nam et al	2011	50	DES	<0.80	20	12 months	2 TVR	10%

FFR: fractional flow reserve; BMS: bare metal stents; DES: drug eluting stents; TLR: target lesion revascularisation; TVR: target vessel revascularisation; SPECT: single photon emission computed tomography.

Important is to outline that none of the available studies have observed an acute myocardial infarction or death related to an FFR-deferred ISR. However, all applicable information on FFR-guidance in the ISR scenario comes from small, observational, non-randomized studies. Indeed, DEFER [15] excluded this entity, and although FAME I [3] and FAME II [4]allowed ISR, no accessible information on this respect has been published, thus emphasizing the need for further studies of stronger designs before definitive recommendations are made.

Can Physiology Help Identify Patients prone to Develop Post-Intervention Adverse events?

The accurate identification of patients that will develop stent failure, ISR and adverse events after successful PCI is a continuing challenge. Consequent efforts have been made, and several studies have explored the prognostic value of adjuvant intracoronary techniques to predict post-PCI events. FFR has shown to be also useful in this regard. This benefit comes from basic physiology, as normal epicardial vessels provide minimum resistance to hyperaemic flow [9]. Hence, optimal coronary stenting --that has been shown to reduce adverse events [23]-- should result in the disappearance of any hyperaemic pressure drop within the respective coronary segment. This hypothesis was explored in the BMS era by Pijls et al., in a large multicenter registry (750 patients), by relating post-stenting FFR to major adverse events [24]. At 6 months of follow-up,76 patients (10.2%) suffered at least 1 adverse event: five deaths, 19 myocardial infarctions, and 52 TVR. By multivariate analysis, post-stenting FFR was the most significant independent variable related to all types of events; and the event rate significantly increased as post-stent FFR decreased throughout the study population. As a matter of fact, the event rate rose steeply from 4.9 to 6.2 to 20.3 and finally to 29.5% as post-stent FFR decreased from >0.95, 0.90, <0.90 to <0.80, respectively. Moreover and specifically, the potential value of post-stent FFR to predict the development of ISR in both BMS and DES eras has also been explored in observational studies. Jensen et al. observed that a suboptimal post-stent FFR value was an independent predictor of binary angiographic ISR at 9 months (44.0% versus 8.1%; p<0.001) in a cohort of patients treated with BMS [25]. Similar findings in patients treated with DES were found by Nam et al., as the rate of ISR at one year was significantly higher (17.5 vs. 2.5%) in vessels with post-stent FFR ≤0.90 when compared to those that achieved a value above [26]. Whilst these studies are of limited size (< 100 patients), further evidence will soon be provided by the on going-PERSPECTIVE registry (Influence of FFR on the Clinical Outcome After Percutaneous Coronary Intervention) that aims to evaluate the influence of physiologic parameters on the clinical outcome after DES implantation [27].

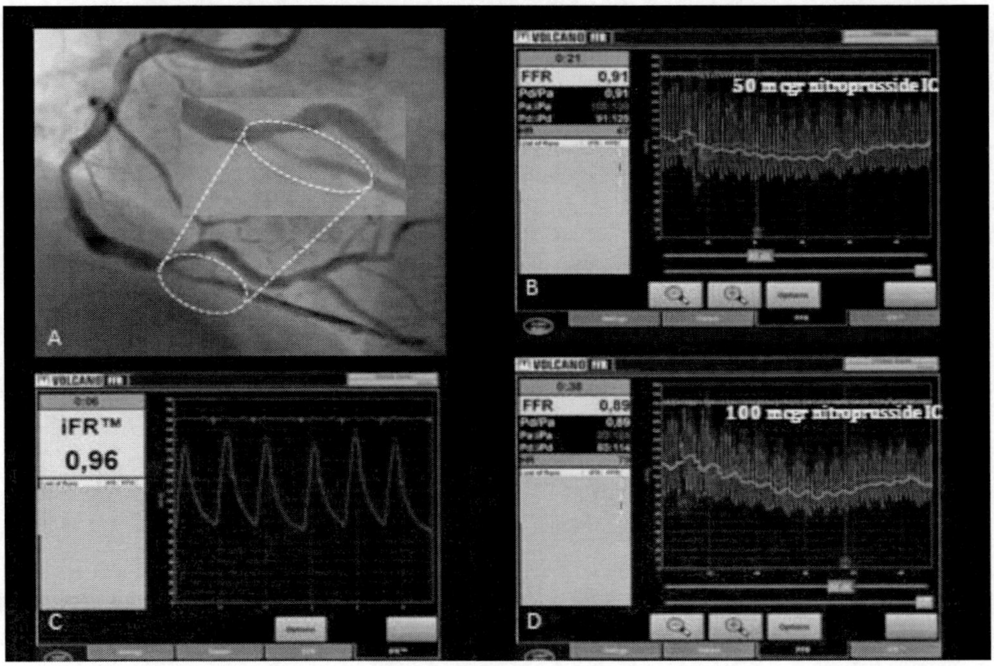

Figure 3. A 75 year-old male patient with history of severe chronic obstructive pulmonary disease was referred for cardiac catheterization because of exertional dyspnea and atypical chest pain. Three years before, a bare metal stent was implanted in the proximal posterior descending artery. New angiograms revealed mild luminal irregularities in the left anterior descending artery and circumflex (not shown) as well as a severe, diffuse-ISR (Panel A). Functional interrogation was done first, with the instantaneous wave free ratio (iFR) (panel C) followed by FFR (panels B and D). Hyperemia was induced with sequential doses of intracoronary nitroprus side. Both iFR and FFR revealed that the restenosis was not functionally significant (values above the 0.90 and 0.80 thresholds for treatment, respectively). No further interventions were performed.

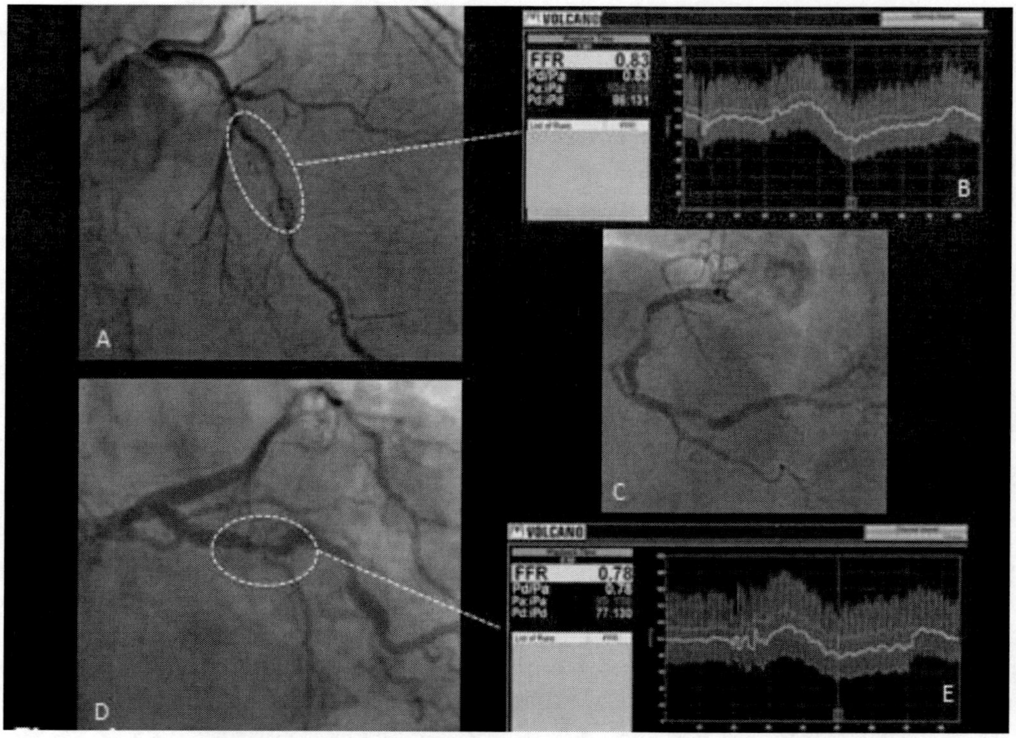

Figure 4. A 66 year-old male patient was referred for cardiac catheterization prior to kidney transplantation. He suffered an acute anterior myocardial infarction 10 years before, treated with 2 BMS in the left anterior descending (LAD) artery at primary PCI. One year later, 1 new BMS was implanted in the LAD because of late stent thrombosis. At a staged procedure, one sirolimus eluting DES was implanted in the right coronary artery. Current angiograms revealed a critical DES-ISR in the RCA with TIMI grade 2 flow (panel C), a severe de novo stenosis in the circumflex (panel D) and a diffuse, severe BMS-ISR in the LAD. FFR was performed in the LAD (panel B) and circumflex (panel E), demonstrating that only the latter was hemodynamically significant.

It is important to underscore the non-randomized design of these studies as well as the fact that whether additional intervention in the case of suboptimal FFR resulted in a decreased adverse event rate was not addressed. Put differently, whether the increase in event rates observed in cases with suboptimal post-stent FFR values was related to suboptimal PCI or to residual atherosclerotic burden within the vessel is unknown; as the post-stent FFR is also a local measurement of residual atherosclerosis; recognizing the latter entity as a systemic disease. Now, one study has evaluated prospectively the feasibility and clinical impact of targeting a post-stent FFR > 0.95, via incremental in-stent inflation pressures [28]. The FROST III investigators included 100 consecutive patients that underwent FFR measurements at baseline, after balloon predilatation, and after stenting with 4 atmospheres (atm) inflation pressure increments from 8 to 20 atmospheres (atm). Inflations were stopped when FFR increased above 0.95, and angiographic stenosis was less than 20%. FFR > 0.95 was achieved in 81% of cases; and this FFR target was reached at 8 atm in 47% of patients, 12 atm in 16 %, 16 atm in 15%, and 20 atm in 3%. Very importantly, final FFR was significantly correlated with anginal status at 6 months. While a logical conclusion from this study is that better physiological results are obtained when stents are deployed at high pressures, caution is advised when using FFR as an endpoint for treatment. This comes from the fact that focal stenosis commonly coexist with diffuse disease, and that in many cases, longer segments of the vessel (including mild segment of stenosis) might require stenting in order to optimize post-stent FFR measurements, increasing therefore the risks associated with this devices. Further studies of stronger design should rigorously address the risk and benefit ratio of including post-stent FFR as an endpoint for percutaneous treatment.

Conclusion

The percutaneous treatment of ischemic heart disease is evolving, and decision-making based on physiology-guided strategies have shown to result in better patients outcomes than angiography-guided strategies. While the treatment of patients with ISR remains a challenge and represents a major clinical problem and available evidence on the advantages of physiology-guided treatment of ISR is still limited, the benefit of physiology-guided strategies seems to expand also to this complex scenario. Further studies are still needed to accurately establish the potential benefit of physiology-guidance of ISR treatment.

References

[1] Montalescot G, Sechtem U, Achenbach S, Andreotti F, Arden C, Budaj A, Bugiardini R, Crea F, Cuisset T, Di Mario C, Ferreira JR, Gersh BJ, Gitt AK, Hulot J-S, Marx N, Opie LH, Pfisterer M, Prescott E, Ruschitzka F, Sabaté M, Senior R, Taggart DP, van der Wall EE, Vrints CJM, Zamorano JL, Baumgartner H, Bax JJ, Bueno H, Dean V, Deaton C, Erol C, Fagard R, Ferrari R, Hasdai D, Hoes AW, Kirchhof P, Knuuti J, Kolh P, Lancellotti P, Linhart A, Nihoyannopoulos P, Piepoli MF, Ponikowski P, Sirnes PA, Tamargo JL, Tendera M, Torbicki A, Wijns W, Windecker S, Valgimigli M, Claeys MJ, Donner-Banzhoff N, Frank H, Funck-Brentano C, Gaemperli O, Gonzalez-Juanatey JR, Hamilos M, Husted S, James SK, Kervinen K, Kristensen SD, Maggioni AP, Pries AR, Romeo F, Rydén L, Simoons ML, Steg PG, Timmis A, Yildirir A. 2013 ESC guidelines on the management of stable coronary artery disease: the Task Force on the management of stable coronary artery disease of the European Society of Cardiology. *Eur. Heart J.* 2013;34:2949-3003.

[2] Echavarria-Pinto M, Escaned J, Macías E, Medina M, Gonzalo N, Petraco R, Sen S, Jimenez-Quevedo P, Hernandez R, Mila R, Ibañez B, Nuñez-Gil IJ, Fernández C, Alfonso F, Bañuelos C, García E, Davies J, Fernández-Ortiz A, Macaya C. Disturbed coronary hemodynamics in vessels with intermediate stenoses evaluated with fractional flow reserve: a combined analysis of epicardial and microcirculatory involvement in ischemic heart disease. *Circulation.* 2013;128:2557-66.

[3] Tonino PAL, De Bruyne B, Pijls NHJ, Siebert U, Ikeno F, van' t Veer M, Klauss V, Manoharan G, Engstrøm T, Oldroyd KG, Ver Lee PN, MacCarthy PA, Fearon WF, FAME Study Investigators. Fractional flow reserve versus angiography for guiding percutaneous coronary intervention. *N. Engl. J. Med.* 2009;360:213-24.

[4] De Bruyne B, Pijls NHJ, Kalesan B, Barbato E, Tonino PAL, Piroth Z, Jagic N, Möbius-Winkler S, Mobius-Winckler S, Rioufol G, Witt N, Kala P, MacCarthy P,

Engström T, Oldroyd KG, Mavromatis K, Manoharan G, Verlee P, Frobert O, Curzen N, Johnson JB, Jüni P, Fearon WF, FAME 2 Trial Investigators. Fractional flow reserve-guided PCI versus medical therapy in stable coronary disease. *N. Engl. J. Med.* 2012;367:991-1001.

[5] van de Hoef TP, Meuwissen M, Escaned J, Davies JE, Siebes M, Spaan JAE, Piek JJ. Fractional flow reserve as a surrogate for inducible myocardial ischaemia. *Nat. Rev. Cardiol.* 2013;10:682.

[6] van de Hoef TP, Nolte F, Rolandi MC, Piek JJ, van den Wijngaard JPHM, Spaan JAE, Siebes M. Coronary pressure-flow relations as basis for the understanding of coronary physiology. *J. Mol. Cell Cardiol.* 2012;52:786-93.

[7] Gould KL, Lipscomb K, Hamilton GW. Physiologic basis for assessing critical coronary stenosis. Instantaneous flow response and regional distribution during coronary hyperemia as measures of coronary flow reserve. *Am. J. Cardiol.* 1974;33:87-94.

[8] Gould KL. Quantification of coronary artery stenosis in vivo. *Circ. Res.* 1985;57:341-53.

[9] Pijls NH, van Son JA, Kirkeeide RL, De Bruyne B, Gould KL. Experimental basis of determining maximum coronary, myocardial, and collateral blood flow by pressure measurements for assessing functional stenosis severity before and after percutaneous transluminal coronary angioplasty. *Circulation.* 1993;87:1354-67.

[10] van de Hoef TP, Nolte F, Damman P, Delewi R, Bax M, Chamuleau SAJ, Voskuil M, Siebes M, Tijssen JGP, Spaan JAE, Piek JJ, Meuwissen M. Diagnostic accuracy of combined intracoronary pressure and flow velocity information during baseline conditions: adenosine-free assessment of functional coronary lesion severity. *Circ. Cardiovasc. Interv.* 2012;5:508-14.

[11] Sen S, Escaned J, Malik IS, Mikhail GW, Foale RA, Mila R, Tarkin J, Petraco R, Broyd C, Jabbour R, Sethi A, Baker CS, Bellamy M, Al-Bustami M, Hackett D, Khan M, Lefroy D, Parker KH, Hughes AD, Francis DP, Di Mario C, Mayet J, Davies JE. Development and validation of a new adenosine-independent index of stenosis severity from coronary wave-intensity analysis: results of the ADVISE (ADenosine Vasodilator Independent Stenosis Evaluation) study. *J. Am. Coll. Cardiol.* 2012;59:1392-402.

[12] Meuwissen M, Siebes M, Chamuleau SAJ, van Eck-Smit BLF, Koch KT, de Winter RJ, Tijssen JGP, Spaan JAE, Piek JJ. Hyperemic stenosis resistance index for evaluation of functional coronary lesion severity. *Circulation.* 2002;106:441-6.

[13] Pijls NH, De Bruyne B, Peels K, Van Der Voort PH, Bonnier HJ, Bartunek J Koolen JJ, Koolen JJ. Measurement of fractional flow reserve to assess the functional severity of coronary-artery stenoses. *N. Engl. J. Med.* 1996;334:1703-8.

[14] Echavarría-Pinto M, Escaned J. Use of fractional flow reserve in contemporary scenarios of coronary revascularization. *Minerva Med.* 2011;102:399-415.

[15] Pijls NHJ, van Schaardenburgh P, Manoharan G, Boersma E, Bech J-W, van't Veer M, Bär F, Hoorntje J, Koolen J, Wijns W, de Bruyne B. Percutaneous coronary intervention of functionally nonsignificant stenosis: 5-year follow-up of the DEFER Study. *J. Am. Coll. Cardiol.* 2007;49:2105-11.

[16] Alfonso F, Pérez-Vizcayno MJ, Cruz A, García J, Jimenez-Quevedo P, Escaned J, Hernandez R. Treatment of patients with in-stent restenosis. *Euro Intervention.* 2009;5 Suppl D:D70-8.

[17] Mohan AV, Fazel R, Huang P-H, Shen Y-C, Howard D. Changes in Geographic Variation in the Use of Percutaneous Coronary Intervention for Stable Ischemic Heart Disease After Publication of the Clinical Outcomes Utilizing Revascularization and Aggressive Drug Evaluation (COURAGE) Trial. *Circ. Cardiovasc. Qual. Outcomes.* 2013.

[18] Pijls NHJ, Sels J-WEM. Functional measurement of coronary stenosis. *J. Am. Coll. Cardiol.* 2012;59:1045-57.

[19] Lopez-Palop R, Pinar E, Lozano I, Saura D, Picó F, Valdés M. Utility of the fractional flow reserve in the evaluation of angiographically moderate in-stent restenosis. *Eur. Heart. J.* 2004;25:2040-7.

[20] Kobori Y, Tanaka N, Takazawa K, Yamashina A. Usefulness of fractional flow reserve in determining the indication of target lesion revascularization. *Catheter. Cardiovasc. Interv.* 2005;65:355-60.

[21] Krüger S, Koch K-C, Kaumanns I, Merx MW, Hanrath P, Hoffmann R. Clinical significance of fractional flow reserve for evaluation of functional lesion severity in stent restenosis and native coronary arteries. *Chest.* 2005;128:1645-9.

[22] Nam C-W, Rha S-W, Koo B-K, Doh J-H, Chung W-Y, Yoon M-H, Tahk S-J, Lee B-K, Lee J-B, Yoo K-D, Cho Y-K, Chung I-S, Hur S-H, Kim K-B, Choi CU, Oh DJ. Usefulness of coronary pressure measurement for functional evaluation of drug-eluting stent restenosis. *Am. J. Cardiol.* 2011;107:1783-6.

[23] . Zhang Y, Farooq V, Garcia-Garcia HM, Bourantas CV, Tian N, Dong S, Li M, Yang S, Serruys PW, Chen S-L. Comparison of intravascular ultrasound versus angiography-guided drug-eluting stent implantation: a meta-analysis of one randomised trial and ten observational studies involving 19,619 patients. *EuroIntervention.* 2012;8:855-65.

[24] Pijls NHJ, Klauss V, Siebert U, Powers E, Takazawa K, Fearon WF, Escaned J, Tsurumi Y, Akasaka T, Samady H, De Bruyne B, Fractional Flow Reserve (FFR) Post-Stent Registry Investigators. Coronary pressure measurement after stenting predicts adverse events at follow-up: a multicenter registry. *Circulation.* 2002;105:2950-4.

[25] Jensen LO, Thayssen P, Thuesen L, Hansen HS, Lassen JF, Kelbaek H, Junker A, Hansen KN, Boetker HE, Krusell LR, Pedersen KE. Influence of a pressure gradient distal to implanted bare-metal stent on in-stent restenosis after percutaneous coronary intervention. *Circulation.* 2007;116:2802-8.

[26] Nam C-W, Hur S-H, Cho Y-K, Park H-S, Yoon H-J, Kim H, Chung I-S, Kim Y-N, Kim K-B, Doh J-H, Koo B-K, Tahk S-J, Fearon WF. Relation of fractional flow reserve after drug-eluting stent implantation to one-year outcomes. *Am. J. Cardiol.* 2011;107:1763-7.

[27] ClinicalTrials.gov: Influence of FFR on the Clinical Outcome After Percutaneous Coronary Intervention (PERSPECTIVE). Identifier: NCT01873560. Last accessed: january 2014.

[28] Dupouy P, Gilard M, Morelle J-F, Furber A, Aptecar E, Cazaux P, Slama M, Feldman L-J, Wittenberg O, Pernès J-M, Huret B, Commeau P, Boschat J, Teiger E, Lafont A, Steg P-G, Dubois Randé J-L. Usefulness and clinical impact of a fractional flow reserve and angiographic targeted strategy for coronary artery stenting: FROST III, a multicenter prospective registry. *Euro Intervention.* 2005;1:85-92.

In: Coronary Artery Restenosis
Editor: Amir S. Lotfi
ISBN: 978-1-63321-346-3

Chapter 8

The Role of Intravascular Ultrasound in Understanding the Mechanism, Prevention and Management of Restenosis

Jaya Mallidi, MD, MHS, Ali Haider, MD and Amir S. Lotfi*, MD
Division of Cardiology, Baystate Medical Center, Springfield, MA, US

Abstract

The prevention and treatment of in-stent restenosis (ISR) even in the era of Drug Eluting Stents (DES) has been challenging because of the high recurrence rates, especially in long and complex lesions. Intravascular ultrasound (IVUS) in addition to traditional angiographic data provides more information regarding the lumen, plaque burden, vessel wall thickness and cross sectional area. This information is useful in preventing suboptimal stent deployment, under expansion, malapposition and obtaining a maximal achievable lumen diameter – all of which have been associated with increased rates of restenosis. Despite these seemingly obvious benefits, routine use of IVUS for every stent deployment is not recommended. Recent randomized controlled trials, involving both drug eluting and bare metal stents showed only a modest benefit in reducing the target vessel revascularization rates without any difference in in rates of myocardial infarction or death. The role of IVUS in the treatment of in-stent restenosis is more well defined and currently supported by the ACC / AHA PCI guidelines. IVUS helps in identifying the mechanisms of re stenosis – whether it is purely neo-intimal hyperplasia or as a result of other mechanical factors (stent under expansion, malapposition, stent fracture, edge restenosis). There are several treatment options for restenosis including balloon angioplasty, cutting / scoring balloon angioplasty, placement of another DES, brachytherapy or surgery. IVUS analysis helps in choosing an appropriate option individualized to each patient. For focal lesions (<10 mm) resulting from stent under expansion or neo intimal hyperplasia, IVUS guided high pressure

* Corresponding Author: Amir Lotfi, Division of Cardiology, Baystate Medical Center, 759 Chestnut Street, Springfield, MA – 01199. Phone: 413 794 4492, Email: amir.lotfi@bhs.org.

balloon angioplasty may be performed. For diffuse proliferative lesions (>10 mm), placement of another DES or surgery may be warranted. This article will provide a comprehensive review of the role of IVUS in understanding the mechanism, prevention and management of restenosis.

Keywords: IVUS, restenosis

Introduction

The prevention and management of in-stent restenosis (ISR) has been a long-standing challenge for interventional cardiologists. The use of drug eluting stents (DES) has helped in significantly reducing the rate of restenosis compared to bare metal stents (BMS). [1] Studies have shown the rate of restenosis among patients with non - complex lesions treated with DES is < 10%. [2, 3] However, higher rates of restenosis are observed in everyday clinical practice given the extensive use of drug eluting stents, especially in complex lesions such as long diffuse lesions, bifurcating lesions, left main lesions, small vessels, calcified lesions and vein grafts. [4-8]

Intravascular Ultrasound (IVUS) is a catheter-based technology providing a detailed, high resolution cross sectional image of the coronary arteries in vivo. [9] A single element transducer is attached to the tip of the imaging catheter. It is rotated with the help of a flexible drive shaft. It sends and receives ultrasound signals from the coronary vessel wall and creates an image from the radial scan lines. [10] It has become an invaluable adjunctive tool in optimal coronary revascularization because of it's unique ability to image both the lumen and the vessel wall simultaneously. This allows a better assessment of the reference vessel size, plaque burden and morphology. It is particularly useful in eccentric lesions to identify the degree of calcification, coronary lesion length and cross sectional area (CSA). Stents are echo reflective. They are easily seen and distinguished from the vessel wall and any tissue growth. Hence IVUS can identify the relationship of the stent struts to the vessel wall. This anatomical and structural information obtained by IVUS provides a better understanding of the mechanism of ISR. [11] This structural information is also helpful for optimal stent deployment when treating complex coronary lesions at the time of initial therapy and in management of ISR. This chapter summarizes the role of IVUS in understanding the mechanism, prevention and management of restenosis.

Role of IVUS in Understanding the Mechanism of Restenosis

Serial two dimensional and volumetric IVUS measurements done in several studies were key to our understanding of the mechanisms of restenosis. [11-16] When angiographic lumen dimensions at time of stent implantation were compared to follow up IVUS studies which showed stent under expansion, chronic stent recoil was thought to be the cause of restenosis. However, subsequent serial IVUS studies proved that the etiology of restenosis was exclusively related to neo intimal hyperplasia rather than stent recoil. [11, 17] Regardless of any predisposing mechanical or structural issues, neo intimal hyperplasia is the predominant feature responsible for in stent restenosis.

Neo Intimal Hyperplasia

Neo intimal hyperplasia (IH) as the cause for delayed restenosis was extensively studied by serial IVUS measurement in several trials, specifically among patients with bare metal stents. [11-14] In a seminal article, Hoffman et al., described serial IVUS measurements (lumen cross sectional area diameters) among 142 Palmaz – Schatz stents in 115 lesions. [11] About 2% of the lesions were found to be restenosed at a mean follow up interval of 5.4 + 3.8 months. [11] IVUS imaging showed that the smallest lumen CSA was located at the central articulation of the stent because of the combination of initial tissue prolapse at the time of implantation and subsequent accumulation of neo intimal hyperplasia. [11] Growth of neo intimal hyperplasia appeared to be greatest in segments with large plaque burden. [11]

IVUS analysis also helped in understanding the differences in neo intimal hyperplasia and vascular remodeling between bare metal and drug eluting stents. Akoi et al. did serial IVUS analysis among 161 patients enrolled in TAXUS II trial comparing the slow release and moderate release TAXUS stents with bare metal stents. [17] At 2 years, the neo intimal area was significantly suppressed in the TAXUS stent group compared to the BMS (1.49 +1.12 mm^2 in BMS Vs. 0.94+0.76 mm^2 in TAXUS, p – 0.02). This difference remained significant despite a small late increase in the IH noted in the DES group. [17] Similar late increase in neo intimal hyperplasia was also noted at 2 years based on the IVUS results in the SPIRIT II trial among patients in the Everolimus group. [18]

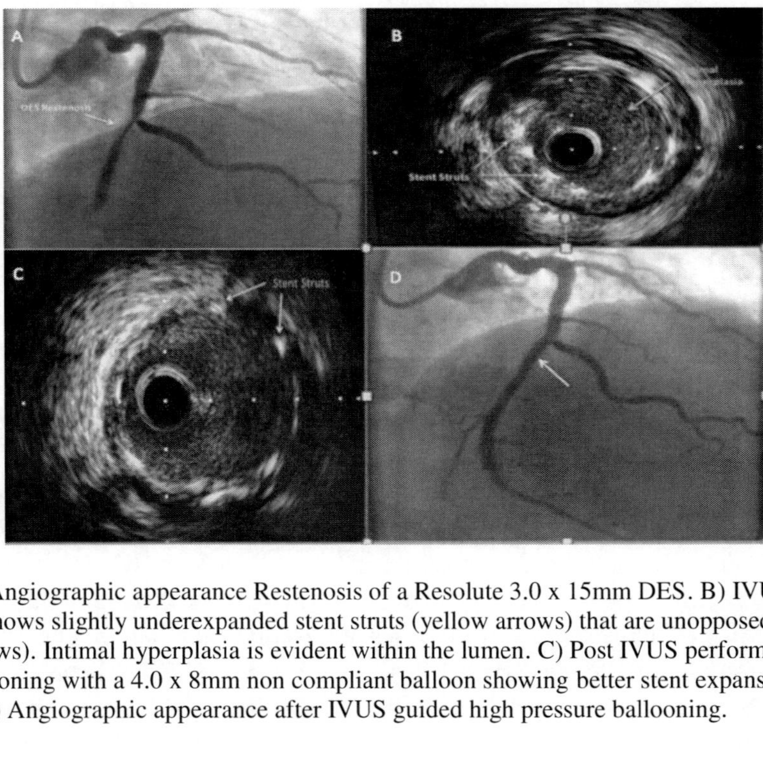

Figure 1. A) Angiographic appearance Restenosis of a Resolute 3.0 x 15mm DES. B) IVUS performed within stent shows slightly underexpanded stent struts (yellow arrows) that are unopposed to the vessel wall (red arrows). Intimal hyperplasia is evident within the lumen. C) Post IVUS performed after high pressure ballooning with a 4.0 x 8mm non compliant balloon showing better stent expansion and apposition. D) Angiographic appearance after IVUS guided high pressure ballooning.

However, this late increase did not result in increased rates of stent thrombosis or target lesion revascularization (TLR). [18] In a retrospective study done among 82 patients with DES restenosis, using an IVUS definition of a luminal narrowing less than 4 mm^2, 93% of the lesions were noted to have intimal hyperplasia. [19] This shows that restenosis in both bare metal and drug eluting stents is due to neo intimal hyperplasia. Figure 1 shows the angiographic and IVUS images of restenosis in a DES secondary to intimal hyperplasia.

Quantitative coronary angiographic measures (QCA - follow up diameter stenosis and binary restenosis) are sometimes used as surrogates for intimal hyperplasia when evaluating for restenosis during the follow up period after primary percutaneous coronary intervention (PCI). This is in contrast to IVUS where intimal hyperplasia (IH) can be visualized and directly quantified. IVUS parameters for IH include intimal hyperplasia volume, percentage of intimal hyperplasia (IH volume divided by stent volume), intimal hyperplasia area and maximum thickness of intimal hyperplasia. [19] In a meta analysis of angiographic vs. IVUS parameters in a subset of 407 patients from TAXUS IV, V and VI studies, the overall incidence of QCA binary restenosis was noted to be 14.0% (9.3% in TAXUS group vs. 19% in BMS group, $p < 0.05$). [20] QCA parameters – late lumen loss and percentage of diameter stenosis correlated only modestly with various IVUS parameters for intimal hyperplasia ($r = 0.52$). [20] None of the QCA parameters had the power to predict IVUS binary restenosis, suggesting that QCA can underestimate ISR when compared to IVUS evaluation. [20]

Mechanical Factors

Restenosis that occurs within a few months after stent deployment is primarily related to mechanical factors during the initial stent deployment, particularly with DES. These factors are usually preventable unlike unprovoked intimal hyperplasia. The stent struts are radiolucent, but highly echo sensitive. Hence, IVUS provides a direct visualization of the stent struts and helps in understanding the underlying mechanical factors that resulted in restenosis by showing the relationship of the stent struts to the vessel wall.

Stent Under Expansion

Stent under expansion is the most common mechanical factor related to restenosis. It has also been associated with stent thrombosis. [21-23] Only about 5% of the ISR lesions are secondary to mechanical complications other than stent under expansion. Studies have shown that stent under expansion is due to poor expansion during initial stent deployment, rather than chronic stent recoil. [24-25] Stent under expansion can be commonly missed angiographically. In some studies, post stent IVUS imaging has demonstrated under expansion of the stents despite an acceptable angiographic appearance. [26, 27] Stent under expansion by IVUS is evident when the stent cross sectional area (CSA) is significantly smaller than the vessel wall CSA and the reference lumen CSA. [28] In a study of 1090 patient with in-stent restenosis, by Castagna et al., 20% of the lesions were noted to have stent under expansion with CSA < 5.0 mm^2 and 38% had CSA < 6.0 mm^2. [24] In a large multicenter study called MUSIC (Multi-center ultrasound stenting in coronaries study), Jaegere et al. used minimal luminal area (MLA) in the stent > 90% of the average reference lumen area as the criteria for optimal expansion. [29] If the desired CSA is not achieved post stenting, larger balloons and higher pressure-inflations can be used to fully expand the stent.

However, this fine-tuning of the final stent dimensions is done most safely with IVUS. In the OSTI (Optimal Stent Implantation) trial, with increasing inflation pressures, IVUS demonstrated stent expansion that could not be visualized well angiographically. [30] This may be particularly relevant in lesions with dense calcifications and high plaque burden making angiography alone less sensitive in evaluating the stent.

Stent Malapposition

Stent malapposition is defined as separation of at least one of the stent struts from the vessel wall. [31] There is evidence of blood speckling between the intimal layer and the stent struts. [31] Malapposition can be extremely difficult to identify angiographically. Malapposition can happen early and could be related to initial stent implantation, or it can be delayed or acquired due to late vessel remodeling. Serial IVUS studies have identified vascular remodeling with increase in the effective membrane size (positive remodeling), without any increase in the plaque and media area, as the possible explanation for late malappostion. [32, 33] In lesions involving infarcted territories, thrombus dissolution can result in subsequent late malapposition. [31] The prognostic importance of both early and late malapposition is still controversial, particularly in the absence of stent under expansion. Among 1580 patients enrolled in the IVUS sub study of TAXUS trial (Treatment of De Novo Coronary Artery Disease using a Single Paclitaxel Eluting Stent), 6% were found to have early incomplete stent opposition on routine evaluation. [34] In this study, there was no association between early or late malapposition and long term clinical outcomes in terms of stent thrombosis, restenosis or major cardiovascular events. [34] In another recent study by Cook et al. involving 194 patients, with a mean follow up of 5 years, presence of incomplete stent apposition assessed by IVUS at 8 months after DES implantation, was associated with very late stent thrombosis and higher rates of myocardial infarction. [35] However, unlike under expansion, the real clinical impact of malapposition in terms of ISR and stent thrombosis remains debatable.

Stent Fracture

The incidence of stent fracture among DES ranges from 1- 8%. [36-39] IVUS is more likely to identify stent fractures compared to angiography. Doi et al. described stent fracture as complete or partial depending on the visibility of the stent struts on the IVUS frames. [36] In complete stent fracture, the stent is divided into greater than 2 pieces, with no visible stent struts seen in between. [36] In partial stent fracture, the struts are not visible in > 1/3rd of the stent circumference. [36] Stent fracture is associated with increased risk of restenosis and target vessel revascularization. [38, 39] In a retrospective cohort analysis of 530 patients who underwent angiography, stent fracture was identified in 10 patients, out of which 7 required repeat revascularization because of restenosis. [38] Predisposing factors for stent fracture include excessive tortuosity, longer stents, saphenous venous graft stents, overlapping stents and aneurysms. [37-39] IVUS is helpful in identify the stent fracture, possible mechanisms and also in optimal subsequent revascularization. The true incidence of stent fracture in the newer generation stents remains to be seen. Newer, more sensitive imaging modalities such as Optical Coherence Tomography (OCT) may be better at assessing this in the future.

Stent Edge Restenosis

IVUS has played an important role in our understanding of the mechanism of stent edge restenosis. Negative arterial remodeling in the proximal part and intimal hyperplasia in the distal part are associated with edge restenosis based on IVUS studies. [40] The reference segment plaque burden was noted to be the strongest predictor of edge restenosis after implantation of both bare and drug eluting stents. [41-43]

Role of IVUS in Prevention of Restenosis

Most interventional cardiologists commonly assess the success of percutaneous intervention based on visual interpretation of the angiographic images. As per the ACC / AHA guidelines 2001 for PCI, angiographic success after PCI is defined as the attainment of 30% or less of residual diameter stenosis or at least 20% improvement in diameter stenosis and relief of ischemia. [44] However, this subjective estimation is often unreliable. Several IVUS studies have shown that visual estimation or quantitative angiographic analysis of vessel dimensions is not entirely accurate. [45-48] In current clinical practice, most interventional cardiologists do not use IVUS routinely for stent deployment. It is commonly reserved for difficult and complex lesions or when angiographic appearance is unclear. This is predominantly due to the time and cost involved in using IVUS. Whether routine IVUS guided optimization of stent deployment will translate into meaningful clinical outcomes and reduce long term restenosis and revascularization rates is still controversial especially in the drug eluting stent era. The following is a brief overview of the studies done to evaluate outcomes among patients with IVUS guided stent placement, both from the BMS and DES eras.

Role of IVUS for Prevention of Restenosis in Bare Metal Stents

In the largest multicenter randomized trial to date, AVID (Angiography versus intravascular ultrasound directed bare metal coronary stent placement), 800 patients were randomized for elective stent placement either to the IVUS guided Vs. Angiographic guided stenting. [49] A 12 month significant reduction in target vessel revascularization (TVR) was noted only for vessels > 2.5 mm by angiography and for high grade stenosis. (10.1% vs. 4.3%, p - 0.01). [49] However, when the entire study population was analyzed, there was no significant difference in TVR rates between the two groups. The rates of restenosis were not mentioned in this study. [49]

In another large study multicenter trial, OPTICUS (Optimization with IVUS to reduce stent restenosis), a total of 550 patients with symptomatic coronary lesions or silent ischemia were randomized to IVUS or angiography guided BMS deployment. [50] At 6 months, a repeat angiography showed no significant differences in restenosis rates (24.5% Vs. 22.8%, p-0.68) and minimal lumen diameter (1.95 + 0.72 mm Vs. 1.91+ 0.68 mm, p=0.52). [50] At 12 months, TVR or major cardiovascular events were not reduced in the IVUS guided arm. [50]

All other randomized studies looking at the effect of IVUS guided PCI in BMS stents are small with less than 300 patients enrolled. [51-55] In the TULIP Study, 73 patients with stenosis > 20 mm were included. In this population, at 6 month follow up, the rate of restenosis was significantly lower in the IVUS guided group (23% Vs. 45%, - <0.05). [53] At 12 months, combined end points of ischemia driven TVR and myocardial infarction (MI) were significantly lower (p – 0.02). [53]

In a meta analysis of all the randomized studies, involving 2193 patients, IVUS guidance was associated with significantly larger post procedure minimal lumen diameter (mean difference of 0.12 mm, 95% CI 0.06 – 0.18 mm Hg, p <0.001), reduced 6 month angiographic restenosis (22% vs. 29%, p - 0.02), reduced revascularization rate (12% vs. 18%, p – 0.004) and reduced overall major cardiac events (19% vs. 23%, p - 0.03). [56] However, there was no significant difference between the groups in myocardial infarction or mortality. [56]

Given the controversial results from various studies and the meta-analysis, it appears that IVUS guided PCI might prevent restenosis and target vessel revascularization in bare metal stents in select group of patients with long and complex lesions by preventing stent under expansion.

Role of IVUS in Preventing Restenosis in Drug Eluting Stent Era

The data supporting the IVUS guided PCI for DES is extremely limited. Table 1 shows all the studies in DES comparing IVUS Vs. Angiographic directed PCI.

In a propensity score matched analysis of 884 patients, Roy et al. found that at 12 months, the patients who underwent IVUS guides PCI with DES had lower rates of sub acute stent thrombosis (0.7 % Vs. 2.0%, p=0.014). [57] There was no significant difference between the groups in late stent thrombosis, major cardiovascular events, myocardial infarction or death. However, statistically non-significant trend in favor of the IVUS group was seen for both target vessel revascularization and restenosis. [57] In another propensity matched observational study involving 1504 patients, at 1 year IVUS guided stenting group has significantly less major adverse cardiac events (9.1 % s 13.9%, p - 0.07) and composite end point of death and myocardial infarction (3.3% Vs. 6.5 %, p<0.01). [50] The rates of restenosis were not mentioned. [58]

IVUS guidance is helpful in complex coronary lesions such as left main stenosis and bifurcation lesions. An analysis of 975 patients with unprotected left main coronary artery stenosis from the MAIN – COMPARE registry, showed a trend towards decreased mortality in the IVUS guided group (6.0% Vs. 12.6%, p=0.06). There was no difference in the rates of myocardial infarction or target vessel revascularization. [59] In an analysis of 1668 patients from a Korean multicenter bifurcation registry, IVUS guidance compared with angiographic guidance for bifurcating lesions was associated with decreased incidence of death and myocardial infarction (3.8% Vs. 7.8%, p - 0.03) [60]

In the first randomized study conducted among 210 patients with DES at a single center, Jakabcin et al. did not find any significant difference in terms of major cardiovascular end points or stent thrombosis between IVUS guided vs. angiographically guided PCI. [61] Kim et al. noted similar findings in another recent randomized study. In this study, 543 patients with long lesions (> 28 mm) were randomly assigned to IVUS guidance or angiographic guidance. Post intervention minimal luminal diameters were similar in both the groups. At 1 year, in an intention to treat analysis there was no difference in the major cardiovascular end points between both the groups (4.5% Vs. 7.3%, p=0.16). [62] A meta analysis of one randomized study and 10 registry studies, showed IVUS guided DES implantation was associated with reduced incidence of death and stent thrombosis. The incidence of myocardial infarction and target vessel revascularization was not significantly different (Table 1). [63]

Given the paucity of data especially in randomized trials, at this time there is no compelling evidence for routine use of IVUS for DES implantations. In a sub group analysis from the randomized trial EXCELLENT, Park et al., found that adjunctive use of IVUS routinely during PCI is associated with more aggressive treatment in terms of using longer stents, larger stent diameter and increased risk of peri-procedural MI without any difference in subsequent cardiac death, myocardial infarction or target vessel revascularization. [64] However, IVUS guidance in left main lesions and bifurcations lesions may be helpful. As per the 2013 ACCF / AHA/ SCAI expert consensus statement, use of IVUS is reasonable for guidance of stent deployment for a left main lesion (Level of Evidence IIb B) and for identifying the mechanisms of stent restenosis (Level of evidence: IIa C). [65] It is not recommended for routine lesion assessment based on limited data. [65]

Table 1. Studies Comparing Angiographhic Vs. IVUS Guidance for Percutaneous Coronary Intervention with Drug Eluting Stents

Study	N (IVUS/Angio)	Death HR (95% CI)	MI HR (95% CI)	Stent thrombosis HR (95% CI)	TVR HR (95% CI)
Roy et al.	884 / 884	0.81 (0.55 – 1.20)	0.69 (0.36 -1.32)	0.59 (0.39 - 0.89)	0.95 (0.68 - 1.32)
Park et al.	145 /145	0.39 (0.15 – 1.20)	0.83 (0.43 – 1.59)	3.00 (0.12 – 76.9)	0.80 (0.35 – 1.84)
Kim et al.	308 /112	0.21 (0.06 – 0.73)	NA	0.28 (0.06 – 1.28)	NA
Jakabein et al.	105 /105	1.50 (0.15 – 15.4)	0.25 (0.02 – 3.97)	0.67 (0.15 – 3.00)	NA
Kim et al.	487 /487	0.58 (0.21 – 1.61)	0.32 (0.09 – 1.16)	0.33 (0.04 – 2.96)	NA
Claessen et al.	631 / 873	0.74 (0.37 – 1.47)	0.18 (0.06 – 0.55)	0.60 (0.10 -3.51)	0.91 (0.63 – 1.31)
Hur et al.	2765 / 1816	0.49 (0.35 – 0.69)	0.50 (0.22 – 1.12)	0.72 (0.44 – 1.17)	0.99 (0.76 – 1.28)
Ahmed et al.	1893 / 6280	0.49 (0.28 – 0.86)	1.78 (1.05 – 3.03)	NA	0.63 (0.26 – 1.53)
Park et al.	619 / 802	1.56 (0.48 – 5.09)	2.77 (1.01 – 7.59)	0.52 (0.10 – 2.68)	0.95 (0.51 – 1.77)
Chen et al	324 / 304	0.55 (0.19 – 1.57)	0.52 (0.26 – 1.03)	0.18 (0.05 – 0.01)	0.66 (0.41 – 1.06)
Overall	8161 /11808	0.59 (0.48 – 0.72)	0.81 (0.63 – 1.06)	0.58 (0.44 – 0.77)	0.90 (0.77 – 1.05)

* Abbreviations: Hazard Ratio (HR); Myocardial Infarction (MI) ; Target vessel Revascularization (TVR). Table copied with permission from Lotfi et al. (Ref 65), original data adapted from Zhang et al. (Ref 63).

IVUS Predictors of in Stent Restenosis

The ability to predict restenosis after an intervention is an ongoing challenge, mainly because of the multiple factors associated with restenosis. These include patient, lesion and procedure related factors. [66] IVUS has been instrumental in our understanding of the procedure and lesion related factors that contribute to restenosis.

The single most important predictor of restenosis is the minimum lumen diameter (MLD) achieved or the final stent Cross sectional Area (CSA). In a multicenter study - CRUISE (Can Routine Ultrasound Influence Stent Expansion), done among 525 patients with BMS, the 9 month target vessel revascularization rate was related to the final stent CSA (27% for CAS

4.0 – 5.9 mm^2; 19% for CSA 6.0- 6.9 mm^2; 12% for CSA 7.0 – 8.9 mm^2 and 4% for final stent CSA > 9mm^2). [67] In a study by Hong et al. among 550 patients with drug eluting stents, final minimum lumen area of < 5.5 cm^2 and stent length > 40mm had the highest rates of restenosis (17%) compared to all other groups. [68] In an IVUS sub-study done among 464 patients enrolled in the HORIZONS AMI, Choi et al. showed that the minimum stent area was an independent predictor of re stenosis after PCI in patients with STEMI. [69]

De Feyter et al., developed a reference chart for predicting restenosis based on a multivariable logistic regression model using the data from 3 registries and 2 randomized trials. [70] The minimum stent CSA and the stent length were the strongest predictors of in stent restenosis. [70] The highest rates of restenosis were found among the lesions with longest stents and smallest CSA. Given this interaction between CSA and lesion length, IVUS can be helpful in long lesions for obtaining the maximum lumen diameter. [70] This is also supported by the results from TULIP study which showed significantly better 12 month angiographic and clinical outcomes in the IVUS guided stent deployment group among patients with long (> 20mm) stenosis. [53]

Another IVUS predictor of restenosis is the plaque burden. While some studies showed that distribution of pre intervention plaque burden was related to restenosis, other studies showed that residual plaque burden rather than pre intervention plaque burden correlated with neo intimal hyperplasia and restenosis. [71, 72] In a recent study by Kang et al., in a cohort of 1668 reference segments with new generation drug eluting stents, 2.8% had edge restenosis at 9 months. [43] Edge restenosis is predicted by post stenting reference plaque burden, residual plaque eccentricity and stent edge asymmetry. [43, 73]

IVUS Criteria for Optimal Stent Deployment

There are no definitive guidelines on the IVUS parameters that determine optimal stent deployment. In routine clinical practice when IVUS is used during PCI, optimization is left to the discretion of the operator. The optimization is aimed at reducing the IVUS related predictors of restenosis and adverse events, i.e., avoiding stent under expansion by maximizing the minimal luminal area, incomplete stent apposition, edge dissection and lesion under coverage. [74]

Though there are no specific guidelines, various studies have suggested and used different IVUS criteria for optimization. In the first large multicenter study, MUSIC (Multicenter Ultrasound stenting in coronaries study) defined optimal stent deployment as complete apposition and symmetric expansion of the stent, in-stent minimal lumen area of >90% of the average reference lumen area or > 100% of lumen area of the reference segment with the lowest lumen area. [29] AVID (Angiographic versus IVUS direct stent placement) is another larger randomized multicenter study that used the following IVUS criteria: the smallest Cross sectional area should be > 90% of the distal reference vessel lumen cross sectional area and full apposition of the stent to the vessel wall without dissections. [49]

Among studies done in the DES era, in the HOME DES study, optimal stent deployment criteria were defined as good apposition, optimal stent expansion with minimal stent area of 5 mm^2 or a CSA > 90% of the distal reference lumen for small vessel and no edge dissection. [61] In a serial IVUS analysis from the SIRIUS trial, the optimal threshold to for minimum stent area (MSA) to prevent in stent restenosis was 5 mm^2 for Sirolimus stents and 6.5 mm^2 for BMS. [75] Adequate stent patency at follow up was defined as MSA > 4 cm^2. [75] Post stent deployment, if the desired MSA is not achieved, additional high pressure inflations with larger balloons can be performed with IVUS guidance. [76] Though there are no specific recommendations, a suggested ideal end point is a be a well expanded stent with complete vessel wall apposition with no plaque prolapse or edge dissections. [76]

Role of IVUS in Treatment of in Stent Restenosis

Every in stent restenosis does not require treatment. The role of IVUS in the decision whether to intervene on an "intermediate" lesion is poorly defined. In a study by Nishioka et al. involving 150 intermediate in stent restenosis lesions (angiographic diameter of 45 – 75%), at 6 months repeat intervention was deferred if the CSA > 3.5 mm^2 regardless of symptoms and non invasive testing. [77] At 2 years the event free survival rate was 96.5%. [77] In another sub study of 635 patients enrolled in TAXUS IV, V and VI trials, Doi et al., observed that at 9 months a MLA > 4 mm^2 predicted a TLR free survival up to 3 years. [78] The ability to predict TLR when MLA < 4 mm^2 is low. [78] The correlations between IVUS anatomic measurements and functional ischemic testing have so far been inconclusive. [78, 79] Hence, if the MLA is < 4 mm^2, without a clinical correlation, FFR or non invasive stress test, a decision to intervene based only IVUS derived anatomic measurements is not recommended. [80]

The optimal treatment option for restenosis is not well defined, particularly in the absence of an identifiable cause such as stent under expansion. There are a variety of treatment options (plain / cutting balloon angioplasty, repeat stenting, drug eluting balloon, vascular brachytherapy) available. IVUS is helpful in identifying the mechanism and pattern of restenosis and hence in guiding therapy. The rate of TLR even after treatment is influenced by the pattern of restenosis. In a study of 288 ISR lesions, TLR in focal, proliferative and totally occluded ISR was noted to be 19%, 50% and 83% respectively. [82]

Balloon / Cutting Balloon Angioplasty

Balloon Angioplasty was one of the first modalities used for management of restenosis. Long before the advent of DES, IVUS guided balloon angioplasty was found to be associated with reduced restenosis rates. In a randomized study of 37 lesions by Skamoto et al., IVUS guided as compared to angiography guided PCI was associated with reduced rates of restenosis (17% vs. 53%, p<0.05). [83]

Data regarding use of IVUS in cutting balloon angioplasty is extremely limited. Most of the data is from very small observational studies. [84-86] In the RESCUT trial - a multicenter randomized study of 428 patients, cutting balloon angioplasty did not reduce recurrent ISR. [87] IVUS analysis was not done in this study.

Now a days, only if there is a contraindication to DES placement, balloon / cutting angioplasty is used for BMS restenosis.

In a randomized controlled trial called RIBS II (Restenosis Intra stent Balloon Angioplasty Vs. Elective Sirolimus Stenting), done among 150 patients with ISR, use of Sirolimus eluting stent was found to be superior to balloon angioplasty in terms of achieving greater minimal lumen diameter, larger lumen volume based on IVUS volumetric analysis and decreased target vessel revascularization. [88] Balloon angioplasty is now reserved for restenosis secondary to under expanded stents and when patient has a contraindication to placement of DES.

Brachytherapy

In the early 21st century, prior to the advent of DES, there were several studies that showed vascular brachytherapy with Gamma or beta radiation to be useful in treating ISR. [89-93] IVUS analysis has been used extensively in these studies to understand the mechanisms as well as complications of intracoronary brachytherapy. IVUS analysis has showed that repeated stenting of a lesion post irradiation causes exaggerated neo intimal growth resulting in late stent thrombosis. [94] In some of these studies, IVUS was also used as a dosimetry tool. [95, 96]

Randomized controlled trials have now proven that DES for in stent stenosis from BMS is superior to brachytherapy in preventing restenosis and has significantly increased event free survival. [97, 98] Also, because of the procedural logistics, and costs involved, brachytherapy is no longer used in the treatment of in-stent restenosis for BMS.

In DES restenosis, the role of brachytherapy is not defined. There are only a few observational studies done among small populations, that reported a possible reduction in target vessel revascularization with brachytherapy compared to restenting with DES. [99. 100]

Repeat Stenting with DES

DES is currently the most common mode of treatment for both BMS and DES restenosis, particularly for the focal pattern of restensosis. [28] If the IVUS analysis reveals focal (< 10 mm) restenosis from edge restenosis, stent fracture or stent gap, DES deployment using IVUS for optimization is the preferred treatment of choice. For diffuse restenosis (>10 mm), the treatment modalities are not as well defined. [28]

In a randomized controlled trial involving a cohort of 48 patients with focal in stent restenosis, sirolimus eluting stent as compared to cutting balloon angioplasty was associated with reduced in segment restenosis rates. [101] In this study patterns of angiographic stenosis were quantitatively assessed by Mehran's classification, which was originally validated by IVUS analysis. [102] There are no randomized controlled trials in patients with restenosis, comparing IVUS guided vs. angiographic guided stent deployment. Figure 2 provides a general approach to treatment of DES based on the IVUS mechanism of restenosis.

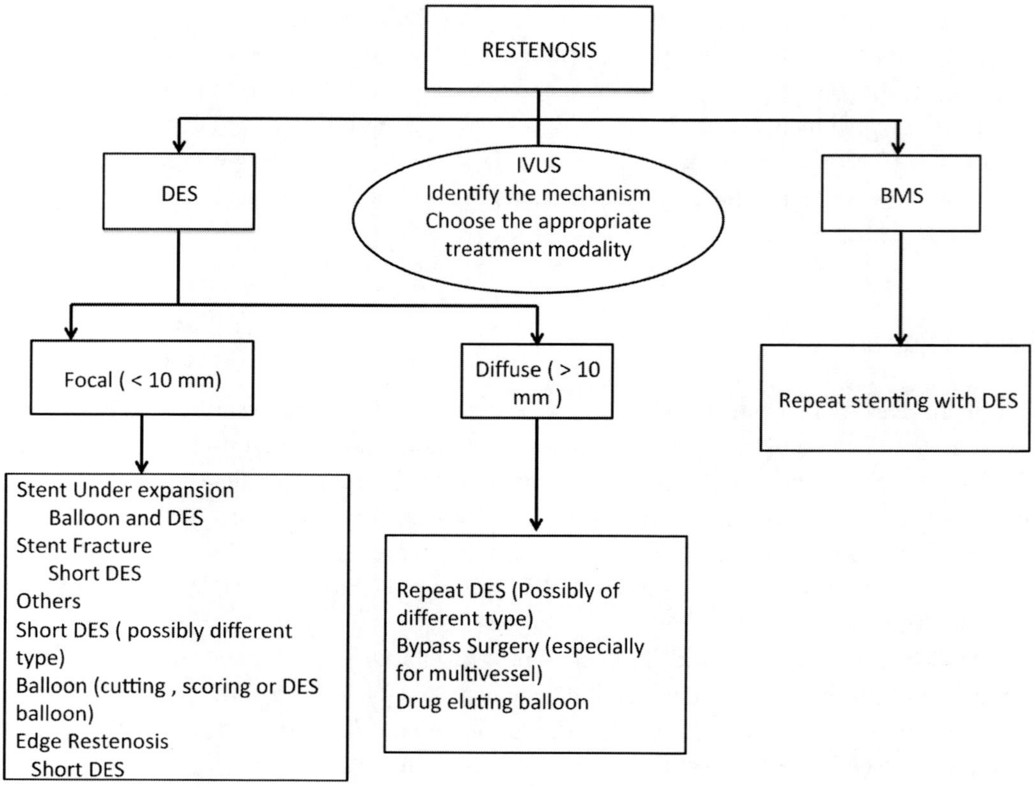

Abbreviations: IVUS (Intravascular Ultrasound); DES (Drug Eluting stent); BMS (Bare Metal Stent).
* Adapted and modified from Dangas et al. (Ref 28).

Figure 2. Algorithm for management of In-stent Restenosis.

Conclusion

In-stent restenosis and its management remains a challenging problem for interventionists, particularly in the DES era. IVUS can help elucidate a predisposing factor for in stent restenosis. It should strongly be considered as a part of the evaluation of in stent restenosis, particularly when dealing with DES, to assist with the treatment strategy. This may impact a decision to perform balloon angioplasty or repeat stenting.

Although routine IVUS for stenting is not recommended for all DES implantations, it should be considered on a case by case basis for complex lesions including left main, bifurcation lesions, and situations where under expansion is more likely such as high plaque burden and heavily calcified vessels in order to minimize future ISR due to mechanical factors.

References

[1] Stettler C, Wandel S, Allemann S, et al. Outcomes associated with drug – eluting and bare-metal stents: a collaborative network meta-analysis. *Lancet;* 2007; 370: 937 – 48.

[2] Stone GW, Ellis SG, Cox DA, et al. A polymer – based paclitaxel – eluting stent in patients with coronary artery disease. *N. Engl. J. Med.* 2004; 350:221 – 231.

[3] Stone GW, Ellis SG, Cannon L, et al. Comparison of a polymer based paclitaxel – eluting stent with a bare metal stent in patient with complex coronary artery disease. *JAMA;* 2005; 294: 1215 – 1223.

[4] Kastrati A, Schomig A, Elezi S, et al. Prognostic value of the modified American College of Cardiology/American heart association stenosis morphology classification for long-term angiographic and clinical outcome after coronary stent placement. *Circulation* 1999; 100:1285–90.

[5] Kastrati A, Elezi S, Dirschinger J, Hadamitzky M, Neumann FJ, Schomig A. Influence of lesion length on restenosis after coronary stent placement. *Am. J. Cardiol.* 1999;83:1617–22.

[6] Kobayashi Y, De Gregorio J, Kobayashi N. et al. Stented segment length as an independent predictor of restenosis. *J. Am. Coll. Cardiol.* 1999;34:651–9.

[7] Reimers B, Moussa I, Akiyama T. et al. Long-term clinical follow-up after successful repeat percutaneous intervention for stent restenosis. *J. Am. Coll. Cardiol.* 1997;30:186–92.

[8] Mehran R, Dangas G, Abizaid AS et al. Angiographic patterns of in-stent restenosis: classification and implications for long-term outcome. *Circulation* 1999;100:1872–8.

[9] Klein LW, McPherson D. The diagnostic potential of intravascular ultrasound in the coronary arteries. *Cardiovasc. Rev. Rep.*1990;11:31–36.

[10] Mintz G. *Intravascular Ultrasound.* 2005; Taylor & Francis. pg 12.

[11] Hoffmann R, Mintz GS, Dussaillant GR et al. Patterns and mechanisms of in-stent restenosis. A serial intravascular ultrasound study. *Circulation.*1996;94:1247–54.

[12] Mudra H, Regar E, Klauss V et al. Serial follow-up after optimized ultrasound-guided deployment of Palmaz-Schatz stents. In-stent neointimal proliferation without significant reference segment response. *Circulation* 1997; 95:363–70.

[13] Hoffmann R, Mintz GS, Kent KM et al. Serial intravascular ultrasound predictors of restenosis at the margins of Palmaz-Schatz stents. *Am. J. Cardiol.* 1997;79:9513.

[14] Hoffmann R, Mintz GS, Pichard AD, Kent KM, Satler LF, Leon MB. Intimal hyperplasia thickness at follow-up is independent of stent size: a serial intravascular ultrasound study. *Am. J. Cardiol.* 1998;82:1168–72.

[15] Weissman NJ, Wilensky RL, Tanguay J. et al. Extent and distribution of in-stent intimal hyperplasia and edge effect in a non-radiation stent population. *Am. J. Cardiol.* 2001;88:248–52.

[16] Hoffmann R, Mintz GS, Popma JJ et al. Chronic arterial responses to stent implantation: a serial intravascular ultrasound analysis of Palmaz-Schatz stents in native coronaryarteries. *J. Am. Coll. Cardiol.* 1996;28:1134–9.

[17] Aoki J, Colombo A, Dudek, et al. Peristent remodeling and neointimal suppression 2 years after polymer-based, paclitaxel-eluting stent implantation: Insights from serial

intravascular ultrasound analysis in the TAXUS II study. *Circulation* 2005; *112*(25): 3876-3883.

[18] Claessen BE, Beijk MA, Legrand V, et al. Two-year clinical, angiographic, and intravascular ultrasound follow-up of the XIENCE V everolimus-eluting stent in the treatment of patients with de novo native coronary artery lesions: the SPIRIT II trial. *Circ. Cardiovasc. Interv.* 2009; 2:339–47.

[19] Kang SJ, Mintz GS, Park DW, et al.. Mechanisms of in-stent restenosis after drug-eluting stent implantation: Intravascular ultrasound analysis. *Cir. Cardiovas. Interv.* 2011 4(1): 9-14.

[20] Escolar E, Mintz GS, Popma J, et al. Meta-analysis of angiographic versus intravascular ultrasound parameters of drug-eluting stent efficacy (from TAXUS IV, V, and VI). *Am. J. of Cardiol.* 2007; 100(4), 621-626.

[21] Fujii K, Carlier SG, Mintz GS, et al. Stent underexpansion and residual reference segment stenosis are related to stent thrombosis after sirolimus-eluting stent implantation: An intravascular ultrasound study. *J. Am. Coll. Cardiol.* 2005; 45(7), 995-998.

[22] Uren NG, Schwarzacher SP, Metz JA, et al. Predictors and outcomes of stent thrombosis: an intravascular ultrasound registry. *Eur. Heart J.* 2002;23:124 –32.

[23] Cheneau E, Leborgne L, Mintz GS, et al. Predictors of subacute stent thrombosis: results of a systematic intravascular ultrasound study. *Circulation* 2003;108:43.

[24] Castagna MT, Mintz GS, Leiboff BO, et al. The contribution of "mechanical" problems to in-stent restenosis: An intravascular ultrasonographic analysis of 1090 consecutive in-stent restenosis lesions. *Am. Heart J.* 2001; 142(6), 970-974.

[25] Mintz GS. Features and parameters of drug-eluting stent deployment discoverable by intravascular ultrasound. *Am. J. Cardiol.* 2007;100: 26M–35M.

[26] Colombo A, Hall P, Nakamura S, et al. Intracoronary stenting without anticoagulation accomplished with intravascular ultrasound guidance. *Circulation* 1995; 91: 1676–88.

[27] Nakamura S, Colombo A, Gaglione A, et al. Intracoronary ultrasound observations during stent implantation. *Circulation* 1994; 89: 2026–34.

[28] Dangas GD, Claessen BE, Caixeta A, Sanidas EA, Mintz G. S, Mehran, R. In-stent restenosis in the drug-eluting stent era. *J. of Am. Col. of Cardiol.* 2010; 56(23): 1897-1907.

[29] de Jaegere P, Mudra H, Figulla H, et al. Intravascular ultrasoundguided optimized stent deployment. Immediate and 6 months clinical and angiographic results from the Multicenter Ultrasound Stenting in Coronaries study (MUSIC study). *Eur. Heart J.* 1998;19:1214 –23.

[30] Stone GW, St Goar FG, Hodgson JM, et al. Analysis of the relation between stent implantation pressure and expansion. optimal stent implantation (OSTI) investigators. *The Am. J. of Cardiol.* 1999; 83(9): 1397-400, A8.

[31] Mintz G. *Intravascular Ultrasound.* 2005; Taylor & Francis. pg 5062 – 63.

[32] Mintz GS, Shah VM, Weissman NJ. Regional remodeling as the cause of late stent malapposition. *Circulation* 2003; 107(21): 2660-2663.

[33] Nakamura M, Kataoka T, Honda Y, et al. Late incomplete stent apposition and focal vessel expansion after bare metal stenting. *The Am. J. of Cardiol.* 2003; 92(10), 1217-1219.

[34] Steinberg DH, Mintz GS, Mandinov L, et al. Long-term impact of routinely detected early and late incomplete stent apposition: An integrated intravascular ultrasound analysis of the TAXUS IV, V, and VI and TAXUS ATLAS workhorse, long lesion, and direct stent studies. *JACC. Cardiovascular Interventions* 2010; 3(5): 486-494.

[35] Cook S, Eshtehardi P, Kalesan B, Raber L, Wenaweser P, Togni M, et al. Impact of incomplete stent apposition on long-term clinical outcome after drug-eluting stent implantation. *Euro Heart J.* 2012; 33(11): 1334-1343.

[36] Doi H, Maehara A, Mintz GS, et al. Classification and potential mechanisms of intravascular ultrasound patterns of stent fracture. *The Am. J. of Cardiol.* 2009, 103(6): 818-823.

[37] Aoki J, Nakazawa G, Tanabe K, et al. Incidence and clinical impact of coronary stent fracture after sirolimus-eluting stent implantation. *Catheter. Cardiovasc. Interv.* 2007; 69(3): 380-386.

[38] Lee MS, Jurewitz D, Aragon J, Forrester J, Makkar RR, Kar S. Stent fracture associated with drug-eluting stents: Clinical characteristics and implications. *Catheter. Cardiovasc. Interv.* 2007; 69(3): 387-394.

[39] Okumura M, Ozaki Y, Ishii J, et al. Restenosis and stent fracture following sirolimus-eluting stent (SES) implantation. *Circulation Journal* 2007, 71(11):1669-1677.

[40] Ichimoto E, Fujimoto Y, Kubo K, et al. Mechanism of Edge Restenosis after Sirolimus – Eluting Stent Implantation. *The Journal of Invasive Cardiology*. February 2012. Vol 24, issue 2. 55- 57.

[41] Morino Y, Tamiya S, Masuda N, et al. Intravascular ultrasound criteria for determination of optimal longitudinal positioning of sirolimus-eluting stents. *Circ. J.* 2010;74:1609e1616.

[42] Liu J, Maehara A, Mintz GS, et al. An integrated TAXUS IV, V, and VI intravascular ultrasound analysis of the predictors of edge restenosis after bare metal or paclitaxel-eluting stents. *Am. J. Cardiol.* 2009;103:501e506.

[43] Kang SJ, Cho YR, Park GM, et al. Intravascular ultrasound predictors for edge restenosis after newer generation drug-eluting stent implantation. *Am. J. Cardiol.* 2013 May 15;111(10):1408-14.

[44] Smith SC Jr, Feldman TE, Hirshfeld JW Jr, et al. ACC/AHA/SCAI 2005 Guideline Update for Percutaneous Coronary Intervention- summary article: a report of the American College of Cardiology/American Heart Association Task Force on Practice Guidelines (ACC/AHA/SCAI Writing Committee to Update the 2001 Guidelines for Percutaneous Coronary Intervention). *Circulation* 2006;113:156-175.

[45] Nakamura S, Colombo A, Gaglione A, et al. Intracoronary ultrasound observations during stent implantation. *Circulation* 1994;89:2026-2034.

[46] Gorge G, Haude M, Ge J, et al. Intravascular ultrasound after low and high inflation pressure coronary artery stent implantation. *J. Am. Coll. Cardiol.* 1995;26:725-730.

[47] Mudra H, Klauss V, Blasini R, et al. Ultrasound guidance of Palmaz-Schatz intracoronary stenting with a combined intravascular ultrasound balloon catheter. *Circulation* 1994;90:1252- 1261.

[48] Brodie BR, Cooper C, Jones M, Fitzgerald P, Cummins F; Postdilatation Clinical Comparative Study (POSTIT) Investigators. Is adjunctive balloon post dilatation necessary after coronary stent deployment? Final results from the POSTIT trial. *Catheter. Cardiovasc. Interv.* 2003;59:184-192.

[49] Russo RJ, Silva PD, Teirstein PS, et al. A randomized controlled trial of angiography versus intravascular ultrasound-directed bare-metal coronary stent placement (the AVID trial). *Circ. Cardiovasc. Interv.* 2009;2:113–123.

[50] Mudra H, di Mario C, de Jaegere P, et al. Randomized comparison of coronary stent implantation under ultrasound or angiographic guidance to reduce stent restenosis (OPTICUS Study). *Circulation* 2001;104:1343–1349.

[51] Gil RJ, Pawłowski T, Dudek D, et al. Comparison of angiographically guided direct stenting technique with direct stenting and optimal balloon angioplasty guided with intravascular ultrasound: the multicenter, randomized trial results (DIPOL). *Am. Heart J.* 2007;154:669–675.

[52] Schiele F, Meneveau N, Seronde MF, et al. Medical costs of intravascular ultrasound optimization of stent deployment. Results of the multicenter randomized "REStenosis after Intravascular ultrasound Stenting" (RESIST) study. *Int. J. Cardiovasc. Interv.* 2000;3:207–213.

[53] Oemrawsingh PV, Mintz GS, Schalij MJ, Zwinderman AH, Jukema JW, van der Wall EE; TULIP Study. Thrombocyte activity evaluation and effects of Ultrasound guidance in Long Intracoronary stent placement: intravascular ultrasound guidance improves angiographic and clinical outcome of stent implantation for long coronary artery stenoses: final results of a randomized comparison with angiographic guidance (TULIP Study). *Circulation* 2003;107:62– 67.

[54] Frey AW, Hodgson JM, Müller C, Bestehorn HP, Roskamm H. Ultrasound-guided strategy for provisional stenting with focal balloon combination catheter: results from the randomized Strategy for Intracoronary Ultrasound-guided PTCA and Stenting (SIPS) trial. *Circulation* 2000;102: 2497–2502.

[55] Gaster AL, Slothuus Skjoldborg U, Larsen J, et al. Continued improvement of clinical outcome and cost effectiveness following intravascular ultrasound guided PCI: insights from a prospective, randomized study. *Heart* 2003;89:1043–1049.

[56] Parise H, Maehara A, Stone GW, Leon MB, Mintz, GS. Meta-analysis of randomized studies comparing intravascular ultrasound versus angiographic guidance of percutaneous coronary intervention in pre-drug-eluting stent era. *American J. of Cardiol.* 2011; 107(3): 374-382.

[57] Roy P, Steinberg DH, Sushinsky SJ, et al. The potential clinical utility of intravascular ultrasound guidance in patients undergoing percutaneous coronary intervention with drug-eluting stents. *Eur. Heart J.* 2008;29:1851-1857.

[58] Claessen BE, Mehran R, Mintz GS, et al. Impact of intravascular ultrasound imaging on early and late clinical outcomes following percutaneous coronary intervention with drug-eluting stents. *JACC Cardiovasc. Interv.* 2011 Sep;4(9):974-81.

[59] Park SJ, Kim YH, Park DW, et al. MAIN-COMPARE Investigators. Impact of intravascular ultrasound guidance on long-term mortality in stenting for unprotected left main coronary artery stenosis. *Circ. Cardiovasc. Interv.* 2009 Jun;2(3):167-77.

[60] Kim JS, Hong MK, Ko YG, et al. Impact of intravascular ultrasound guidance on long-term clinical outcomes in patients treated with drug-eluting stent for bifurcation lesions: data from a Korean multi-center bifurcation registry. *Am. Heart* 2011;161:180–7.

[61] Jakabcin J, Spacek R, Bystron M, et al. Long-term health outcome and mortality evaluation after invasive coronary treatment using drug eluting stents with or without

the IVUS guidance. Randomized control trial. HOME DES IVUS. *Catheter. Cardiovasc. Interv.* 2010;75:578–83.

[62] Kim JS, Kang TS, Mintz GS, et al. Randomized Comparison of Clinical Outcomes Between Intravascular Ultrasound and Angiography-Guided Drug-Eluting Stent Implantation for Long Coronary Artery Stenoses. *J. Am. Coll. Cardiol. Intv.* 2013;6:369–76.

[63] Zhang Y, Farooq V, Garcia-Garcia HM, et al. Comparison of intravascular ultrasound versus angiography-guided drug-eluting stent implantation: a meta-analysis of one randomised trial and ten observational studies involving 19,619 patients. *Euro Intervention.* 2012 Nov 22;8(7):855-65.

[64] Park KW, Kang SH, Yang HM, et al. Impact of intravascular ultrasound guidance in routine percutaneous coronary intervention for conventional lesions: data from the EXCELLENT trial. *Int. J. Cardiol.* 2013 Aug 10;167(3):721-6.

[65] Lotfi A, Jeremias A, Fearon WF, et al. Expert consensus statement on the use of fractional flow reserve, intravascular ultrasound, and optical coherence tomography: A consensus statement of the society of cardiovascular angiography and interventions. *Catheter. Cardiovasc. Interv.* 2013; Oct 6: Epub Ahead of Print.

[66] Hoffman R, Mintz GS. Coronary in-stent restenosis — predictors, treatment and Prevention. *European Heart Journal* 2000; 21: 1739–1749.

[67] Fitzgerald PJ, Oshima A, Hayase M, et al. Final results of the Can Routine Ultrasound Influence Stent Expansion (CRUISE) study. *Circulation.* 2000 Aug 1;102(5):523-30.

[68] Hong MK, Mintz GS, Lee CW, et al. Intravascular ultrasound predictors of angiographic restenosis after sirolimus-eluting stent implantation. *Eur. Heart J.* 2006 Jun;27(11):1305-10. Epub 2006 Apr 27.

[69] Choi SY, Witzenbichler B, Maehara A, et al. Intravascular ultrasound findings of early stent thrombosis after primary percutaneous intervention in acute myocardial infarction: a Harmonizing Outcomes with Revascularization and Stents in Acute Myocardial Infarction (HORIZONS-AMI) substudy. *Circ. Cardiovasc. Interv.* 2011;4:239-247.

[70] De Feyter PJ, Kay C, Disco and P. W. Serruys Reference Chart Derived From Post□Stent-Implantation Intravascular Ultrasound Predictors of 6-Month Expected Restenosis on Quantitative Coronary Angiography. *Circulation.* 1999;100:1777-178.

[71] Hoffmann R, Mintz GS, Mehran R, et al. Intravascular ultrasound predictors of angiographic restenosis in lesions treated with Palmaz-Schatz stents. *J. Am. Coll. Cardiol.* 1998; 31: 43–9.

[72] Prati F, Di Mario C, Moussa I, et al. In-stent neointimal proliferation correlates with the amount of residual plaque burden outside the stent. *Circulation* 1999; 99: 1011–14.

[73] Liu X, Doi H, Maehara A, et al. A volumetric intravascular ultrasound comparison of early drug-eluting stent thrombosis versus restenosis. *JACC Cardiovasc. Interv.* 2009;2:428–434.

[74] Yoon HJ, Hur SH. Optimization of stent deployment by intravascular ultrasound. *The Korean Journal of Internal Medicine* 2012; 27(1): 30-38.

[75] Sonoda S, Morino Y, Ako J, et al. Impact of final stent dimensions on long-term results following sirolimus-eluting stent implantation: serial intravascular ultrasound analysis from the sirius trial. *J. Am. Coll. Cardiol.* 2004;43:1959-1963.

[76] Mintz G. (2005). Intravascular Ultrasound: Taylor & Francis. Pg 3533 – 37.

[77] Nishioka H, Shimada K, Fukuda S, et al. Long- term follow up of intermediate in-stent restenosis lesions following deferral of re-intervention on the basis of intravascular ultrasound findings. *Circulation* 2003; 106:11-587.

[78] Doi H, Maehara A, Mintz GS, et al. Impact of in-stent minimal lumen area at 9 months poststent implantation on 3-year target lesion revascularization–free survival: a serial intravascular ultrasound analysis from the TAXUS IV, V, and VI trials. *Circ. Cardiovasc. Intervent.* 2008;1:111–118.

[79] Nishioka T, Amanullah AM, Luo H, et al. Clinical validation of intravascular ultrasound imaging for assessment of coronary stenosis severity. Comparison with stress myocardial perfusion imaging. *J. Am. Coll. Cardiol.* 1999;33:1870 –1878.

[80] Takagi A, Tsurumi Y, Ishii Y, Suzuki K, Kawana M, Kasanuki H. Clinical potential of intravascular ultrasound for physiological assessment of coronary stenosis: relationship between quantitative ultrasound tomography and pressure-derived fractional flow reserve. *Circulation.* 1999;100:250 –255.

[81] Bass T, Caprazano P. Managing Patients With Intermediate In-Stent Restenotic Lesions Is It "Prime Time" for Intravascular Ultrasound Imaging? *Circ. Cardiovasc. Intervent.* 2008;1:90-92.

[82] Mehran R, Dangas G, Abizaid AS et al. Angiographic patterns of in-stent restenosis: classification and implications for long-term outcome. *Circulation* 1999;100:1872–8.

[83] Sakamoto T, Kawarabayashi T, Taguchi H et al. Intravascular ultrasound-guided balloon angioplasty for treatment of in-stent restenosis. *Catheter. Cardiovasc. Interv.* 1999;47:298–303.

[84] Kinoshita Y, Matsuno Y, Ohta T. et al. Dilatation mechanism of Cutting Balloon Angioplasty for in-stent restenosis: comparison with Plain Old Balloon Angioplasty using volumetric intravascular ultrasound analysis. *Am. J. Cardiol.* 2000;(Suppl);8A.

[85] Ahmed JM, Mintz GS, Castagna M. et al. Intravascular ultrasound assessment of the mechanism of lumen enlargement during cutting balloon angioplasty treatment of in-stent restenosis. *Am. J. Cardiol.* 2001;88:1032–4.

[86] Muramatsu T, Tsukahara R, Ho M. et al. Efficacy of cutting balloon angioplasty for in-stent restenosis: an intravascular ultrasound evaluation. *J. Invasive Cardiol.* 2001; 13:439–44.

[87] Albiero R, Silber S, Di Mario C, Cernigliaro C, Battaglia S, Reimers B, Frasheri A, Klauss V, Auge JM, Rubartelli P, Morice MC, Cremonesi A, Schofer J, Bortone A, Colombo A; RESCUT Investigators. Cutting balloon versus conventional balloon angioplasty for the treatment of in-stent restenosis: results of the restenosis cutting balloon evaluation trial (RESCUT). *J. Am. Coll. Cardiol.* 2004 Mar 17;43(6):943-9.

[88] Alfonso F, Pérez-Vizcayno MJ, Hernandez R, Bethencourt A, Martí V, López-Mínguez JR, Angel J, Mantilla R, Morís C, Cequier A, Sabaté M, Escaned J, Moreno R, Bañuelos C, Suárez A, Macaya C; RIBS-II Investigators. A randomized comparison of sirolimus-eluting stent with balloon angioplasty in patients with in-stent restenosis: results of the Restenosis Intrastent: Balloon Angioplasty Versus Elective Sirolimus-Eluting Stenting (RIBS-II) trial. *J. Am. Coll. Cardiol.* 2006 Jun 6;47(11):2152-60.

[89] Mintz GS, Weissman NJ, Teirstein PS et al. Effect of intracoronary gamma-radiation therapy on in-stent restenosis: an intravascular ultrasound analysis from the gamma-1 study. *Circulation* 2000;102:2915–8.

[90] Waksman R, White RL, Chan RC et al. Intracoronary gamma radiation therapy after angioplasty inhibits recurrence in patients with in-stent restenosis. *Circulation* 2000;101: 2165–71.

[91] Ahmed JM, Mintz GS, Leiboff B, Jackson M, Harrington D, Pichard A. A serial intravascular ultrasound study to assess the efficacy of intracoronary _-radiation in preventing recurrent diffuse in-stent restenosis in long lesions. *Circulation* 2000;102:II-692.

[92] Waksman R, Bhargava B, White L et al. Intracoronary beta radiation therapy inhibits recurrence of in-stent restenosis. *Circulation* 2000;101:1895–8.

[93] Takagi A, Morino Y, Fox T. Efficacy of intracoronary -irradiation for the treatment on in-stent restenosis: volumetric analysis by intravascular ultrasound. *Circulation* 2000;102:II-422.

[94] Morino Y, Limpijankit T, Honda Y, Lansky AJ, Waksman R, Bonneau HN, Yock PG, Mintz GS, Fitzgerald PJ. Late vascular response to repeat stenting for in-stent restenosis with and without radiation: an intravascular ultrasound volumetric analysis. *Circulation*. 2002 May 28;105(21):2465-8.

[95] Arbab – Zadeh A, Bhargava V, Russo RJ, et al. Centered versus non centered source for intracoronary artery radiation therapy: a model based on the SCRIPPS trial. *Am. Heart J.* 2002. 143: 3342 – 8.

[96] Maehara A, Patel NS, Harrison LB, et al. Dose heterogeneity may not affect the neointimal proliferation after gamma radiation for in-stent restenosis: a volumetric intravascular ultrasound dosimetric study. *J. Am. Coll. Cardiol.* 2002, 39: 1937 – 42.

[97] Stone G, Ellis S, O'Shaughnessy CD, Martin SL, Satler LS, McGarry T, Turco MA, Kerieakes D, Kelley L, Popma JJ, Russell M. Prospective, randomized evaluation of paclitaxel-eluting stents compared to vascular brachytherapy for treatment of in-stent restenosis: the TAXUS-V ISR trial. *JAMA* 2006;295: 1253–1263.

[98] Holmes DR, Teirstein PS, Satler LF, et al. Sirolimus – eluting stents vs. vascular brachytherapy for in-stent restenosis within bare-metal stents: the SISR randomized trial. *JAMA* 2006; 295 (11):1264 -73.

[99] Torguson R, Sabate M, Deible R, et al. Intravascular brachytherapy versus drug-eluting stents for the treatment of patients with drug eluting stent restenosis. *Am. J. Cardiol.* 2006;98:1340–4.

[100] Bonello L, Kaneshige K, De Labriolle A, et al. Vascular brachytherapy for patients with drug-eluting stent restenosis. *J. Interv. Cardiol.* 2008;21:528 –34.

[101] Song HG, Park DW, Kim YH, et al. Randomized trial of optimal treatment strategies for in-stent restenosis after drug-eluting stent implantation. *J. Am. Coll. Cardiol.* 2012 Mar 20;59(12):1093-100.

[102] Mehran R, Dangas G, Abizaid AS et al. Angiographic patterns of in-stent restenosis: classification and implications for long-term outcome. *Circulation* 1999;100:1872–8.

In: Coronary Artery Restenosis
Editor: Amir S. Lotfi

ISBN: 978-1-63321-346-3

Chapter 9

Optical Coherence Tomography: Current Utility and Future Potential for Management of In-Stent Restenosis

Talla A. Rousan, MD and Faisal Latif*, MD, FACC, FSCAI
Department of Medicine, Cardiovascular Section,
VA Medical Center and University of Oklahoma Health Sciences Center,
Oklahoma City, Oklahoma, US

Abstract

Optical coherence tomography relies on the backscattering of light wavelength to obtain cross-sectional images of tissue. In-stent restenosis is a complex process and OCT, due to its image resolution, can be very useful to evaluate the causes for stent failure. In this chapter the technical aspects and clinical utility of OCT in patient with bare metal and drug eluting stents will be discussed in detail.

Introduction

After being utilized in ophthalmology and gastrointestinal systems, Optical Coherence Tomography (OCT) has created a significant impact in intravascular imaging. It is a system which utilizes near infrared light to generate cross sectional tomographic images of the blood vessels. [1] OCT is similar to intravascular ultrasound (IVUS); however it uses light instead of ultrasound. Essentially, the light beam is directed toward the target (the vessel wall for intravascular imaging) and the magnitude and echo time delay of the reflected time signal is measured. [2, 3] There are multiple applications of OCT. It has been utilized in studying the

* Corresponding Author: Faisal Latif MD, FACC, FSCAI, Assistant Professor of Medicine, Department of Medicine, Cardiovascular Section, VA Medical Center and University of Oklahoma Health Sciences Center, Oklahoma City, Oklahoma, USA. Phone: 405-323-9115. Fax: 405-456-1576. Email: Faisal-latif@ouhsc.edu.

culprit lesions in acute coronary syndrome as well as in the imaging of vulnerable plaques. OCT can also be used to define the tissue characteristics and the lipid content of the atherosclerotic plaque. In interventional cardiology, OCT is being increasingly utilized as a method in determining the reference vessel diameter and minimal luminal area of coronary arteries, although definitive studies to establish standardized measurements are underway. Because of its peculiar ability to image the stent struts and the stent strut-vessel wall interface, OCT can be used to ascertain stent apposition and rule out stent edge dissection after percutaneous coronary intervention (PCI). In the longer term follow up, OCT is being utilized for measuring the degree and nature of in-stent restenosis (ISR). [1, 3, 4]

Technical Characteristics of OCT

The OCT system consists of three major components; a light source, reference mirror, and a photodetector. [4] The light source is monochromic and emits wavelengths between 1,250 and 1,350 nm in a continuous sweep. [3] The two technologies utilized to obtain images by OCT are: time domain and frequency domain, with the latter being a faster method in acquiring images as it has an improved signal-to-noise ratio. [2, 4] Both methods involve flushing the blood from the coronary artery using a transparent media flush (crystalloid solution infused at a rate of 0.5-1.0 mL/s in the case of the time-domain technique and a viscous iso-osmolar solution such as iodixanol infused at a rate of 1-3 mL/s in the frequency domain technique. Time-domain (TD-OCT) was the first generation OCT (M2CV OCT Imaging System, LightLab Imaging, Westford, Massachusetts): It required occlusion of the proximal vessel with a balloon to create a bloodless area for imaging. It was technically challenging, not very well tolerated by the patients all the time and was plagued with underestimation of luminal area as well as reference vessel diameter when compared to IVUS. [5] However, with the advent of frequency domain (FD-OCT) (C7XR Imaging System, LightLab Imaging), some of these issues have been resolved with improved patient tolerance along with an improved imaging quality, and luminal measurements have a better correlation with IVUS-derived measurements. [6] The pullback speed of OCT is up to 20 mm/second with a scanning length up to 50 mm. [4] OCT generates images with up to 10 μm axial resolution and a lateral resolution of 20 μm. [1, 3] OCT offers an anatomic resolution of 0.02 mm when compared to 0.2 mm and 0.1 mm for angiography and IVUS, respectively. [7] The imaging depth (which is the axial range over which an OCT image can be obtained) is 4-6 mm. [8] An important limitation of OCT is its limited tissue penetration of 2-3 mm, which is significantly less than that of IVUS. [3] Resolution of the images acquired by OCT depends on several factors including the intrinsic wavelength range, the light source used, the detection efficiency, and tissue scattering and absorption properties. [2] The higher resolution of OCT allows for a more discrete imaging of vessel lumen and vessel wall, tissue composition of atherosclerotic plaque in the coronary arteries and intravascular stents. It can distinguish lipid-rich plaques from fibrous and fibro-calcific plaques better than IVUS. [9] Similar to IVUS, patients need to be anticoagulated prior to inserting the guidewire into the coronary artery. It is recommended to administer intracoronary nitroglycerin to minimize catheter-induced vasospasm prior to image acquisition. [8]

Mechanism of ISR and Its Relevance to OCT

In-stent restenosis is a complex process. Neointimal hyperplasia seems to be the predominant mechanism early on due mainly to the "healing" process of the vessel wall after stent implantation. Autopsy studies from the era of bare metal stents (BMS) showed that within the first two weeks after stent implantation, microthrombi form within the stents with formation of neointima. After 2 months of implantation, smooth muscle cells are present in the tissue within the stents along with a distinct layer of neointima, which is significantly thicker in restenotic lesions. [10]

Insights into very late ISR have led to the discovery of another phenomenon, namely neoatherosclerosis. Neoatherosclerosis occurs by infiltration of foamy macrophages, re-endothelialization with deposition of neointima within the stented lumen. [11] This tissue undergoes deposition of extracellular matrix and smooth cells migrate into it. [12] Neoatherosclerosis occurs much earlier within drug-eluting stent (DES), when compared to BMS. [13] Before OCT, IVUS with virtual histology (IVUS-VH) capability has been in use to characterize restenotic tissue with variable accuracy. Whether the restenosis is within DES or BMS, as time from implantation progresses, necrotic core and dense calcification continue to increase within the restenotic tissue. [14] These changes render the restenotic tissue more prone to stent thrombosis as well. Hence, in-stent neoatherosclerosis is considered the common mechanism for late stent restenosis and thrombosis. [12] Neoatherosclerotic lesions in ISR are also prone to rupture particularly when they have a "thin-cap" neoatheroma which renders these plaques more "vulnerable". Development of significant calcification in the neoatherosclerotic plaques seems to be a very late phenomenon occurring >6 years after stent implantation. [15]

The Patterns of In-Stent Restenosis Using OCT

ISR has been the major limitation in the long term patency of stents. [16] Several advances have been made in the last two decades in coronary stenting with ISR rates declining to approximately 5% with the advent of DES. [17] Coronary angiography has been the gold standard method in the detection and quantification of coronary artery disease as well as ISR. However, given the limitations of angiography, intravascular imaging with IVUS and now OCT are more reliable methods to ascertain the degree of ISR. Several techniques have been used for the quantitative as well as the qualitative assessment of the extent of ISR including fractional flow reserve (FFR), IVUS, and OCT. The latter provides the highest spatial resolution albeit it has limited tissue penetration. [8] OCT has the ability to identify different patterns of restenotic tissue after stenting allowing for better understanding of the mechanisms involved in this process. [18] ISR patterns based on OCT findings have been classified based on the structure of restenotic tissue (homogenous, heterogeneous, and layered), backscatter from the tissue (high vs. low), the presence of visible microvessels within the tissue, the lumen shape (regular vs. irregular), and the presence of intraluminal material. [18] In the study by Gonzalo et al., the heterogeneous pattern of ISR was more prevalent in angiographically focal versus angiographically diffuse ISR (45.5% vs. 0%; $p = 0.005$). Additionally, irregular lumen shape was observed more commonly in patients with unstable angina compared to patients with stable angina (60 vs. 6.7%, p = 0.007). [18] It was proposed that certain restenosis patterns could be associated with the clinical presentation (stable versus unstable) as well as the time from stent implantation (less or more than 12 months) which adds to the utility of this technology in the management of ISR. [18]

In a BMS, neointima within the restenotic tissue appears homogeneous on OCT. [19] The tissue in the homogeneous pattern could be in the form of a single band or two-layered. [20] The single band pattern is because of the highly compact smooth muscle cells concentrated on the luminal border. [20] Neoatherosclerotic tissue, on the other hand, appears as a heterogeneous structure with a low-intensity area. [11] Heterogeneous intima and intimal disruption are present more frequently in neoatherosclerosis when compared to intimal hyperplasia. Moreover, intraintimal neovascularization is also present in the neoatherosclerotic restenotic plaques, which in case of rupture can lead to intramural hemorrhage. [21]

Pattern of ISR in DES is more varied than that of BMS, and the size of thrombi are larger. [20] Yamamoto et al. [20] studied 25 patients with ISR of DES, 8% of DES contained large thrombi which were much larger than thrombi seen in BMS previously.

OCT Use in the Evaluation of ISR in Bare Metal Stents

OCT has helped improve our understanding of the composition of the restenotic tissue. Without the polymer and the drug, bare metal stents (BMS) tend to endothelialize faster than DES. In a study on 82 patients, 43 patients experienced very late ISR (>5 years after implantation of BMS) while 39 experienced early ISR (within the first year after implantation): OCT allowed tissue characterization (heterogeneous vs. homogeneous), as well as evaluation for the presence of microvasculature, and intimal disruption. Heterogeneous intima was present significantly more often in very late ISR compared to early ISR (60.5±28.5% versus 5.8±11.5%, P<0.0001), as was disrupted intima (18.6% versus 0%, P<0.03). They also demonstrated that the incidence of neoatherosclerosis is much lower (17.9%) in early BMS restenosis when compared to 90.7% in very late ISR in BMS. [11] Heterogeneous intima was more frequently present in the most severely stenotic segment of the ISR. This shows that neoatherosclerosis occurs very late in the well endothelialized bare metal stents. [11] Presence of neoatherosclerosis not only causes ISR, but also makes the stents more prone to thrombosis.

In another study evaluating ISR in bare metal stents, 51 patients were enrolled between 2009 and 2011. [22] Thirty patients had stable angina while 21 had unstable coronary syndromes. Patients with unstable angina showed a trend toward a thin-cap neoatheroma (50 μm vs. 60 μm, p = 0.056). In 13 lesions, neointimal rupture was identified, and in 12 out of those 13 lesions, intramural thrombi were also identified.

OCT Use in the Evaluation of ISR of Drug-Eluting Stents

In the era of BMS, ISR was considered to be a complex process secondary to neointimal hyperplasia, inflammatory changes, and neovascularization. [10] DES were introduced to prevent or slow down this process and its associated complications. [16] ISR in DES is a relatively less frequent complication occurring in 5-10% of the cases. [16] Different studies showed that the OCT findings of DES ISR correlated with the pattern of presentation (unstable vs. stable) in addition to the time from stent implantation. [20, 23, 24] IVUS has been the standard for the identification of and characterization of ISR; however with the advent of a higher resolution technology, OCT is being increasingly used. [24]

ISR in DES has been shown to present as a spectrum of histopathological changes. [23, 24] In a study by Lee et al., [24] OCT analysis performed approximately one year after different types of DES implantation showed higher frequency of heterogeneous or layered tissue (78.8% vs. 22.9%, P <0.001) and micorovessels (48.5% vs. 5.7%, P<0.001), and a lower backscatter (60.6% vs. 20.8%, P<0.001) compared to non-ISR lesions. In this study, which included 33 ISR lesions (4 Sirolimus-eluting, 17 Paclitaxel-eluting, 10 Zotarolimus-eluting, and 2 Everolimus-eluting stents), Paclitaxel-eluting stents had the highest frequency of ISR with less homogenous tissue and higher backscatter as demonstrated by OCT. Multiple logistic regression analysis showed that the increased burden of neointimal tissue, lumen area, and hypertension were independent predictors for heterogeneous or layered neointimal tissue in these restenotic tissues.

ISR in DES can occur early (less than 12 months after stent implantation) or late (more than 12 months after stent implantation). Similar to ISR in BMS, the mechanism of early ISR is thought to be neointimal hyperplasia with diabetes mellitus, long lesions, ostial or bifurcation locations, and underexpansion of the stent having been identified as the predictors for acceleration of this process. [25] Late stent ISR, on the other hand, remains an interesting phenomenon with mechanisms not entirely understood. [26] OCT has been utilized in the identification of the early and late ISR. [26] In the study by Ino et al., the OCT pattern of early and late ISR after sirolimus-eluting stent implantation was studied on 57 patients (48 patients were eventually included in the analysis; 30 patients with early ISR and 18 patients with late ISR). The mean duration from stent implantation was 8 ± 1 month in the early ISR group and 34 ± 14 months in the late ISR group. The frequency of unstable angina was relatively higher in the late ISR group (33% vs. 10%, p = 0.094). It was noted that the late ISR group had a higher frequency of heterogeneous neointima (89% vs. 43%, P = 0.002), lipid-rich neointima (83% vs. 27%, p < 0.001), microchannels within the neointimal tissue (67% vs. 27%, p = 0.007), thin-cap fibroatheroma-like neointima (39% vs. 10%, p = 0.028), and neointimal disruption (33% vs. 3%, p = 0.008) compared to the early ISR group. The frequency of intraluminal thrombus was similar in both groups. [26] The mechanism of later ISR after DES implantation is very likely related to chronic inflammation leading to progression of neoatherosclerosis. [27]

DES also suffers from delayed endothelialization and incomplete stent coverage which makes them prone to late adverse events, stent thrombosis being significantly more morbid than ISR. Miyazki et al. studied the OCT characteristics of 58 treated lesions (6 with very late stent thrombosis, 32 with late ISR, and 20 with no events). [28] In this study, a total of 9,763 stent struts were analyzed. The proportion of uncovered struts per stented segment was significantly higher in the very late in-stent thrombosis group compared to the late ISR and the no event groups (29.2 ± 22.8% vs. 7.9 ± 9.7% vs. 7.6 ± 8.0%, p = 0.002). The proportion of malapposed struts per total number of struts per stented segment was significantly higher in the very late stent thrombosis group compared to the other two groups. In two out of the six patients in the very late stent thrombosis group, OCT showed lipid-laden neointima with disruption. These findings suggest that although they might be the major contributors, uncovered and malapposed struts are not solely responsible for stent thrombosis, the presence of lipid-laden intima leading to rupture also contributes to this process. [28]

The utility of OCT in the characterization of lesions depending on the clinical presentation (stable vs. unstable angina) was studied by Kang et al. [23] Fifty patients with ISR (30 with stable angina and 20 with unstable angina) were included (25 with Sirolimus-eluting stents, 10 with Paclitaxel-eluting stents, 3 with Zotarolimus-eluting stents, 2 with Everolimus-eluting stents, and 10 with other drug-eluting stents). Compared to the stable angina group, the unstable angina group had a thinner fibrous cap (55 vs. 100 μm, P 0.006), higher incidence of thin-cap fibroatheroma (TCFA) containing neointima (15% vs. 11%, P = 0.008), and intimal rupture (15% vs. 14%, P = 0.044). Thrombi were identified more frequently in the unstable angina group (80% vs. 43%, P = 0.010). Interestingly, the lesions containing TCFA neointima presented later that those without this finding (42.3 months vs. 11.6 months). The duration of twenty months since stent implantation was the best predictor of the presence of TCFA-containing neointima with a sensitivity of 73% and a specificity of 67%. The ISR lesions in patients presenting later than 20 months after stent implantation had a thinner fibrous cap, higher incidence of thrombus and TCFA-containing neointima, and had a trend towards a higher frequency of clinical presentation with unstable angina (50% vs. 29%, p = 0.112). Interestingly, when compared to IVUS, OCT was superior in detecting intimal rupture and thrombus, with the agreement between the two technologies being <50%.

OCT Findings in DES versus BMS In-Stent Restenosis

Development of neoatherosclerosis is not only affected by the duration of stent implantation, but also by the type of stents implanted, as well as many clinical characteristics. [15] In an OCT study on 138 implanted stents (18 BMSs and 43 DESs), it was found that restenotic tissue in DES had a higher concentration of lipid-rich plaque when compared to BMS (12.9 ± 25.1% vs. 1.2 ± 4.3%, p = 0.01) within the first 9 months after implantation. Between 9 and 48 months, DES continues to have a greater percentage of lipid-rich plaque (24.8 ± 28.1% vs. 4.1 ± 7.3%, p <0.01). However, in the late phase (>4 years after implantation), lipid-laden plaque was the predominant type in both DES and BMS. [13] Additionally, neovascularization of the restenotic tissue occurs earlier in BMS than DES. [13] This early neovascularization in BMS could be the reason for a more diffuse neoatherosclerosis in the very late phase.

Yonetsu et al. conducted another OCT study on patients with neoatherosclerosis >100 μm neointimal thickness in 179 lesions from a pool of 1,080 patients. Uni- and multi-variate analyses showed that longer duration of stent implantation (>4 years), any type of DES (OR,

2.66; P=0.004), chronic kidney disease (OR, 4.17; P=0.009), smoking and interestingly, use of angiotensin-converting enzyme inhibitors or angiotensin II receptor blockers were independent predictors of these vulnerable neoatherosclerotic plaques. [15] This indicates that factors which lead to recurrent events in patients with implanted coronary stents are the same as the well-known risk factors for development of native coronary artery disease.

Comparison of OCT with Other Technologies

OCT versus IVUS in In-Stent Restenosis

Over the last two decades, IVUS has been widely used to elucidate plaque structure and luminal area in coronary arteries, to determine appropriateness for surgical versus percutaneous revascularization. Standard IVUS measurements with a good correlation with ischemia-producing thresholds have been identified, which have also been associated with improved outcomes after PCI. [29] The prime example of this was left main coronary artery disease. Before IVUS, in the coronary artery surgery study (CASS), a threshold of 50% angiographic left main disease was utilized to refer patient for coronary artery bypass grafting (CABG) surgery. [30] With the use of IVUS, threshold of an MLA of <6 mm^2 has been established to identify significant left main disease when CABG should be considered. [31, 32]

With a resolution 10 times higher than that of IVUS, and an imaging acquisition speed of 40 times faster than that of IVUS, OCT promises to be a superior imaging system than IVUS for ISR as well. Comparative studies have been performed between OCT and IVUS. [5, 33, 34] It is important to realize that the pullback speed of IVUS at 0.5-1 mm/sec is markedly slower than that of FD-OCT (20 mm/sec). Therefore, IVUS images the vessel lumen over many cardiac cycles, while FD-OCT has much less transition between the two phases of cardiac cycle. The difference in lumen size can vary up to 12% between systole and diastole, as shown in IVUS studies. [35] Moreover, inter-scan reproducibility of frequency domain OCT has been well established, lending itself as an excellent tool for longitudinal studies of coronary artery disease. [36]

In a study to compare the technical aspects of TD-OCT and FD-OCT with IVUS, 227 matched pullback runs were compared. [5] In the non-stented vessels, FD-OCT depicted more severe native coronary artery disease than IVUS (MLA 2.33 ± 1.56 mm^2 vs. 3.32 ± 1.92 mm^2; p<0.001), whereas the reference vessel diameter was similar in both previously stented and non-stented vessels. On the other hand, TD-OCT depicted smaller reference lumen size than IVUS. In the previously stented vessels, both varieties of OCT depicted a smaller MLA than IVUS, owing largely to the fact that OCT detects neointimal hyperplasia better in ISR. Because OCT uses light instead of ultrasound (in IVUS), it delineates lumen-wall interface better allowing improved detection of malapposition of stent struts and also, a more precise estimation of MLA in non-stented arteries. Additionally, the smaller profile of the OCT catheter than IVUS may cause less vessel wall stretch in regions of high-grade stenosis, yielding a smaller MLA.

The utility of OCT-guided PCI versus IVUS-guided PCI is evident from the finding that OCT detects malapposition of stents and inter-strut tissue prolapse significantly better than

IVUS. [5] OCT enables detection of individual strut-level malapposition, a luxury only affordable by OCT due to its much higher resolution. Besides stent thrombosis, malapposition of stent struts has been associated with stent restenosis as well. [37] Therefore, OCT-guided stent placement has the potential to decrease in-stent restenosis as well, above and beyond IVUS-guided stent placement. OCT is less susceptible to the blooming artifact of calcification than IVUS. [5] Therefore, the stent-lumen interface is well delineated even in calcified plaques. However, this advantage does not persist with stent struts, as they produce a blooming artifact with both IVUS and OCT. It is important to mention that even though OCT offers potential advantages over IVUS as stated above, prospective studies comparing patient outcomes for OCT-guided PCI versus IVUS-guided PCI have not been performed.

OCT versus FFR in In-Stent Restenosis

Invasive functional assessment of native coronary lesions using FFR has been strongly correlated with ischemia on stress testing. [38] FFR-guided PCI has been shown to yield improved outcomes including the combined endpoint of death/myocardial infarction, when compared to angiography-guided PCI. [29, 39] However, studies on the utility of FFR for ISR are few and far between. But, nevertheless, correlation between abnormal FFR and ischemia on myocardial scintigraphy has been proven to be strong even for ISR. [40]

In a study comparing FFR for ISR versus FFR for native coronary arteries, 42 patients with intermediate ISR (40-70%) were compared with 57 patients with intermediate native coronary artery disease. [41] At a similar degree of angiographic stenosis, FFR in the restenotic lesions was lower when compared to the native coronary arteries (0.77 +/- 0.15 vs. 0.82 +/- 0.12, $p < 0.05$) and was more frequently hemodynamically significant (<0.75) in restenotic lesions versus the native coronary arteries (48% vs. 26%, $p < 0.05$). Additionally, patients with restenotic lesions without hemodynamic significance (FFR >0.75) did not experience any adverse coronary events over a 6-month follow-up with conservative medical management. [41]

The correlation between a >50% ISR and a significant FFR (<0.75) is poor. In a study on 65 in-stent restenotic lesions, the correlation between an intermediate ISR (40-70%) and FFR <0.75 was <0.5. [42] Conservative management of lesions with FFR >0.75 was not associated with any adverse outcome (combined endpoint of death by any cause, non-fatal myocardial infarction, and revascularization of the evaluated lesion).

In the past IVUS-derived measurements have been correlated with physiologically significant lesions (FFR ≤0.8). [43, 44] Certain studies showed an MLA of 3-4 mm^2 to correlate with an FFR <0.75, however a more recent study showed an MLA of 2.4 mm^2 to have a correlation with FFR ≤0.8 (a more widely accepted FFR value nowadays). [44] Similarly, recent studies have been performed to identify potential cut-off MLA values on OCT which correlate with functional significance of a lesion. [45]. Forty-six patients with diabetes mellitus type with stable coronary artery disease with intermediate (40-70%) coronary stenosis were enrolled and both OCT and FFR were performed on 62 lesions. OCT-derived MLA of <1.59 mm^2 and minimal luminal diameter of <1.31 mm were found to be the optimal cut-off values to predict an FFR of ≤0.80. [45]

Applications of OCT to Decrease the Incidence of In-stent Restenosis

OCT is being extensively studied, but limited studies have been performed in the arena of ISR. Based on the findings of various studies, we have teased out potential advantages OCT can offer to decrease incidence of ISR, as well as its treatment. Studies to determine patient outcomes of these potential benefits are hereto lacking.

Determination of Adequacy of PCI

Malapposition of stent struts can cause ISR as well as stent thrombosis. [37] OCT allows for discrete identification of stent struts. [5] Moreover, it can identify milder degree of malapposition of stent struts after deployment, because it can visualize the strut-intima interface clearly. In heavily calcified lesions, malapposition of stent struts occurs more frequently, as the calcified portion of the lesion does not expand as well by PCI as does the non-calcified portion. This is an area where OCT can help because, as opposed to IVUS, it does not suffer from the blooming artifact from calcification. [4]

Due to its ability to differentiate stent strut- neointimal hyperplasia interface better, OCT can be utilized to optimize sizing of devices also. In a study on ISR lesions, cutting balloon angioplasty was first performed based on angiographic guidance, followed by OCT to help detect the percentage of remaining neointimal hyperplasia. [46] With OCT guidance, a cutting balloon 0.5mm size bigger could be utilized leading to a significant increase in minimal stent area (4.9 ± 0.42 to 6.35 ± 0.92 mm^2) with a reduction in neointimal hyperplasia from 41% to 27%. [46] OCT could help achieve a better final minimal stent area, which has been shown to predict improved long-term stent patency. [47]

Selection of Type of Treatment

Even though DES has been shown to reduce ISR remarkably in de novo as well as restenotic lesions of BMS, when compared to BMS, it still remains a less than satisfactory treatment for restenotic lesions of DES. DES ISR is an inflammatory process to begin with a re-implantation of a new DES might just compound such an inflammatory reaction, and therefore, limit the success of the newer DES. [48] Whether the use of bioabsorbale stents could mitigate this problem, remains to be seen and OCT-guided tissue characterization could provide further insights.

Nagoshi et al. conducted a study on 122 ISR lesions (79 DES and 43 BMS) using OCT. [49] The lesions were classified as homogeneous, layered or heterogeneous. The layered type was predominant with DES, whereas lesions were homogeneous with BMS ($P<0.001$). Backscatter and signal intensity were significantly higher with BMS ($P<0.05$ and $P<0.001$ respectively). Interestingly, with balloon angioplasty alone, reduction of neointimal hyperplasia was higher in the layered and heterogeneous groups than in the homogeneous group ($P<0.01$). Larger studies with clinical outcomes based on OCT patterns of ISR could lead to further insights into the appropriate therapy for patients.

Assessment of Vulnerability of Plaque

Owing to its high resolution, OCT allows measurement of fibrous cap thickness of the neoatherosclerotic plaques in the restenotic tissue. TCFA has been associated with higher incidence of cardiovascular events in de novo coronary lesions. [50] Atherosclerotic plaques in coronary arteries with TCFA are deemed to be the vulnerable plaques, which despite the relatively milder stenosis, can actually lead to unstable coronary syndromes including myocardial infarction. In a study on diabetic patients, fibrous cap thickness of <80μm was associated with an FFR of ≤0.80. [45] In a recent large study, it was determined that attenuated plaque, and tissue protrusion through stent struts is a predictor of stent thrombosis. [51] Attenuated plaque on IVUS is considered a determinant of plaques with a larger necrotic core and thin fibrous cap, measures which can be better assessed by OCT which predicts a more important role for OCT in future in areas of stent thrombosis and in-stent restenosis. As opposed to heavy calcification which is more often present in patients with stable angina when compared to patients with acute coronary syndromes, sporadic superficial calcification has been found to be present more frequently in patients with acute myocardial infarction. With OCT, this superficial calcification is better visualized and additionally, the distance between lumen and inner surface of the calcium deposit can be measured more accurately. [52]

Moreover, OCT allows for volumetric assessment of lesion severity, as it constructs a tomographic image of the coronary artery. For volumetric assessment, vascular resistance ratio is calculated taking into account the epicardial and microvascular resistances, as well as the flow redistribution into side branches. [53] Following PCI, the microvascular resistance decreases besides the epicardial resistance due to the stenosis. [54] Volumetric assessment of the coronary artery by OCT has been shown to have a better correlation with FFR than MLA alone. [53] Although not tested yet, in coronary restenosis, this volumetric assessment holds promise as its correlation with functional significance of the lesion could be higher than simply measuring the MLA within the restenotic stent.

Reduction in Target-vessel Revascularization

OCT-guided PCI has the potential to reduce the need for target vessel revascularization due to restenosis. In a retrospective study on 670 patients, outcomes of 335 patients who underwent angiography + OCT-guided PCI with 335 patients who underwent angiography-only guided PCI were better at one year. [55] The combined endpoint of cardiac death and MI occurred significantly less in patients undergoing angiography + OCT-guided PCI versus angiography only (OR=0.49[0.25-0.96], p=0.037). Interestingly, OCT-guidance led to additional interventions during the PCI in more than one-third of the patients (34.7%). Although this could just be an early success story for OCT, it is in sharp contrast to some of the larger trials on IVUS-guided PCI. [56, 57] In the Optimization with Intracoronary Ultrasound to reduce Stent Restenosis (OPTICUS) trial, angiographic follow-up did not demonstrate any reduction in binary restenosis at 6 months (p=0.68), or minimal lumen diameter (p=0.52). Additionally, major adverse clinical events were not different at one year. [56]

OCT can differentiate neoatherosclerosis from neointimal hyperplasia, which could have ramifications in terms of whether to treat restenotic lesions with a new stent versus angioplasty alone. With bare metal stents, late ISR >5 years after implantation is more attributable to neoatherosclerosis, when compared to early ISR (<1 year) which is more due to neo-intimal hyperplasia. [58] On the other hand, with DES, neoatherosclerosis occurs earlier (<2 years) and might contribute to very late stent thrombosis. [23]

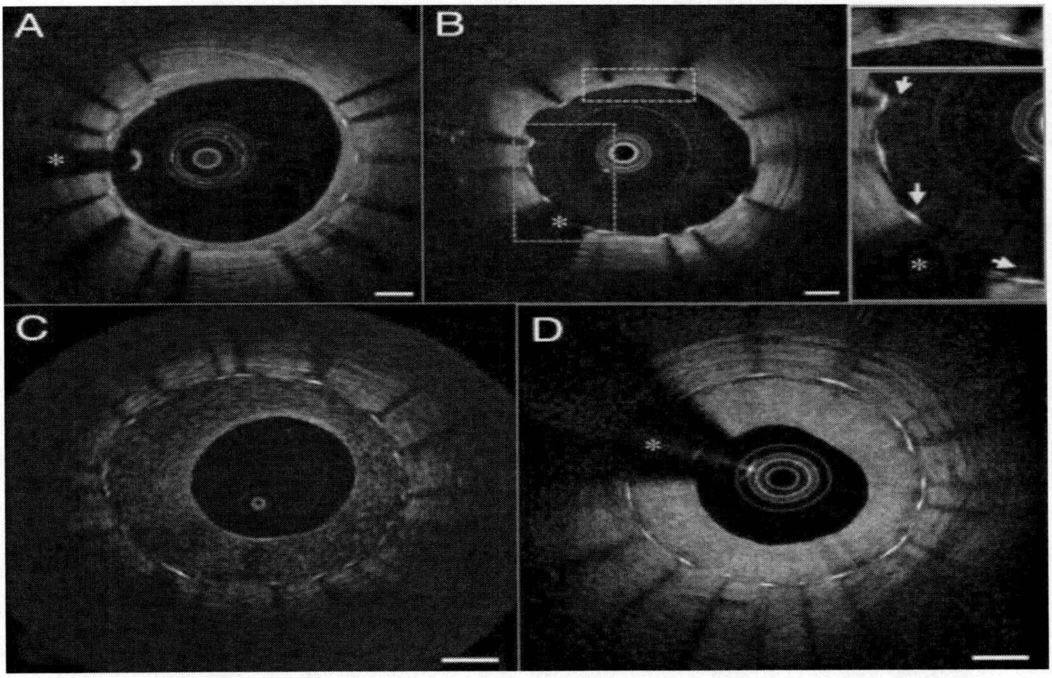

Figure 1. (A) Covered stent struts. Varying degrees of tissue seen overlying all stent struts. (B) Covered and uncovered stent struts. Upper inset shows covered and lower inset shows uncovered stent struts. (C) In-stent restenosis with a low-intensity signal. (D) In-stent restenosis with homogeneous tissue. (Reproduced with permission from Elsevier Publishers: Tearney et al. JACC 2012;59:1058-1072).

Tissue Coverage of Stent Struts

Because of diminished susceptibility of OCT to artifacts at the stent-strut interface, it can visualize presence of tissue overlying the stent struts.[8] If tissue is seen overlying a strut, it is "covered" (Figure 1A), while the lack thereof is an "uncovered" strut (Figure 1B). The restenotic tissue could be seen as signal-poor tissue (Figure 1C), or layered tissue (Figure 1D) overlying the stent struts. OCT was utilized in the Limus-Eluted from a Durable vs. Erodable Stent Coating (LEADERS) trial, to compare strut coverage of a biolimus-eluting stent with biodegradable polymer with a sirolimus-eluting stent using a durable polymer. [59] OCT showed that strut coverage was more complete in biolimus eluting stents with biodegradable polymer.

Future Applications of OCT

The resolution of OCT is being enhanced to <10 μm. Physiological assessment of the lesion with simultaneous coronary pressure measurement (using FFR) could increase the accuracy of detecting hemodynamically severe coronary lesions as it has been shown that FFR has higher specificity in the detection of these lesions compared to OCT. [60]

Since OCT has the capability to evaluate atherosclerotic plaque characteristics significantly better than older imaging modalities, it can be used to evaluate effects of medications such statins on plaque characteristics over a period of time. [3] Statins have been shown to increase fibrous cap thickness, leading to more stable plaques which are less prone to rupture. [61] The effects of newer anti-hyperlipidemia medications such as Proprotein Convertase Subtilisin/Kexin type 9 (PCSK9) could also be evaluated using OCT.

The technology of OCT will continue to evolve to overcome limitations such as limited tissue penetration (2-3mm) which can make characterization of thick plaques more difficult. Additionally, evaluation of left main disease and saphenous vein graft disease is not as distinct as the other coronary arteries because of their larger size.[3] Three-dimensional OCT is in development as well. [4] It will have higher frame rates and will allow longer segments of coronary arteries being imaged especially the "full metal-jacket" coronaries. This along with tissue characterization in restenotic lesions might offer insights into optimal treatment strategies in future.

The recently published consensus document by the Society for Cardiovascular Angiography and Interventions (SCAI) states that use of OCT could have an advantage over IVUS to optimize stent deployment by determination of stent apposition and better identification of stent edge dissection, due to its higher resolution. [62] Additionally, it could be useful in assessment of plaque morphology, however, it cautions against using it to determine whether a PCI should be performed or not, as the measurement criteria for minimal luminal area criteria have not been validated yet.

In an era where there is an ever-increasing focus on characterization of plaques, whether in the native coronary lesions or restenotic lesions, imaging modalities such as near-infrared spectroscopy (NIRS) which determines the amount of lipid content, and OCT which can determine the fibrous cap thickness and characterize tissue, might be used as adjunctive techniques to determine the vulnerability of plaques and help advance medical as well as endovascular therapy to reduce incidence of major adverse cardiovascular events. It has been observed that patients with unstable coronary syndromes have a higher incidence of vulnerable restenotic tissue with thin-cap neoatheroma, neointimal rupture and thrombus based on OCT findings. [23]

Limitations

With respect to coronary stent restenosis, it is important to keep in mind that tissue penetration of OCT is limited to 2-3mm. This is usually appropriate to adjudicate the restenotic tissue within a pre-existing stent, but it limits the ability to see much beyond the stent struts into the true vessel wall and its characteristics for example, degree of calcification.

Conclusion

OCT is an exciting technology which is likely to have a significant impact on our treatment strategies for ISR, due to improved imaging resolution than other imaging techniques particularly IVUS. Through improved optimization of stent deployment in the first place, it can reduce the incidence of restenosis. Secondly, when ISR occurs, it might provide better insight into management strategy based on tissue characterization. Studies with clinical outcomes are needed to ascertain the role of OCT in the treatment of ISR.

References

[1] McCabe JM, Croce KJ. Optical coherence tomography. *Circulation.* Oct 23 2012;126:2140-2143.

[2] Prati F, Regar E, Mintz GS, et al. Expert review document on methodology, terminology, and clinical applications of optical coherence tomography: physical principles, methodology of image acquisition, and clinical application for assessment of coronary arteries and atherosclerosis. *Eur. Heart J.* Feb 2010;31:401-415.

[3] Abtahian F, Jang IK. Optical coherence tomography: basics, current application and future potential. *Current opinion in pharmacology.* Oct 2012;12:583-591.

[4] Kubo T, Tanaka A, Kitabata H, Ino Y, Tanimoto T, Akasaka T. Application of optical coherence tomography in percutaneous coronary intervention. *Circulation journal: official journal of the Japanese Circulation Society.* 2012;76:2076-2083.

[5] Bezerra HG, Attizzani GF, Sirbu V, et al. Optical coherence tomography versus intravascular ultrasound to evaluate coronary artery disease and percutaneous coronary intervention. *JACC. Cardiovascular interventions.* Mar 2013;6:228-236.

[6] Takarada S, Imanishi T, Liu Y, et al. Advantage of next-generation frequency-domain optical coherence tomography compared with conventional time-domain system in the assessment of coronary lesion. *Catheter Cardiovasc Interv.* Feb 1 2010;75:202-206.

[7] Johnson NP, Kirkeeide RL, Gould KL. Coronary anatomy to predict physiology: fundamental limits. *Circulation. Cardiovascular imaging.* Sep 2013;6:817-832.

[8] Tearney GJ, Regar E, Akasaka T, et al. Consensus standards for acquisition, measurement, and reporting of intravascular optical coherence tomography studies: a report from the International Working Group for Intravascular Optical Coherence Tomography Standardization and Validation. *J. Am. Coll. Cardiol.* Mar 20 2012;59: 1058-1072.

[9] Kawasaki M, Bouma BE, Bressner J, et al. Diagnostic accuracy of optical coherence tomography and integrated backscatter intravascular ultrasound images for tissue characterization of human coronary plaques. *J. Am. Coll. Cardiol.* Jul 4 2006;48:81-88.

[10] Komatsu R, Ueda M, Naruko T, Kojima A, Becker AE. Neointimal tissue response at sites of coronary stenting in humans: macroscopic, histological, and immunohistochemical analyses. *Circulation.* Jul 21 1998;98:224-233.

[11] Habara M, Terashima M, Nasu K, et al. Difference of tissue characteristics between early and very late restenosis lesions after bare-metal stent implantation: an optical

coherence tomography study. *Circulation. Cardiovascular interventions.* Jun 2011;4:232-238.

[12] Park SJ, Kang SJ, Virmani R, Nakano M, Ueda Y. In-stent neoatherosclerosis: a final common pathway of late stent failure. *J. Am. Coll. Cardiol.* Jun 5 2012;59:2051-2057.

[13] Yonetsu T, Kim JS, Kato K, et al. Comparison of incidence and time course of neoatherosclerosis between bare metal stents and drug-eluting stents using optical coherence tomography. *Am. J. Cardiol.* Oct 1 2012;110:933-939.

[14] Kang SJ, Mintz GS, Park DW, et al. Tissue characterization of in-stent neointima using intravascular ultrasound radiofrequency data analysis. *Am. J. Cardiol.* Dec 1 2010;106:1561-1565.

[15] Yonetsu T, Kato K, Kim SJ, et al. Predictors for neoatherosclerosis: a retrospective observational study from the optical coherence tomography registry. *Circulation. Cardiovascular imaging.* Sep 1 2012;5:660-666.

[16] Serruys PW, Kutryk MJ, Ong AT. Coronary-artery stents. *The New England journal of medicine.* Feb 2 2006;354:483-495.

[17] Simonton CA, Brodie B, Cheek B, et al. Comparative clinical outcomes of paclitaxel- and sirolimus-eluting stents: results from a large prospective multicenter registry--STENT Group. *J. Am. Coll. Cardiol.* Sep 25 2007;50:1214-1222.

[18] Gonzalo N, Serruys PW, Okamura T, et al. Optical coherence tomography patterns of stent restenosis. *Am. Heart J.* Aug 2009;158:284-293.

[19] Kume T, Akasaka T, Kawamoto T, et al. Visualization of neointima formation by optical coherence tomography. *International heart journal.* Nov 2005;46:1133-1136.

[20] Yamamoto M, Takano M, Murakami D, et al. Optical coherence tomography analysis for restenosis of drug-eluting stents. *Int. J. Cardiol.* Jan 7 2011;146:100-103.

[21] Takano M, Yamamoto M, Inami S, et al. Appearance of lipid-laden intima and neovascularization after implantation of bare-metal stents extended late-phase observation by intracoronary optical coherence tomography. *J. Am. Coll. Cardiol.* Dec 29 2009;55:26-32.

[22] Kang SJ, Song HG, Ahn JM, et al. OCT-verified neoatherosclerosis in BMS restenosis at 10 years. *JACC. Cardiovascular imaging.* Dec 2012;5:1267-1268.

[23] Kang SJ, Mintz GS, Akasaka T, et al. Optical coherence tomographic analysis of in-stent neoatherosclerosis after drug-eluting stent implantation. *Circulation.* Jun 28 2011;123:2954-2963.

[24] Lee SJ, Kim BK, Kim JS, et al. Evaluation of neointimal morphology of lesions with or without in-stent restenosis: an optical coherence tomography study. *Clinical cardiology.* Oct 2011;34:633-639.

[25] Lemos PA, Saia F, Ligthart JM, et al. Coronary restenosis after sirolimus-eluting stent implantation: morphological description and mechanistic analysis from a consecutive series of cases. *Circulation.* Jul 22 2003;108:257-260.

[26] Ino Y, Kubo T, Kitabata H, et al. Difference in neointimal appearance between early and late restenosis after sirolimus-eluting stent implantation assessed by optical coherence tomography. *Coronary artery disease.* Mar 2013;24:95-101.

[27] Virmani R, Liistro F, Stankovic G, et al. Mechanism of late in-stent restenosis after implantation of a paclitaxel derivate-eluting polymer stent system in humans. *Circulation.* Nov 19 2002;106:2649-2651.

[28] Miyazaki S, Hiasa Y, Takahashi T, et al. In vivo optical coherence tomography of very late drug-eluting stent thrombosis compared with late in-stent restenosis. *Circulation journal: official journal of the Japanese Circulation Society.* 2012;76:390-398.

[29] Tonino PA, De Bruyne B, Pijls NH, et al. Fractional flow reserve versus angiography for guiding percutaneous coronary intervention. *The New England journal of medicine.* Jan 15 2009;360:213-224.

[30] Coronary artery surgery study (CASS): a randomized trial of coronary artery bypass surgery. Comparability of entry characteristics and survival in randomized patients and nonrandomized patients meeting randomization criteria. *J. Am. Coll. Cardiol.* Jan 1984;3:114-128.

[31] Sano K, Mintz GS, Carlier SG, et al. Assessing intermediate left main coronary lesions using intravascular ultrasound. *Am. Heart J.* Nov 2007;154:983-988.

[32] Gil RJ, Gziut AI, Prati F, Witkowski A, Kubica J. Threshold parameters of left main coronary artery stem stenosis based on intracoronary ultrasound examination. *Kardiologia polska.* Sep 2005;63:223-231; discussion 232-223.

[33] Jang IK, Bouma BE, Kang DH, et al. Visualization of coronary atherosclerotic plaques in patients using optical coherence tomography: comparison with intravascular ultrasound. *J. Am. Coll. Cardiol.* Feb 20 2002;39:604-609.

[34] Suzuki Y, Ikeno F, Koizumi T, et al. In vivo comparison between optical coherence tomography and intravascular ultrasound for detecting small degrees of in-stent neointima after stent implantation. *JACC. Cardiovascular interventions.* Apr 2008;1:168-173.

[35] Tsutsui H, Schoenhagen P, Crowe TD, et al. Influence of coronary pulsation on volumetric intravascular ultrasound measurements performed without ECG-gating. Validation in vessel segments with minimal disease. *The international journal of cardiovascular imaging.* Feb 2003;19:51-57.

[36] Orii M, Kubo T, Tanaka A, et al. Inter-scan reproducibility of geometric coronary artery measurements using frequency-domain optical coherence tomography. *International heart journal.* 2013;54:64-67.

[37] Santos MC, Lin T, Barlis P. In-stent restenosis associated with stent malapposition: seven year optical coherence tomography findings. *Int. J. Cardiol.* Feb 17 2011;147:149-151.

[38] Pijls NH, De Bruyne B, Peels K, et al. Measurement of fractional flow reserve to assess the functional severity of coronary-artery stenoses. *The New England journal of medicine.* Jun 27 1996;334:1703-1708.

[39] De Bruyne B, Pijls NH, Kalesan B, et al. Fractional flow reserve-guided PCI versus medical therapy in stable coronary disease. *The New England journal of medicine.* Sep 13 2012;367:991-1001.

[40] Kruger S, Koch KC, Kaumanns I, et al. Use of fractional flow reserve versus stress perfusion scintigraphy in stent restenosis. *European journal of internal medicine.* Oct 2005;16:429-431.

[41] Kruger S, Koch KC, Kaumanns I, Merx MW, Hanrath P, Hoffmann R. Clinical significance of fractional flow reserve for evaluation of functional lesion severity in stent restenosis and native coronary arteries. *Chest.* Sep 2005;128:1645-1649.

[42] Lopez-Palop R, Pinar E, Lozano I, Saura D, Pico F, Valdes M. Utility of the fractional flow reserve in the evaluation of angiographically moderate in-stent restenosis. *Eur. Heart J.* Nov 2004;25:2040-2047.

[43] Takagi A, Tsurumi Y, Ishii Y, Suzuki K, Kawana M, Kasanuki H. Clinical potential of intravascular ultrasound for physiological assessment of coronary stenosis: relationship between quantitative ultrasound tomography and pressure-derived fractional flow reserve. *Circulation.* Jul 20 1999;100:250-255.

[44] Kang SJ, Ahn JM, Song H, et al. Usefulness of minimal luminal coronary area determined by intravascular ultrasound to predict functional significance in stable and unstable angina pectoris. *Am. J. Cardiol.* Apr 1 2012;109:947-953.

[45] Reith S, Battermann S, Jaskolka A, et al. Relationship between optical coherence tomography derived intraluminal and intramural criteria and haemodynamic relevance as determined by fractional flow reserve in intermediate coronary stenoses of patients with diabetes mellitus type. *Heart.* May 2013;99:700-707.

[46] Secco GG, Foin N, Viceconte N, Borgia F, De Luca G, Di Mario C. Optical coherence tomography for guidance of treatment of in-stent restenosis with cutting balloons. *EuroIntervention: journal of EuroPCR in collaboration with the Working Group on Interventional Cardiology of the European Society of Cardiology.* Nov 2011;7:828-834.

[47] Sonoda S, Morino Y, Ako J, et al. Impact of final stent dimensions on long-term results following sirolimus-eluting stent implantation: serial intravascular ultrasound analysis from the sirius trial. *J. Am. Coll. Cardiol.* Jun 2 2004;43:1959-1963.

[48] van Beusekom HM, Saia F, Zindler JD, et al. Drug-eluting stents show delayed healing: paclitaxel more pronounced than sirolimus. *Eur. Heart J.* Apr 2007;28:974-979.

[49] Nagoshi R, Shinke T, Otake H, et al. Qualitative and quantitative assessment of stent restenosis by optical coherence tomography: comparison between drug-eluting and bare-metal stents. *Circulation journal: official journal of the Japanese Circulation Society.* 2013;77:652-660.

[50] Kubo T, Imanishi T, Takarada S, et al. Assessment of culprit lesion morphology in acute myocardial infarction: ability of optical coherence tomography compared with intravascular ultrasound and coronary angioscopy. *J. Am. Coll. Cardiol.* Sep 4 2007;50:933-939.

[51] Maehara A, Mintz G, Witzenbichler B, et al. IVUS Predictors of Stent Thrombosis: Results From the Prospective, Multicenter ADAPT-DES Study. *J. Am. Coll. Cardiol.* 2012;60.

[52] Mizukoshi M, Kubo T, Takarada S, et al. Coronary superficial and spotty calcium deposits in culprit coronary lesions of acute coronary syndrome as determined by optical coherence tomography. *Am. J. Cardiol.* Jul 1 2013;112:34-40.

[53] Guagliumi G, Sirbu V, Petroff C, et al. Volumetric assessment of lesion severity with optical coherence tomography: relationship with fractional flow. *EuroIntervention: journal of EuroPCR in collaboration with the Working Group on Interventional Cardiology of the European Society of Cardiology.* Feb 22 2013;8:1172-1181.

[54] Verhoeff BJ, Siebes M, Meuwissen M, et al. Influence of percutaneous coronary intervention on coronary microvascular resistance index. *Circulation.* Jan 4 2005;111:76-82.

[55] Prati F, Di Vito L, Biondi-Zoccai G, et al. Angiography alone versus angiography plus optical coherence tomography to guide decision-making during percutaneous coronary

intervention: the Centro per la Lotta contro l'Infarto-Optimisation of Percutaneous Coronary Intervention (CLI-OPCI) study. *EuroIntervention: journal of EuroPCR in collaboration with the Working Group on Interventional Cardiology of the European Society of Cardiology.* Nov 22 2012;8:823-829.

[56] Mudra H, di Mario C, de Jaegere P, et al. Randomized comparison of coronary stent implantation under ultrasound or angiographic guidance to reduce stent restenosis (OPTICUS Study). *Circulation.* Sep 18 2001;104:1343-1349.

[57] Fitzgerald PJ, Oshima A, Hayase M, et al. Final results of the Can Routine Ultrasound Influence Stent Expansion (CRUISE) study. *Circulation.* Aug 1 2000;102:523-530.

[58] Hou J, Qi H, Zhang M, et al. Development of lipid-rich plaque inside bare metal stent: possible mechanism of late stent thrombosis? An optical coherence tomography study. *Heart.* Aug 2010;96:1187-1190.

[59] Barlis P, Regar E, Serruys PW, et al. An optical coherence tomography study of a biodegradable vs. durable polymer-coated limus-eluting stent: a LEADERS trial sub-study. *Eur. Heart J.* Jan 2010;31:165-176.

[60] Gonzalo N, Escaned J, Alfonso F, et al. Morphometric assessment of coronary stenosis relevance with optical coherence tomography: a comparison with fractional flow reserve and intravascular ultrasound. *J. Am. Coll. Cardiol.* Mar 20 2012;59:1080-1089.

[61] Takarada S, Imanishi T, Kubo T, et al. Effect of statin therapy on coronary fibrous-cap thickness in patients with acute coronary syndrome: assessment by optical coherence tomography study. *Atherosclerosis.* Feb 2009;202:491-497.

[62] Lotfi A, Jeremias A, Fearon WF, et al. Expert consensus statement on the use of fractional flow reserve, intravascular ultrasound, and optical coherence tomography: A consensus statement of the society of cardiovascular angiography and interventions. *Catheter Cardiovasc. Interv.* Oct 6 2013.

In: Coronary Artery Restenosis
Editor: Amir S. Lotfi

ISBN: 978-1-63321-346-3

Chapter 10

Coronary CTA for the Evaluation of In-Stent Restenosis

Jaspreet Singh, MD, Amgad N. Makaryus, MD and Avneet Singh, MD*

North Shore-LIJ Health System, NuHealth, Nassau University Medical Center, East Meadow, NY, US

Abstract

Diagnosis of in-stent restenosis requires anatomic and physiological assessment of the stenosis. Compared to conventional angiography, Coronary Cardiac Computed Tomography (CTA) is a non-invasive tool that can provide valuable information to guide treatment. Over the last decade rapid advancements in acquisition technology and processing techniques have led to the utilization of Coronary CTA for quantitative evaluation of luminal area and also physiological parameters such as Fractional Flow Reserve and myocardial perfusion. In this chapter we will discuss the technical aspects of CTA, the clinical utilization, limitations and other factors that influence the use of CTA for assessment of native vessels and stents for stenosis.

Introduction

Despite advances in coronary revascularization techniques for coronary artery disease, in-stent restenosis (ISR) defined as stenosis within the stent and 5mm on either side of the stent edge, leads to patient morbidity, ischemia and need for repeat target lesion revascularization (TLR). Incidence of ISR varies from 3% to 20% for drug-eluting stents (DES) and 16% to 44% for bare-metal stents (BMS). There are number of clinical, anatomic and procedural factors that may influence the risk of restenosis after PCI. [1, 2] As described elsewhere ISR can be evaluated using multiple modalities to assess for functional and anatomic significance.

* Corresponding Author: Avneet Singh, MD. North Shore-LIJ Health System NuHealth, Nassau University Medical Center, 2201 Hempstead Turnpike, East Meadow, NY 11554. Tel: 516-296-4949, e-mail: asingh1@numc.edu.

Clinical application of Coronary computed tomography angiography (CCTA) for evaluation of ISR has been limited due to limitations of CT scan for temporal and spatial resolution especially when vessel luminal diameter is less than 3mm. But with recent advancements and application of CT for assessment of myocardial perfusion, CT is emerging as a promising non-invasive modality for anatomic and physiological evaluation for stent patency.

Historically, EBCT was used to assess for vessel patency indirectly from presence or absence of contrast in the stent lumen distal to the stent. [4] Stent related artifacts, Stent size and type, orientation, and surrounding tissue can influence the lumen visibility, thus confounding the utility of CCTA for direct visualization for ISR. [3]

Over the last decade there has been a tremendous technological enhancement with development of 16 and 64- slice CT scanners followed by newer generation dual source, 256 and 320-slice high-definition multislice/multidetector computed tomography (MSCT/MDCT) hardware with improved spatial and temporal resolution, shorter scan times, and iterative reconstruction techniques permitting more accurate detection of in-stent restenosis. [5]

Coronary Computed Tomography Technical Considerations

Modern day multislice/multidetector CT (MSCT/MDCT) techniques allow noninvasive evaluation of coronary vessels and bypass grafts. These continue to evolve as alternatives to invasive coronary angiography with respect to two main parameters: temporal resolution and spatial resolution. Modern systems provide ECG-gated acquisition with excellent temporal resolution (100-220ms) and the sub millimeter spatial resolution needed to visualize the lumen of the coronary arteries. More recent modern dual source systems have further improved temporal resolution (~80-90 ms). Conventional fluoroscopic angiography is able to acquire 30 frames per second and therefore has a temporal resolution of approximately 33 milliseconds, adequate for motion-free cardiac imaging. Currently, latest generation MDCT has a spatial resolution in the range of 0.35-0.5 mm in all three dimensions (compared with 0.16 mm for conventional fluoroscopic angiography). For all practical purposes spatial resolution of 1.0 mm is sufficient for imaging most of the coronary vascular tree, except for distal and calcified segments that require a higher spatial resolution of 0.5 mm or less. [6, 7]

Appropriateness of CT for Evaluation of Stents and Assessment of ISR

As per the ACCF/AHA/ASE/ASNC/HFSA/HRS/SCAI/SCCT/SCMR/STS 2013 multimodality Appropriate Use Criteria for the detection and risk assessment of stable ischemic heart disease, use of CCTA in symptomatic patients post PCI and asymptomatic patients post left main coronary stent has been given a “may be appropriate” indication [8].

According to the ACCF/SCCT/ACR/AHA/ASE/ASNC/NASCI /SCAI/SCMR 2010 Appropriate Use Criteria for Cardiac Computed Tomography, utilization of CCTA in patients with the evaluation of coronary stents is based on symptoms, time from revascularization, and stent size. CCTA was considered uncertain (U) with stents ≥3 mm in diameter ≥2 year post PCI. Imaging of stents in the left main coronary artery is considered appropriate (A). [9]

Artifacts in Coronary Stent Evaluation

Blooming, partial volume, and motion artifacts, and lastly patient`s body habitus can pose significant challenges in evaluating the stent patency Blooming artifact is particularly more pronounced with smaller stent diameter and metallic stent struts (Figure 1 and 2). Metal composition of the stent struts with higher atomic number causes more blooming artifact but bot as much with Magnesium. Blooming causes the stent struts to appear thicker causing inadequate visualization of stent lumen. Blooming is more prominent with overlapping stents. In the area of high density material such as stents, surgical clips and calcifications, lower energy X-ray photons are more completely absorbed than high energy photons resulting in beam hardening artifact. Increasing the spatial resolution and data filtering techniques can decrease beam hardening. Also lower tube voltage can worsen beam hardening [10].

Partial volume averaging results in a CT number that represents average attenuation of the materials within a voxel. In larger blood vessels such as aorta, partial volume artifact is limited to the vessel wall as compared to the coronary arteries where it tends to encroach on the lumen. Partial volume averaging in smaller coronary arteries can worsen beam hardening artifact and make the stent lumen more difficult to visualize. Utilizing thinner detector width and therefore greater spatial resolution on newer generation scanners can reduce this artifact. [11] Stents made of lower density material, especially magnesium appear to cause fewer artifacts. [12] Cardiac motion exacerbates blooming artifact and can be reduced by using scanners with higher gantry rotation speed, novel reconstruction techniques, and lowering heart rate with beta-blockers.

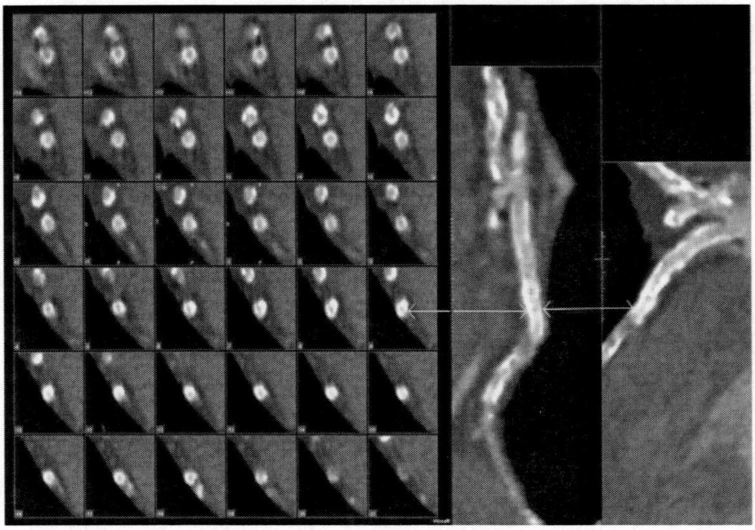

Figure 1. Coronary CTA showing images from the left anterior descending artery of a 62-year-old man with history of LAD stent. Cross sectional images (left) and the curved multi-planar reformatted images show blooming effect (arrows).

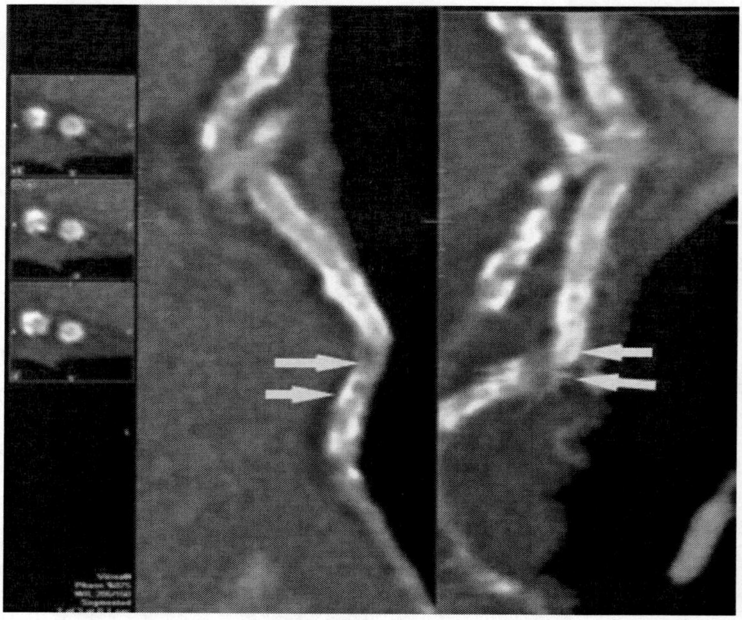

Figure 2. Blooming artifact occurs in the presence of motion artifact (arrows) limits accurate assessment of the stent lumen.

Recent Advances in CT Techniques

Current CT algorithms aim to achieve lower radiation doses in accordance with the As Low As Reasonably Achievable (ALARA) practices implemented in all imaging tests.

With the advent of prospective EKG triggering techniques and dose modulation techniques, radiation dose has significantly decreased and is nearly similar to invasive coronary angiography. [2] Prospective EKG gating techniques have shown high diagnostic accuracy in the evaluation of ISR. [13, 14] The use of iterative reconstruction (IR) techniques along with prospective gating has also allowed for reduction in radiation dose, image noise and increased spatial resolution without affecting diagnostic accuracy. [15] IR reconstruction also reduces beam hardening artifacts.

Multiplan reformatted images (MPR) and cross-sectional images of the stent are recommended to assess ISR. Adequate windowing (window width, 1500 HU; window center, 300 HU) provides better visualization of stent lumen than narrow window settings, which increase image noise. [11] Sharper edge enhancing reconstruction kernels also aid to reduce stent artifacts and improve stent lumen visualization (Figure 3) [16].

Newer research techniques employing 128, 256 and 320 multi-slice CT scanners are promising to improve image quality, reduce artifacts, especially motion artifacts secondary to reduced breath holding time, and to improve temporal resolution, lowering the radiation dose in combination with prospective imaging protocols and reduction in contrast dose [17-19].

Dual source CT (DSCT) imaging with high pitch spiral mode has also resulted in better diagnostic accuracy with improved image quality and markedly reduced radiation dosage. [20]

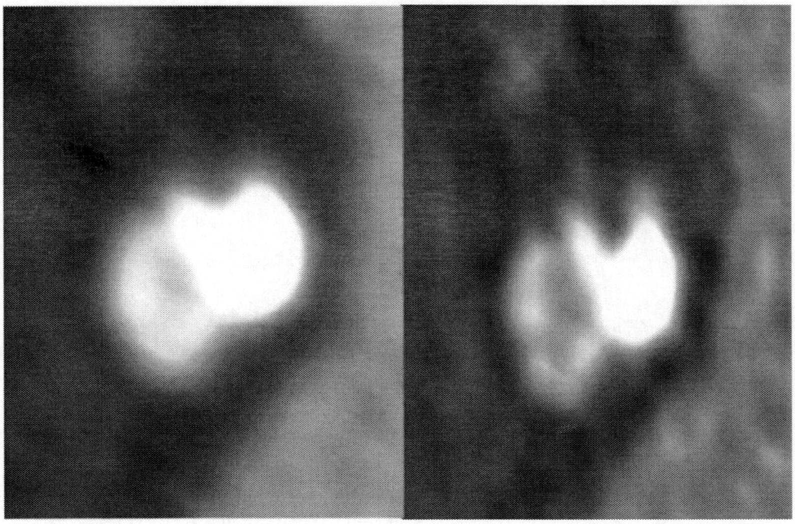

a b

Figure 3. Smooth-kernel-filtered cross-sectional image (A), obtained at the level of the yellow arrows in Figure 1, is more affected by blooming than is the sharp-kernel-filtered cross-sectional image (B).

Clinical Utilization and Literature Review in Evaluation of In-Stent Restenosis

Andreini et al. performed a meta-analyses for detection of binary ISR (>50% stenosis) from a segment-based analysis against the standard invasive coronary angiography. 4,16 and 40-slice scanners had sensitivity and specificity of approximately 90% for detection of ISR. Newer generation scanners including 64-slice and DSCT provide overall feasibility and diagnostic accuracy of 90.4% and 91.9%, respectively. [24] In a meta-analysis performed by Sun et al., the diagnostic sensitivity and specificity of 64 multislice CCTA for detecting ISR as compared to conventional coronary angiography was 90% and 91% respectively [25].

Mieghem et al. evaluated use of both 16 and 64 slice multislice CT (MSCT) in detecting left main coronary artery (LMCA) ISR. Their analysis showed sensitivity, specificity, and positive and negative predictive values of 100%, 91%, 67%, and 100% respectively for the 64 slice MSCT. This was attributed to relatively larger size of stents used in LMCA, axial plane of LMCA corresponding to scan direction and less motion artifact in the LMCA. [26] Meta-analysis performed by Kumbhani et al. for diagnostic value of 64 slice CCTA against invasive coronary angiography for detection of ISR (considered if the vessel distal to the stent was occluded or >50% in stenosis) showed a sensitivity, specificity, positive, and negative predictive value of 91%, 91%, 68% and 98% respectively. [27] (Figure 4) Presence of contrast distal to the stent may indicate stent patency, however, this finding is not specific as collaterals can allow filling of coronary arteries in a retrograde fashion.

In another study MSCT was correlated with IVUS for detecting ISR after LMCA PCI.

The study showed a good agreement for detecting ISR with a cut off value of 4.7 mm^2 for minimum luminal area on MSCT. This may represent an expanding area of indication for CCTA for post LMCA PCI patients (Figure 5, 6). [28] Similarly coronary bypass graft stents can be better visualized due to their larger size and relative lack of motion artifact [29].

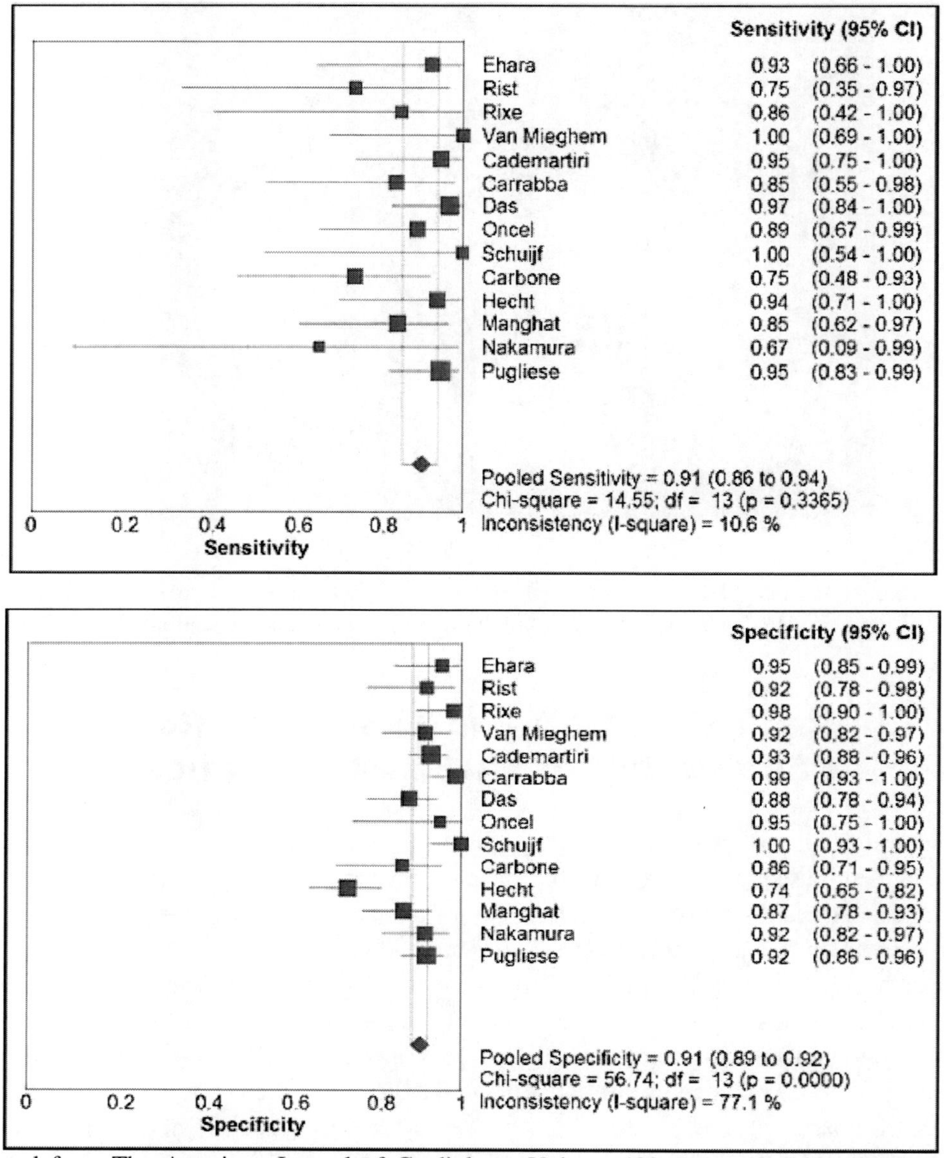

Reprinted from The American Journal of Cardiology, Volume 103, Issue 12, 2009, 1675 – 1681. Dharam J. Kumbhani, Christopher P. Ingelmo, Paul Schoenhagen, Ronan J. Curtin, Scott D. Flamm, Milind Y. Meta-Analysis of Diagnostic Efficacy of 64-Slice Computed Tomography in the Evaluation of Coronary In-Stent Restenosis, 2009. with permission from Elsevier.

Plot showing sensitivity and specificiy of 64-slice CT for diagnosis of ISR compared with conventional coronary angiography. df = degrees of freedom.

Figure 4. Meta-Analysis of Diagnostic Efficacy of 64-Slice Computed Tomography in the Evaluation of Coronary In-Stent Restenosis.

Pugliese et al. demonstrated that dual source CT (DSCT) can reliably rule out ISR irrespective of stent size, but higher false positive rate with stent size ≤2.75mm. The sensitivity, specificity, PPV and NPV in detecting >50% restenosis irrespective of stent size was 94%, 92%, 77% and 98%, respectively.

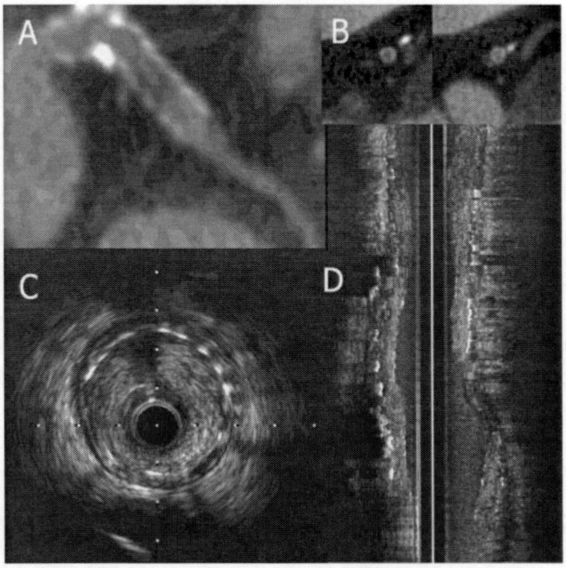

"Reproduced from [Multislice CT for assessing in-stent dimensions after left main coronary artery stenting: a comparison with three dimensional intravascular ultrasound, Gerard Roura, Josep Gomez-Lara, José L. Ferreiro, Joan A. Gomez-Hospital, Rafael Romaguera, Luís M. Teruel, Elena Carreño, Enric Esplugas, Fernando Alfonso, Angel Cequier, Heart. 2013 Aug;99(15):1106-12. doi: 10.1136/heartjnl-2013-303679. Epub. 2013 May 30] with permission from BMJ Publishing Group Ltd."

Figure 5. CCTA images showing a widely patent left main stent and with ISR respectively.

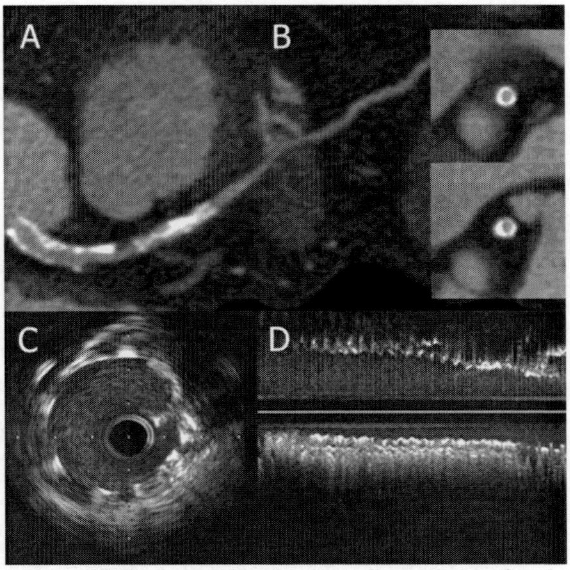

"Reproduced from [Multislice CT for assessing in-stent dimensions after left main coronary artery stenting: a comparison with three dimensional intravascular ultrasound, Gerard Roura, Josep Gomez-Lara, José L. Ferreiro, Joan A. Gomez-Hospital, Rafael Romaguera, Luís M. Teruel, Elena Carreño, Enric Esplugas, Fernando Alfonso, Angel Cequier, Heart. 2013 Aug;99(15):1106-12. doi: 10.1136/heartjnl-2013-303679. Epub. 2013 May 30] with permission from BMJ Publishing Group Ltd."

Figure 6. CCTA images showing a widely patent left main stent and with ISR respectively.

Additionally, the diagnostic performance of DSCT-CA at heart rates <70 beats per minute (bpm) did not differ significantly from that obtained at heart rates >70 bpm. The specificity and PPV of DSCT in bifurcation stenting and overlapping stents was slightly lower than those obtained in single stents. [30] DSCT in combination with prospective gating techniques and iterative reconstruction has also resulted in lowering of radiation dose.

256-slice and 320- slice CT scanners provide higher temporal resolution resulting in improved image quality, reduction in blooming, motion and stair-step artifacts, shorter scan times, reduction in contrast volume and lower radiation exposure as compared to 64- slice CT scanners. [31, 32] 64- slice High definition CT provides significant reduction in partial volume attenuation artifact with improved spatial resolution as compared to standard 64-slice CT. [33] Stent fracture is an important, yet underappreciated mechanism for ISR due to the limited sensitivity of conventional angiography and intravascular ultrasound to detect stent strut disruption. CCTA inherently provides superior image resolution and detect stent fractures that may be associated with the development of ISR and associated with adverse MACE outcomes (Figure 7). [34, 35] In-vitro study by Pang et al. demonstrated that 64-slice MDCT was more accurate than conventional cine-angiography, and IVUS for the evaluation of coronary stent fractures. [36]

Physiological Assessment of In-Stent Restenosis: Myocardial Perfusion, CT-FFR and Myocardial Tagging Techniques

Artifacts from the metallic stent struts may limit accurate assessment of stent lumen. Recent improvement in the assessment of myocardial perfusion on Computed Tomography perfusion (CTP) have shown to provide additive value in assessment of coronary artery stenosis (Figure 8).

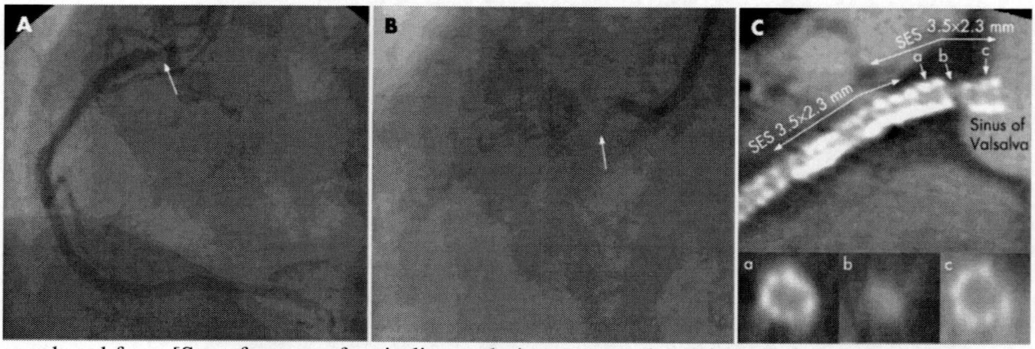

Reproduced from [Strut fracture of a sirolimus-eluting stent at the ostium of the right coronary artery, Osamu Kuboyama, Hidenobu Takei, Takeshi Tokunaga, Heart. 2007 Dec;93(12):1608.] with permission from BMJ Publishing Group Ltd] License number: 3386050911759.

Figure 7. Coronary angiography showed in-stent restenosis at the ostial lesion of the RCA (panel A) and obscurity of the stent strut (panel B). A 16-slice multidetector CT scan was performed after injection of 100 ml of non-iodinated contrast. The scan showed the strut fracture of the sirolimus-eluting stent at the ostium of the right coronary artery and protrusion of the fractured stent into the right sinus of Valsalva (panel C).

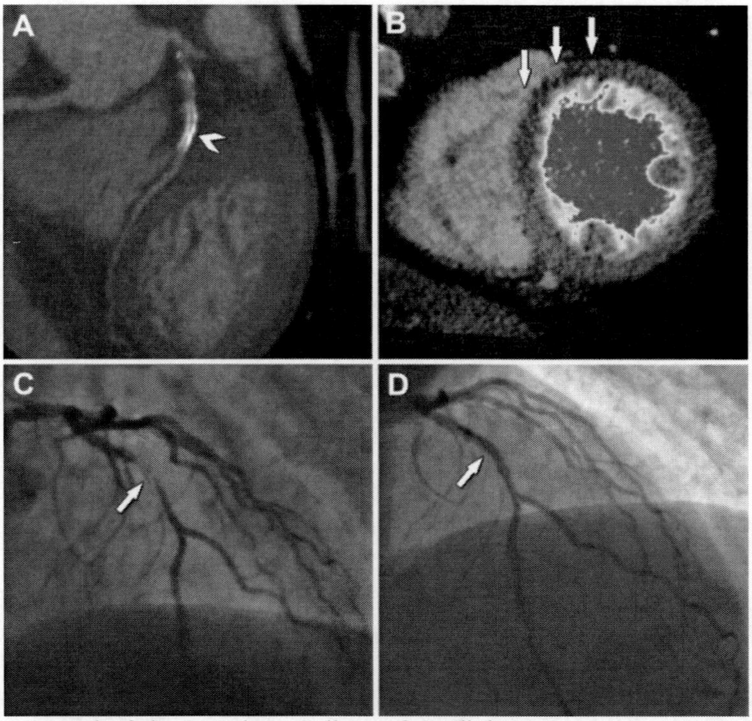

"Reprinted from Journal of the American College of Cardiology, 2013 Oct 15;62(16):1476-85. doi: 10.1016/j.jacc.2013.03.088. Epub 2013 Jun 19, Matthias Rief, Elke Zimmermann, Fabian Stenzel, Peter Martus, Karl Stangl, Johannes Greupner, Fabian Knebel, Anisha Kranz, Peter Schlattmann, Michael Laule, Marc Dewey. Computed Tomography Angiography and Myocardial Computed Tomography Perfusion in Patients With Coronary Stents: Prospective Intraindividual Comparison With Conventional Coronary Angiography, Copyright 2013 with permission from Elsevier.
LAD= left anterior descending coronary artery.

Figure 8. Coronary ISR in a 75-Year-Old Man With a 3-mm Stent in LAD. (A) Nondiagnostic CTA was performed because of artifacts related to metallic stent material (arrowhead), which were pronounced because of the small stent diameter and precluded identification of ISR. (B) CTP in the cardiac short axis identifies stress-induced anteroseptal myocardial ischemia(arrows) resulting from 80% coronary ISR confirmed on CCA (arrow in C). (D) During the same invasive angiography, percutaneous coronary intervention with drug-eluting balloon was performed (arrow).

Similar to nuclear perfusion imaging, the myocardial perfusion assessment utilizing quantitative and qualitative methods for evaluating iodinated contrast enhancement in the segments supplied by stenotic vessels, has been shown to correlate with physiologically significant lesions when assessed by FFR on invasive angiography M. Rielf et al. used CCTA/CTP in patient population suspected to have ISR and correlated results of CT with coronary angiography.

They demonstrated that using CCTA/CTP in combination had sensitivity and specificity of 78% and 90%, respectively, versus 56% ($p = 0.13$) and 78% ($p < 0.001$) for CCTA alone with associated significant reduction in non-diagnostic tests [38].

Stress CT myocardial perfusion has been found to have higher sensitivity in predicting ISR rather than anatomical CCTA evaluation only. Studies were performed for both native CAD and ISR using stress agents commonly used in nuclear cardiology [39].

Recently there has been interest in calculation of FFR from CCTA based on the principles of blood flow dynamics and meticulous but time-consuming computation to derive FFR from non-invasive CCTA images. In two large multi-center trials including DISCOVER-FLOW and DEFACTO, FFRct added significant value in determining severity of coronary artery stenosis. [40-42] Another emerging technique for physiological assessment of coronary stenosis is transluminal contrast attenuation gradient (TAG). This technique utilizes the difference in contrast opacification at evenly placed region of interests along the length of the coronary vessel and comparative analysis of contrast opacification (Hounsfield units) to compute severity of stenosis reported as TAG. [43] *At this time the application of FFRct and TAG for ISR is limited as current evidence is based on native vessel disease and patients with prior revascularization were excluded.* But these may find wider application in the future to provide us with physiologically significant information about stenosis.

Emerging Utilization for Newer Generation Stents

CCTA is expected to have a more frontline place in the assessment for ISR for the next generation bioabsorbable polymeric stents (Figure 9).

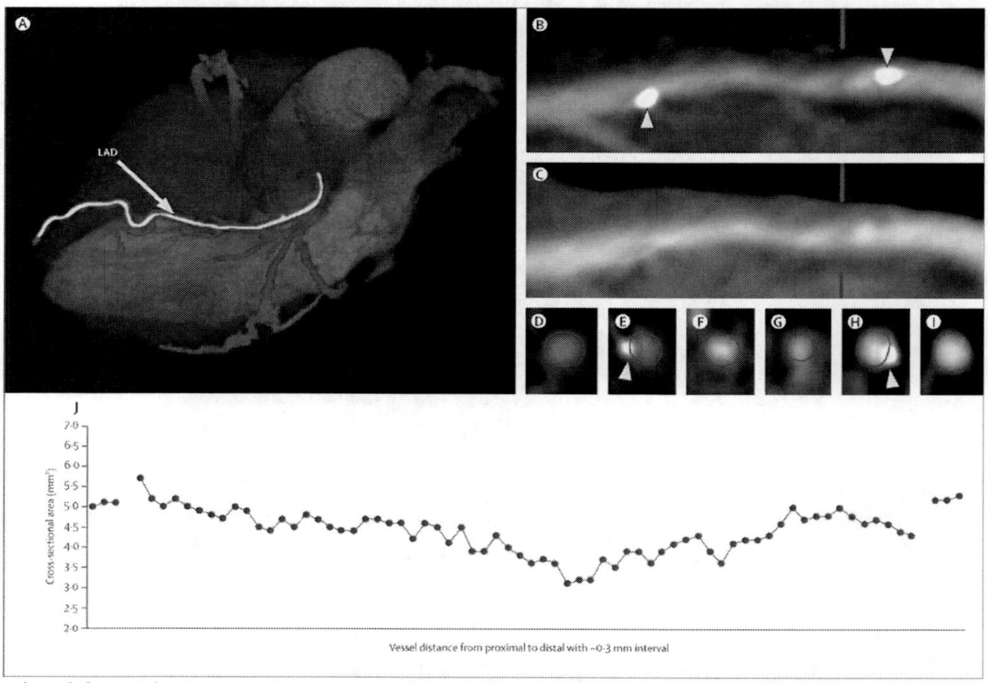

"Reprinted from The Lancet, 2009 Mar 14;373(9667):897-910. doi: 10.1016/S0140-6736(09)60325-1., Patrick W. Serruys, John A. Ormiston, Yoshinobu Onuma, Evelyn Regar, Nieves Gonzalo, Hector M. Garcia-Garcia, Koen Nieman, Nico Bruining, Cécile Dorange, Karine Miquel-Hébert, Susan Veldhof, Mark Webster, Leif Thuesen, Dariusz Dudek. A bioabsorbable everolimus-eluting coronary stent system (ABSORB): 2-year outcomes and results from multiple imaging methods, Pages No 897-910, Copyright 2009, with permission from Elsevier."

Figure 9. Site of prior Bioabsorbable stent implantation. The stent is radiolucent and therefore undetected by multislice CT, apart from the platinum markers at each end of the stent.

In the ABSORB trial, MSCT was found to be feasible in evaluating stents at 18 months due to absence of metallic beam hardening artifact, and dissolution, and incorporation of the polylactide stent struts into the vessel wall. [44] In the future, with advent of routine clinical use of the polymeric bioabsorbable, vascular scaffold, CCTA may become a well accepted modality for the detecting vessel patency, neointimal growth and ISR.

Limitations of CT in Evaluating In-Stent Restenosis

Blooming, beam hardening and partial volume averaging artifacts still pose a significant challenge in stents, especially with diameter less than 3 mm. Current CT technology aims to overcome this by improvement in scanning hardware including multislice CT and dual source CT and development of iterative reconstruction techniques.

Use of edge enhancing convolution filters can also result in higher degree of image noise. In these cases, high degree of contrast enhancement by utilizing appropriate contrast injection parameters is essential in reducing image noise. Additionally, it may be difficult to obtain adequate imaging in patients with Atrial fibrillation and contraindications to using beta-blockers. Radiation dose in CT has been significantly lowered and is comparable to conventional coronary angiography with the development of prospective gating techniques, tube voltage modulation and shorter scan time. Prior history of severe contrast related allergic reaction and renal insufficiency may also prohibit use Iodinated contrast.

Conclusion

Advances in CCTA technology with higher spatial and temporal resolution, prospective gating techniques, iterative reconstruction algorithms, use of sharper kernels for image reconstruction, optimal contrast agents, CT stress myocardial perfusion imaging, introduction of absorbable polymer stents and lastly careful patient selection hold a promising future for the role of coronary CTA in detection of ISR despite the current challenges highlighted in this chapter.

References

[1] Stettler, C., Wandel, S., Allemann, S., et al. Outcomes associated with drug-eluting and bare-metal stents: a collaborative network meta-analysis. *Lancet* 2007;370:937-48.

[2] Schlosser, T., Scheuermann, T., Ulzheimer, S., et al. In-vitro evaluation of coronary stents and 64-detector-row computed tomography using a newly developed model of coronary artery stenosis. *Acta Radiol*. 2008;49:56-64.

[3] De Graaf, F. R., Schuijf, J. D., van Velzen, J. E., et al. Diagnostic accuracy of 320-row multidetector computed tomography coronary angiography to noninvasively assess in-stent restenosis. *Invest. Radiol*. 2010;45:331-40.

[4] Schmermund, A., Haude, M., Baumgart, D., et al. Non-invasive assessment of coronary Palmaz-Schatz stents by contrast enhanced electron beam computed tomography. *Eur. Heart J.* 1996;17:1546-53.

[5] Min, J. K., Swaminathan, R. V., Vass, M., Gallagher, S., Weinsaft, J. W. High-definition multidetector computed tomography for evaluation of coronary artery stents: comparison to standard-definition 64-detector row computed tomography. *J. Cardiovasc. Comput. Tomogr.* 2009;3:246-51.

[6] Kohsaka, S., Makaryus, A. N. Coronary Angiography Using Noninvasive Imaging Techniques of Cardiac CT and MRI. *Curr. Cardiol. Rev.* 2008;4:323-30.

[7] Otero, H. J., Steigner, M. L., Rybicki, F. J. The "post-64" era of coronary CT angiography: understanding new technology from physical principles. *Radiol. Clin. North Am.* 2009;47:79-90.

[8] Wolk, M. J., Bailey, S. R., Doherty, J. U., et al. ACCF/AHA/ASE/ASNC/HFSA/HRS/SCAI/SCCT/SCMR/STS 2013 multimodality appropriate use criteria for the detection and risk assessment of stable ischemic heart disease: a report of the American College of Cardiology Foundation Appropriate Use Criteria Task Force, American Heart Association, American Society of Echocardiography, American Society of Nuclear Cardiology, Heart Failure Society of America, Heart Rhythm Society, Society for Cardiovascular Angiography and Interventions, Society of Cardiovascular Computed Tomography, Society for Cardiovascular Magnetic Resonance, and Society of Thoracic Surgeons. *J. Card. Fail.* 2014;20:65-90.

[9] Taylor, A. J., Cerqueira, M., Hodgson, J. M., et al. ACCF/SCCT/ACR/AHA/ASE/ASNC/NASCI/SCAI/SCMR 2010 Appropriate Use Criteria for Cardiac Computed Tomography. A Report of the American College of Cardiology Foundation Appropriate Use Criteria Task Force, the Society of Cardiovascular Computed Tomography, the American College of Radiology, the American Heart Association, the American Society of Echocardiography, the American Society of Nuclear Cardiology, the North American Society for Cardiovascular Imaging, the Society for Cardiovascular Angiography and Interventions, and the Society for Cardiovascular Magnetic Resonance. *J. Cardiovasc. Comput. Tomogr.* 2010;4:407 e1-33.

[10] Horiguchi, J., Fujioka, C., Kiguchi, M., et al. Prospective ECG-triggered axial CT at 140-kV tube voltage improves coronary in-stent restenosis visibility at a lower radiation dose compared with conventional retrospective ECG-gated helical CT. *Eur. Radiol.* 2009;19:2363-72.

[11] Pugliese, F., Cademartiri, F., van Mieghem, C., et al. Multidetector CT for visualization of coronary stents. *Radiographics* 2006;26:887-904.

[12] Maintz, D., Burg, M. C., Seifarth, H., et al. Update on multidetector coronary CT angiography of coronary stents: in vitro evaluation of 29 different stent types with dual-source CT. *Eur. Radiol.* 2009;19:42-9.

[13] Sun, Z. Coronary CT angiography with prospective ECG-triggering: an effective alternative to invasive coronary angiography. *Cardiovasc. Diagn. Ther.* 2012;2:28-37.

[14] Andreini, D., Pontone, G., Bartorelli, A. L., et al. High diagnostic accuracy of prospective ECG-gating 64-slice computed tomography coronary angiography for the detection of in-stent restenosis: in-stent restenosis assessment by low-dose MDCT. *Eur. Radiol.* 2011;21:1430-8.

[15] Eisentopf, J., Achenbach, S., Ulzheimer, S., et al. Low-dose dual-source CT angiography with iterative reconstruction for coronary artery stent evaluation. *JACC Cardiovasc. Imaging* 2013;6:458-65.

[16] Ulrich, A., Burg, M. C., Raupach, R., et al. Coronary stent imaging with dual-source CT: assessment of lumen visibility using different convolution kernels and postprocessing filters. *Acta Radiol.* 2014.

[17] Andre, F., Muller, D., Korosoglou, G., et al. In-vitro assessment of coronary artery stents in 256-multislice computed tomography angiography. *BMC Res. Notes* 2014;7: 38.

[18] De Graaf, F. R., Schuijf, J. D., van Velzen, J. E., et al. Diagnostic accuracy of 320-row multidetector computed tomography coronary angiography in the non-invasive evaluation of significant coronary artery disease. *Eur. Heart J.* 2010;31:1908-15.

[19] Thai, W. E., Meredith, I. T., Seneviratne, S. Complex bifurcation left main coronary artery in-stent restenosis diagnosed with dynamic volume 320-slice computed tomography. *Heart Lung Circ.* 2010;19:684-6.

[20] Xia, Y., Junjie, Y., Ying, Z., et al. Accuracy of 128-slice dual-source CT using high-pitch spiral mode for the assessment of coronary stents: first in vivo experience. *Eur. J. Radiol.* 2013;82:617-22.

[21] Kitagawa, T., Yamamoto, H., Horiguchi, J., et al. Usefulness of measuring coronary lumen density with multi-slice computed tomography to detect in-stent restenosis. *Int. J. Cardiol.* 2008;124:239-43.

[22] Abdelkarim, M. J., Ahmadi, N., Gopal, A., Hamirani, Y., Karlsberg, R. P., Budoff, M. J. Noninvasive quantitative evaluation of coronary artery stent patency using 64-row multidetector computed tomography. *J. Cardiovasc. Comput. Tomogr.* 2010;4:29-37.

[23] Andreini, D., Pontone, G., Mushtaq, S., et al. Coronary stent evaluation with coronary computed tomographic angiography: comparison between low-osmolar, high-iodine concentration iomeprol-400 and iso-osmolar, lower-iodine concentration iodixanol-320. *J. Cardiovasc. Comput. Tomogr.* 2014;8:44-51.

[24] Andreini, D., Pontone, G., Mushtaq, S., Pepi, M., Bartorelli, A. L. Multidetector computed tomography coronary angiography for the assessment of coronary in-stent restenosis. *Am. J. Cardiol.* 2010;105:645-55.

[25] Sun, Z., Almutairi, A. M. Diagnostic accuracy of 64 multislice CT angiography in the assessment of coronary in-stent restenosis: a meta-analysis. *Eur. J. Radiol.* 2010;73: 266-73.

[26] Van Mieghem, C. A., Cademartiri, F., Mollet, N. R., et al. Multislice spiral computed tomography for the evaluation of stent patency after left main coronary artery stenting: a comparison with conventional coronary angiography and intravascular ultrasound. *Circulation* 2006;114:645-53.

[27] Kumbhani, D. J., Ingelmo, C. P., Schoenhagen, P., Curtin, R. J., Flamm, S. D., Desai, M. Y. Meta-analysis of diagnostic efficacy of 64-slice computed tomography in the evaluation of coronary in-stent restenosis. *Am. J. Cardiol.* 2009;103:1675-81.

[28] Roura, G., Gomez-Lara, J., Ferreiro, J. L., et al. Multislice CT for assessing in-stent dimensions after left main coronary artery stenting: a comparison with three dimensional intravascular ultrasound. *Heart* 2013;99:1106-12.

[29] Muhlenbruch, G., Mahnken, A. H., Das, M., et al. Evaluation of aortocoronary bypass stents with cardiac MDCT compared with conventional catheter angiography. *AJR Am. J. Roentgenol.* 2007;188:361-9.

[30] Pugliese, F., Weustink, A. C., Van Mieghem, C., et al. Dual source coronary computed tomography angiography for detecting in-stent restenosis. *Heart* 2008;94:848-54.

[31] Klass, O., Walker, M., Siebach, A., et al. Prospectively gated axial CT coronary angiography: comparison of image quality and effective radiation dose between 64- and 256-slice CT. *Eur. Radiol.* 2010;20:1124-31.

[32] Dewey, M., Zimmermann, E., Deissenrieder, F., et al. Noninvasive coronary angiography by 320-row computed tomography with lower radiation exposure and maintained diagnostic accuracy: comparison of results with cardiac catheterization in a head-to-head pilot investigation. *Circulation* 2009;120:867-75.

[33] Fuchs, T. A., Stehli, J., Fiechter, M., et al. First in vivo head-to-head comparison of high-definition versus standard-definition stent imaging with 64-slice computed tomography. *Int. J. Cardiovasc. Imaging* 2013;29:1409-16.

[34] Kim, J. S., Lee, S. Y., Lee, J. M., et al. Significant association of coronary stent fracture with in-stent restenosis in sirolimus-eluting stents. *Coron. Artery Dis.* 2009;20:59-63.

[35] Ito, T., Kimura, M., Ehara, M., et al. Impact of sirolimus-eluting stent fractures without early cardiac events on long-term clinical outcomes: A multislice computed tomography study. *Eur. Radiol.* 2014.

[36] Pang, J. H., Kim, D., Beohar, N., Meyers, S. N., Lloyd-Jones, D., Yaghmai, V. Detection of stent fractures: a comparison of 64-slice CT, conventional cine-angiography, and intravascular ultrasonography. *Acad. Radiol.* 2009;16:412-7.

[37] Ko, B. S., Cameron, J. D., Leung, M., et al. Combined CT coronary angiography and stress myocardial perfusion imaging for hemodynamically significant stenoses in patients with suspected coronary artery disease: a comparison with fractional flow reserve. *JACC Cardiovasc. Imaging* 2012;5:1097-111.

[38] Rief, M., Zimmermann, E., Stenzel, F., et al. Computed tomography angiography and myocardial computed tomography perfusion in patients with coronary stents: prospective intraindividual comparison with conventional coronary angiography. *J. Am. Coll. Cardiol.* 2013;62:1476-85.

[39] Magalhaes, T. A., Cury, R. C., Pereira, A. C., et al. Additional value of dipyridamole stress myocardial perfusion by 64-row computed tomography in patients with coronary stents. *J. Cardiovasc. Comput. Tomogr.* 2011;5:449-58.

[40] Koo, B. K., Erglis, A., Doh, J. H., et al. Diagnosis of ischemia-causing coronary stenoses by noninvasive fractional flow reserve computed from coronary computed tomographic angiograms. Results from the prospective multicenter DISCOVER-FLOW (Diagnosis of Ischemia-Causing Stenoses Obtained Via Noninvasive Fractional Flow Reserve) study. *J. Am. Coll. Cardiol.* 2011;58:1989-97.

[41] Nakazato, R., Park, H. B., Berman, D. S., et al. Noninvasive fractional flow reserve derived from computed tomography angiography for coronary lesions of intermediate stenosis severity: results from the DeFACTO study. *Circ. Cardiovasc. Imaging* 2013;6: 881-9.

[42] Min, J. K., Leipsic, J., Pencina, M. J., et al. Diagnostic accuracy of fractional flow reserve from anatomic CT angiography. *JAMA* 2012;308:1237-45.

[43] Stuijfzand, W. J., Danad, I., Raijmakers, P. G., et al. Additional Value of Transluminal Attenuation Gradient in CT Angiography to Predict Hemodynamic Significance of Coronary Artery Stenosis. *JACC Cardiovasc. Imaging* 2014;7:374-86.
[44] Onuma, Y., Dudek, D., Thuesen, L., et al. Five-year clinical and functional multislice computed tomography angiographic results after coronary implantation of the fully resorbable polymeric everolimus-eluting scaffold in patients with de novo coronary artery disease: the ABSORB cohort A trial. *JACC Cardiovasc. Interv.* 2013;6:999-1009.

Part III. Treatment of Restenosis

In: Coronary Artery Restenosis
Editor: Amir S. Lotfi
ISBN: 978-1-63321-346-3

Chapter 11

Pharmacotherapy of Coronary In-Stent Restenosis

Girish R. Sabnis[1,*], MD
and Prafulla G. Kerkar, MD, DM, FACC
[1]Fellow, Dept. of Cardiology, Seth GS Medical College & KEM Hospital, Mumbai, India
[2]Professor & Head, Dept. of Cardiology, Seth GS Medical College & KEM Hospital, Mumbai, India

Abstract

Coronary artery restenosis management continues to be challenging despite the significant technological advances. Drug eluting stents have decreased the incidence of coronary artery restenosis; however, restenosis rates are higher in more complex lesion subsets, such as long lesions, bifurcations, and small vessels. In this chapter, the use of systemic drug therapy to prevent restenosis will be reviewed.

Introduction

Recommendations for the treatment of in-stent restenosis (ISR), currently the Achilles' heel of percutaneous coronary intervention (PCI), are so far based mainly on small non-randomized patient series. A number of long-term pharmacologic approaches have been evaluated in an attempt to prevent restenosis after PCI. For many of these therapies, initial positive results in animal models and/or preliminary human studies were not confirmed in large randomized trials. No medical therapy is in current use other than dual antiplatelet therapy to prevent stent thrombosis. A major limitation to all of the trials is that none has

* Corresponding Author: Dr Prafulla Kerkar; Address: Dept. of Cardiology, 4th floor, CVTC Building, KEM Hospital, Parel, Mumbai-400012, MH- India. Phone: 91-22-2410 7636; Fax: 91-22-2414 3435; Email:prafullakerkar@rediffmail.com.

been performed with drug-eluting stents, with the exception of celecoxib, cilostazol and corticosteroids.

Medical therapy can be considered for asymptomatic restenosis not producing myocardial ischemia, in cases of angiographically proven borderline restenosis with well-collateralized distal territories, and in patients with minimal angina or without proven myocardial ischemia, especially if detected 4 to 6 months after stent implantation [1]. This approach is supported by the fact that there is rarely any progression in lesion severity after 6 months of stent implantation. Moreover, there is late angiographic improvement of minimal luminal diameter between 6 months to 3 years, while repeat interventional procedures might reinitiate the process of intimal hyperplasia and lumen loss.

Why have most of these studies been so disappointing? Of the many potential explanations, the inability to achieve adequate local drug levels has been most commonly cited. Animal studies have supported this, as efficacy is usually demonstrated only when high dosages are used (sometimes 10 times the clinical dose). Such high doses would cause systemic drug intolerance. It was the recognition of this fact that has led to the development of local drug delivery systems and drug-eluting stents. The use of oral agents in combination with standard metal stents may offer a potentially cheaper and more effective means of dealing with restenosis [2].

The following sections review the research that has been done on potential therapeutics (tables 1, 2) and explore their role in treatment and prevention of ISR:

Table 1. Potential therapeutics for coronary restenosis

A. Possibly effective

- Colchicine
- Cilostazol
- Thiazolidinedione
- Oral sirolimus
- Calcium channel blockers
- Corticosteroid therapy
- Probucol
- Celecoxib

B. Probably ineffective

- Statins
- Angiotensin Converting Enzyme (ACE) inhibitors
- Homocysteine reduction, folate therapy
- Fish oil
- Carvedilol
- Tranilast
- Trapidil
- Somatostatin analogues

C. On the horizon

- Nanotechnology
- Gene therapy

Table 2. Mechanism of action, side effects, safety, recommended dosage and contraindications of oral therapies possibly effective to prevent restenosis

Drugs	Pertinent trials	Mechanism of action	Common side effects	Recommended dosage	Contraindication
Colchicine	[3]	Antimitotic effect, anti-inflammatory effect, antiproliferative properties	Abdominal cramps, diarrhoea	0.5mg bid	Renal failure
Cilostazol	DECLARE LONG II [4] CREST [5]	Oral phosphodiesterase III inhibition with pleiotropic effects; as inhibition of platelet function and neointimal hyperplasia	Safety well established, none or minor side effects (headache)	Triple therapy (80 – 325 mg aspirin + 75 mg clopidogrel + 200 mg cilostazol) a day for 6 months	Hypersensitivity to the drug or derivations; CHF AMI
Thiazolidinedione	[6], [7], [8]	Binding to PPAR-γ, induced proliferation of vascular smooth muscle cells and smooth muscle cell migration	Respiratory infection, headache, sinusitis	30 mg/day	Hypersensitivity to the drug or derivations
Sirolimus	ORAR II [9], OSIRIS [10]	mTOR inhibition, blocking phase G1 to S of the cellular cycle and inhibiting cellular proliferation	Gum sores, angio-edema, leucopenia	10 mg loading dose of sirolimus before stent implantation followed by 3 mg + 180 mg of diltiazem/day for 14 days	Hypersensitivity to the drug or derivations
Calcium channel blockers	CAPARES [11], VESPA [12]	Vasodilatory, antianginal properties	Headache, hypo-tension, Anti – inotropic effects, pedal oedema, worsening bradycardia	Amlodipine 10 mg od for 6 months Or Diltiazem 120 mg SR for 6 months	Advanced AV block, heart failure
Prednisone	IMPRESS [13], IMPRESS 2 [14], CEREA-DES[15]	Binding to glucocorticoid receptors, resulting in the inhibition of IL-1, IL-2 and IL-6 production, impairing lymphocyte proliferation	Hypertension, obesity, hyper-glycemia, Cushing's syndrome	1 mg/kg for the first 10 days; 0.5 mg/kg from day 11 – 30; 0.25 mg/kg from day 31 – 45	Diabetes, severe hypertension, poor ejection fraction
Probucol, AGI-1067	[16], CART I [17], CART II [18]	Antioxidant properties, increasing the rate of LDL catabolism, powerful antioxidant	Nausea, headache, Reduction in HDL, prolongation of QTc	T. Probucol 500 mg bid for 6 months	Prolonged baseline QTc
Celecoxib	COREA – TAXUS [19]	Selective COX-2 inhibitor, anti-inflammatory and antiproliferative properties	Potential for adverse cardio-vascular side effects, heart failure	200 mg bid	Allergy to sulfa or NSAIDs

A. Possibly Effective

1. Colchicine

In a recent trial [3], 196 diabetic patients with contraindication to a DES, undergoing PCI with a BMS, were randomized to receive colchicine 0.5 mg twice daily or placebo for 6 months. The use of 0.5 mg twice daily was shown to reduce the angiographic ISR rate from 33% in the control group to 16 % in the treatment group. The number needed to treat to avoid 1 case of ISR was 6. Lumen area loss was 1.6 mm^2 in colchicine-treated patients and 2.9 mm^2 in the control group. Treatment-related adverse events were largely limited to gastrointestinal symptoms.

Colchicine has an antimitotic effect, obviously useful for preventing a process characterized by cellular hyperplasia, as well as an anti-inflammatory effect. This should inhibit the very important contribution of inflammation to in-stent neointima formation. Moreover, it does not seem to share the undesirable immunologic and metabolic adverse effects of other classes of anti-inflammatory agents that render them unsafe for use in patients with cardiovascular disease. This observation may prove useful in patients undergoing PCI in whom implantation of a drug-eluting stent is contraindicated or undesirable.

2. Cilostazol

Cilostazol, a phosphodiesterase III inhibitor and a potent antiplatelet agent used in the management of claudication, has been shown to be beneficial as systemic therapy in prevention of ISR in both BMS and DES. The proposed mechanisms include inhibition of platelet derived growth factor (PDGF), inhibition of smooth muscle cell proliferation with elevated cAMP and inhibition of the mitogen activated protein kinase cascade. The efficacy of cilostazol was recently studied in the DECLARE LONG II trial [4] wherein the use of cilostazol in combination with aspirin and clopidogrel in zotarolimus eluting stents for long (>25mm) native coronary lesions significantly reduced the late luminal loss, angiographic in-stent restenosis and need of target vessel revascularization at 8 months.

The CREST trial [5], showed that use of cilostazol 100 mg twice daily as an additional therapy to dual antiplatelet significantly reduced late luminal loss (0.57 mm vs. 0.75 mm) and angiographic restenosis (22% vs. 35 %).

3. Thiazolidinedione

In a randomised placebo controlled double blind study in 50 non-diabetic patients with BMS, the use of pioglitazone 30 mg daily was associated with significant reduction in angiographic ISR and late luminal loss. The experimental observations that these drugs inhibit vascular smooth muscle cell proliferation and migration and reduce intimal proliferation after vascular injury provided the rationale for assessing their effect on limiting in-stent restenosis. These benefits were seen without significant changes in blood glucose, fasting plasma insulin, or hemoglobin A1c levels [6]. Two small randomised studies demonstrated similar benefit of pioglitazone and rosiglitazone in patients with diabetes mellitus type [7, 8].

4. Oral Sirolimus

Sirolimus (rapamycin) is an immunosuppressive macrolide majorly used in management of renal allograft recipients. The potential efficacy of oral sirolimus was illustrated in the ORAR II trial in which 100 patients who underwent PCI with BMS were randomly assigned to sirolimus (6 mg loading dose before PCI followed by 3 mg/day for 14 days) plus diltiazem or to placebo [9]. Sirolimus was associated with marked reductions in primary end point of angiographic ISR (12% vs. 35% with placebo) and late lumen loss (0.66 mm vs. 1.13 mm) at nine months and in the secondary end point of target lesion revascularization (8% vs. 38%) at one year. Benefit was also noted in the OSIRIS trial in which 300 patients with ISR were randomly assigned to placebo or one of two regimens of oral sirolimus given prior to and for one week after repeat PCI [10]. At six months, angiographic restenosis was less frequent with the high loading dose of sirolimus than with either the low loading dose or placebo (22% vs. 39% and 42%, respectively). Similar effects were seen in the rate of target vessel revascularization at one year (15% vs. 24% and 26%, respectively).

However, oral sirolimus can have significant systemic side effects that do not occur with sirolimus-eluting stents. In addition, the degree of late lumen loss in ORAR II, although less than seen with bare metal stents alone, was greater than that noted in major trials of drug-eluting stents (0.66 mm vs. 0.24 mm and 0.23 mm in SIRIUS and TAXUS IV, respectively). Oral sirolimus therefore, is not approved for the prevention of restenosis.

5. Calcium Channel Blockers

Multiple trials in the balloon angioplasty era have revealed the reduced need of target vessel revascularization with use of calcium channel blockers. However their role in treatment of ISR is still uncertain. The CAPARES study [11] used Amlodipine (10 mg/day) two weeks prior to PCI (predominantly balloon angioplasty) and then four months following the procedure was shown to significantly reduce the need of repeat angioplasty. However there was no significant difference in the mean lumen diameter. In The Randomized, Double-Blind, Placebo-Controlled, Multicenter Verapamil Slow-Release for Prevention of Cardiovascular Events After Angioplasty (VESPA) Trial [12], 240 mg of sustained release verapamil significantly reduced the target vessel revascularization when given over 6 months after PCI. However, these studies could not exclude the possibility that the reduced rate of revascularization with calcium channel blockade was due, at least in part, to their antianginal effect. Another limitation of the VESPA trial is that beta blockers, which have beneficial effects in patients with coronary disease, were withheld to reduce the risk of bradyarrhythmias with verapamil.

6. Corticosteroids

The cytokines IL-1 and -6 secreted by activated macrophages are powerful stimuli for smooth muscle cell proliferation and restenosis. These are the rationale for the use of corticosteroids in clinical settings in the prevention of restenosis.

In recent years, two multi-center studies (IMPRESS I and II) were conducted with oral prednisone therapy in patients undergoing coronary BMS implantation.

The Immunosuppressive Therapy for the Prevention of Restenosis After Coronary Artery Stent Implantation Study (IMPRESS) [13] study included 83 non-diabetic patients with single discrete de novo stenosis in patients with elevated C-reactive protein (CRP) after PCI. Prednisone was given orally during 45 days after stent deployment. The major findings of this study showed that patients treated with oral prednisone had a significantly lower risk of major adverse cardiovascular events (MACE, $p = 0.0063$), TVR ($p = 0.001$) and binary restenosis ($p = 0.001$) than those allocated in the placebo group. Twelve-month, event-free survival rates were 93% and 65% in patients treated with prednisone and placebo respectively. The 6-month restenosis rate and late loss were also significantly improved with oral prednisone therapy. The same group of investigators carried out the Immunosuppressive Therapy for the Prevention of Restenosis After Coronary Artery Stent Implantation Study Multivessel

DIsease (IMPRESS-2/MVD) study [14], which included 86 consecutive patients with multi-vessel disease requiring multiple interventions with elevated CRP levels 48 h after the PCI procedure were included in the study. 43 patients received prednisone for 45 days. The major findings of this study were a significant reduction of TVR, MACE and restenosis. Event-free survival at 12 months was 93% in prednisone-treated patients vs. 69.8% in controls (p = 0.006). Both studies showed an angiographic amount of late loss of ~ 0.61 mm and these benefits in clinical outcome were sustained at 5 years of follow-up. However, these two studies had the following limitations: a relatively small sample size, high selected population, reference vessel size > 2.8 mm and the results applied only to patients with persistently high CRP levels and to non-diabetic populations. Therefore, patients at high risk for restenosis, for example, diabetics, cannot be candidates for prednisone treatment.

In the Cortisone plus BMS or DES veRsus BMS alone to EliminAte Restenosis (CEREA-DES) study [15], 375 non-diabetic patients without contra-indications to corticosteroid therapy were randomised to one of three study arms: BMS implantation (control group), BMS implantation followed by medical treatment with oral prednisone, (prednisone group) or DES. The primary endpoint was the event-free survival of cardiovascular death, myocardial infarction, and recurrence of ischemia needing repeated target vessel revascularization at 1 year, and this was significantly lower in the BMS group (80.8%) compared with the prednisone (88.0%) and DES group (88.8%, P = 0.04 and 0.006, respectively). The four year long-term analysis of the primary endpoint showed that patients receiving BMS alone had significantly lower event-free survival (75.3%) compared with 84.1% in the prednisone group (HR: 0.447; P = 0.007) and 80.6% in DES patients (HR: 0.519; P = 0.03). Prednisone-treated patients did not develop new treatment-related clinical problems. The need for target vessel revascularization remained lower in the prednisone and DES groups (13.6 and 15.2%, respectively), compared with BMS (23.2%).

7. Probucol

Small studies in humans with the antioxidant probucol were promising and were confirmed in a large randomized study [16]. Three hundred seventeen patients were treated with probucol starting 1 month before angioplasty and continued for 6 months post procedure. An extra dose of 1000 mg probucol was also administered 12 h before angioplasty. Significant reduction in restenosis rate was observed (20.7% vs. 38.9%, p = 0.003) as well as in the need for repeated angioplasty (11.2% vs. 26.6%, p = 0.009) in the probucol group. Unfortunately, unwanted side effects, such as 40% reduction in the high-density lipoprotein levels, and the prolongation of the QTc interval, led to the abandon of this pharmacological approach and probucol was not marketed.

AGI-1067 is a metabolically stable compound of probucol with proposed safer profile compared with probucol. A randomized study, the CART (Canadian antioxidant restenosis trial)-1, investigated the efficacy of AGI-1067 in 305 patients post angioplasty (stents were used in 85% of the patients) [17]. Indeed, AGI-1067 reduced the restenosis rate, although it did not prolong the QTc interval, it caused significant reduction in HDL levels varying from 4.4 to 18.7% with increasing dosages. A new trial, the CART-2 should provide a more definite answer regarding the safety and efficacy of this new compound [18].

8. Celecoxib

The selective cyclooxygenase 2 (COX-2) inhibitors have anti-inflammatory and antiproliferative properties, both of which might be useful in the prevention of intracoronary stent restenosis. In the Effect of Celecoxib on Restenosis after Coronary Angioplasty with Taxus stent (COREA-TAXUS) trial, one of the very few trials evaluating systemic pharmacotherapy in management of restenosis in PCI with DES, 274 stable patients with native coronary artery stenoses were randomly assigned to treatment for six months with either celecoxib (200 mg twice daily) or no treatment (open label) after placement of one or more paclitaxel drug-eluting stents [19]. At six months, there were significant reductions in the celecoxib group in the primary endpoint of mean in-stent late lumen loss (0.49 mm vs. 0.75 mm) and in the secondary endpoint of major adverse cardiac events that was entirely due to reduced target lesion revascularization (5% versus 15 %).

This is the first such report and must be viewed with caution given the potential for an increase in adverse cardiovascular events in patients taking COX-2 inhibitors.

B. Probably ineffective

1. Statins (HMG-CoA Reductase Inhibitors)

Statins, because of their lipid lowering properties, have been an indispensible part of treatment in patients with coronary artery disease. The 3-hydroxy-3-methylglutaryl coenzyme A (HMG CoA) reductase inhibitors competitively inhibit biosynthesis of mevalonate, a precursor of non-sterol compounds involved in cell proliferation. Their role in the management of ISR was evaluated in a few trials. However, the exact role of statins remains to be defined.

The fluvastatin angioplasty restenosis (FLARE) study [20], 1054 patients were randomized to fluvastatin 40 mg twice daily staring 2-4 weeks prior to coronary intervention versus placebo. Fluvastatin 80 mg daily did not affect the process of restenosis in patients undergoing PCI without stenting. However, a significantly lower incidence of death and MI was observed in the treatment group.

The Lovastatin Restenosis trial [21], 404 patients were randomized to lovastatin 40mg twice a day versus placebo. The results indicated lovastatin did not prevent or delay the process of restenosis in the first six months after the procedure.

2. Tranilast

Tranilast, an anti-inflammatory agent, interferes with the proliferation and migration of vascular smooth muscle cells. Tranilast was shown to be effective for the reduction of restenosis in a small angiographic trial [22]. The much larger PREvention of reStenosis with Tranilast and its Outcomes (PRESTO) trial investigated the efficacy of Tranilast 600 or 900 mg daily for 1 or 3 months for the prevention of death, myocardial infarction, or ischemia-driven target vessel revascularization (combined end point) at 9 months after PCI [23]. In about 85% of the 11,484 study patients, a stent was implanted. The primary end point occurred in 15.8% of the patients in the placebo group, and in 15.5% and 16% of the patients in the 1 month and 3 month Tranilast groups, respectively.

3. Angiotensin-Converting Enzyme (ACE) Inhibitors

The role of ACE inhibitors has been periodically evaluated in the management of restenosis with varying conclusions. The Multicenter European Research Trial with Cilazapril after Angioplasty to Prevent Transluminal Coronary Obstruction and Restenosis (MERCATOR) Study Group enrolled 735 patients [24] randomized to long-term ACE inhibition with cilazapril in a dose of 5 mg twice a day versus placebo. There was no significant decrease in the rate of restenosis over a six month period. However, in an observational study [25] of patients undergoing PCI with stenting from 1994 to 1997 with a prospective follow up period of 6 months for clinical events, it was found that ACE inhibitor usage remained significantly protective against revascularization (odds ratio[OR]0.46, $p = 0.001$). Protection was not observed in patients treated with balloon angioplasty alone during the same period (OR 1.06, $p = 0.33$), which is consistent with the results of prior randomized trials. ACE inhibitors appear to decrease late revascularization, possibly due to a reduction in restenosis after coronary stenting [26]. However, currently there is no role for ACE inhibitors to reduce restenosis in patients with coronary intervention or patients with angiotensin converting enzyme gene insertion/deletion polymorphism [27].

4. Homocysteine Lowering Agents and Folate Therapy

In a randomised study [28], 636 patients who had undergone successful coronary stenting were assigned to receive 1 mg of folic acid, 5 mg of vitamin B6, and 1 mg of vitamin B12 intravenously, followed by daily oral doses of 1.2 mg of folic acid, 48 mg of vitamin B6, and 60 μg of vitamin B12 for six months, or to receive placebo. The angiographic end points (minimal luminal diameter, late loss, and restenosis rate) were assessed at six months by means of quantitative coronary angiography. At follow-up, the mean minimal luminal diameter was significantly smaller in the folate group than in the placebo group (1.59 ± 0.62 mm vs. 1.74 ± 0.64 mm, $P=0.008$), and the extent of late luminal loss was greater (0.90 ± 0.55 mm vs. 0.76 ± 0.58 mm, $P=0.004$). The restenosis rate was higher in the folate group than in the placebo group (34.5 % vs. 26.5%, $P=0.05$), and a higher percentage of patients in the folate group required repeated target-vessel revascularization (15.8 % vs. 10.6%, $P=0.05$). Folate therapy had adverse effects on the risk of restenosis in all subgroups except for women, patients with diabetes, and patients with markedly elevated homocysteine levels (15 μmol/liter or more) at baseline.

Mild hyperhomocystinemia does not appear to be a major determinant of in-stent restenosis. It does appear, however, to be an independent risk factor for cerebrovascular, peripheral arterial disease, coronary heart disease, and for venous thromboembolic disease. It should be remembered that homocysteine-lowering therapy might have a deleterious effect in patients treated with stent implantation, with paradoxically more neointimal proliferation and in-stent restenosis, particularly in patients with a homocysteine level within the normal range. Additional studies are needed to investigate the impact of moderate to severe hyperhomocystinemia and vitamin therapy on restenosis in the era of drug-eluting stents. Accordingly, use of multivitamins for management of restenosis is not recommended until further studies [29].

5. Fish Oil

Administration of omega-3 polyunsaturated fatty acids, which possess both lipid-lowering and antiplatelet activities, has been investigated in the prevention of restenosis. Although early studies suggested a therapeutic benefit, two large randomized multicenter trials — FORT (Fish Oil Restenosis Trial) involving 551 patients and CART (Coronary Artery Restenosis Trial) involving 500 patients — found that fish oil supplementation (5 to 8 g/day) produced no reduction in restenosis (52% versus 46% for control patients treated with corn oil in FORT and 41% vs. 34% in CART) [30, 31].

6. Carvedilol

Carvedilol is a competitive, non-selective beta and alpha-1 receptor blocker. Carvedilol directly inhibits vascular myocyte migration and proliferation and exerts antioxidant effects that are considerably greater than those of vitamin E or probucol. This provided the basis for evaluation of carvedilol for the prevention of coronary restenosis. In the European carvedilol atherectomy restenosis (EUROCARE) trial [32], The maximum recommended daily dose (25mg twice daily) failed to reduce angiographic restenosis rate (23.4% vs. 23.9%), target lesion revascularization (16.2 versus 14.5), or event-free survival (79.2% vs. 79.7%) at 7 months follow up.

7. Triazolopyrimidine (Trapidil)

Triazolopyrimidine antagonizes platelet-derived growth factor (PDGF), and may therefore interfere with smooth muscle cell proliferation and migration following angioplasty.

Two relatively small human clinical trials with triazolopyrimidine showed some benefit for the prevention of restenosis (33, 34). In one, the frequency of restenosis (defined as ≥50 percent lumen loss index) fell from 40% to 24% in patients receiving triazolopyrimidine. In contrast, the TRAPIST Study, a multicentre randomized placebo controlled clinical trial of trapidil for prevention of restenosis after coronary stenting, measured by 3-D intravascular ultrasound, failed to demonstrate any benefit from triazolopyrimidine (600 mg daily for six months) in 312 patients who underwent Wallstent implantation; there was no significant difference in the primary endpoint (neointimal volume within the stent based on intracoronary ultrasound), in quantitative coronary angiographic analysis, or in clinical events [35].

8. Somatostatin Analogues

Animal studies suggest that treatment with angiopeptin, a somatostatin analogue and insulin-like growth factor (IGF)-I inhibitor, reduces lesion formation after arterial injury. However, evidence of benefit in humans is uncertain. In one trial, 553 patients were randomly assigned to angiopeptin or placebo after PCI [36]. After a one year follow-up, patients treated with angiopeptin had a significantly reduced frequency of clinical events (death, MI, coronary artery bypass graft surgery [CABG], or repeat PCI) and improved survival. However, there was no effect on angiographic findings or the rate of restenosis (37 %). In a second trial, octreotide, another somatostatin analogue, had no effect on either clinical events or restenosis [37].

C. On the Horizon

1. Nanotechnology

Potential developments with nanotechnology include experimental transport vehicles for therapeutic agents which may be used in the near future with immunosuppressive drugs to enhance their local vessel wall concentration. New agents systemically delivered after stent implantation will have the potential to reduce the required level of active immunosuppressive agents, thereby improving the safety profile of these devices and lowering the overall toxicity associated with the higher levels of anti-proliferative drugs as in current formulations. A promising approach to inhibit restenosis is the controlled release of paclitaxel [38]. Paclitaxel, a very potent anti-proliferative and lipohilic drug that binds to the β-subunits of tubulin, promotes the formation of extremely stable and non-functional microtubule bundles and, therefore, it is an attractive method to form nanoparticles. Various types of biodegradable polymers have been used to formulate sustained release nanoparticles. Local administration of paclitaxel nanoparticles in preclinical animal studies was associated with a significant decrease in neointimal formation [39]. These findings support the rationale for the design of colloidal drug delivery systems based on biodegradable nanoparticles, which offer attractive features for the prevention of restenosis after angioplasty. In the first ever In-Human clinical trial using nanotechnology for the delivery of Paclitaxel, the SNAPIST – I study, 23 patients undergoing stenting of a single de novo lesion at least 3 mm in diameter were treated with a novel 130 nm, albumin-bound particle form of paclitaxel (nab-paclitaxel) in various dosages (10, 30, 70, or 100 mg/ m^2 intravenously) [40]. No significant adverse events were attributable to nab-paclitaxel at 10 or 30 mg/ m^2. Doses of 70 mg/ m^2 or higher were considered unacceptable due to moderate neutropenia, moderate sensory neuropathy, and mild to moderate, reversible alopecia. No MACE was reported at 2 months. At 6 months, 4 target lesion revascularizations (TLR) for restenosis were reported (2 each in the 10- and 100-mg/ m^2-dose groups). However, the long-term effects of studied nanoparticle formulations are not known and further studies are required.

2. Gene Therapy

The expression profile of a large number of known genes was identified in human in-stent restenotic tissue at the time of revascularization. This raises the possibility that key mediators of neointimal formation are upregulated in ISR and can be systematically targeted with gene-specific strategies.

Nucleic acid-based drugs provide novel therapeutic options for the treatment of restenosis as well as other conditions [41]. The broad principal behind nucleic acid-based drugs is to specifically target and inhibit a regulatory gene that plays an important role in a pathogenic process, classically by creating a molecule of ribonucleic acid (RNA) or DNA that undergoes complementary base pairing with its endogenous target.

Gene transfer is defined as the direct introduction of a desirable gene into a local environment, with the aim of increasing the function of that gene to gain pathophysiologic benefit. These genes have been selected to attempt modification of a number of processes focusing on smooth muscle proliferation but including cell migration, thrombosis and endothelial function. Animal studies have shown a generally consistent effect in the order of 30% to 70% inhibition of NI formation. Delivery agents include adenoviruses, naked plasmid DNA and recently DNA-Eluting polylactic-polyglycolic acid-coated stent. In particular, transfer of the vascular endothelial growth factor (VEGF) gene may stimulate endothelial repair, which in turn improves coronary physiology through release of nitric oxide and prostaglandin I 2, ultimately resulting in lower incidence of subacute thrombosis and intimal thickening [42]. However, studies are still at an early stage for any recommendation.

Conculsion

In conclusion, is there a potential role for systemic anti-restenotic therapy today? Given the superior performance of current DES platforms, there is no evidence that systemic approaches alone have a bright future for the prevention of restenosis, provided no concerns exist about the long term safety and performance of DES. However, a synergistic inhibitory effect on restenosis may become apparent, especially in high-risk patients, when both therapeutic strategies (local and systemic) are combined, targeting different mechanisms of neointima formation. This hypothesis must be confirmed by randomized trials. Also, if an oral agent were effective, it would allow more flexibility in the choice of the type of stent to be used. It could even be used as an adjunct in very high risk cases or in recurrent restenosis. From the current perspective and based on the experience of more than two decades of intensive research on restenosis therapy, it appears unlikely that systemic pharmacotherapy will challenge the performance of DES within the foreseeable future.

References

[1] Hoffmann R, Mintz GS. Coronary in-stent restenosis — predictors, treatment and prevention. *European Heart Journal* 2000; 21: 1739–49.

[2] Faxon D P. Systemic Drug Therapy for Restenosis: "Déjà Vu All Over Again". *Circulation* 2002;106:2296-8.

[3] Deftereos S, Giannopoulos G, Raisakis K, et al. Colchicine Treatment for the Prevention of Bare-Metal Stent Restenosis in Diabetic Patients. *J Am Coll Cardiol* 2013; 61(16):1679-85.

[4] Lee SW, Park SW, Kim YH, et al. A randomized, double-blind, multicenter comparison study of triple antiplatelet therapy with dual antiplatelet therapy to reduce restenosis after drug-eluting stent implantation in long coronary lesions: results from the DECLARE-LONG II (Drug-Eluting Stenting Followed by Cilostazol Treatment Reduces Late Restenosis in Patients with Long Coronary Lesions) trial. *J Am Coll Cardiol* 2011; 57:1264.

[5] Douglas JS Jr, Holmes DR Jr, Kereiakes DJ, et al. Coronary stent restenosis in patients treated with cilostazol. *Circulation* 2005; 112:2826.

[6] Marx N, Wöhrle J, Nusser T, et al. Pioglitazone reduces neointima volume after coronary stent implantation: a randomized, placebo-controlled, double-blind trial in nondiabetic patients. *Circulation* 2005; 112:2792.

[7] Nishio K, Sakurai M, Kusuyama T, et al. A randomized comparison of pioglitazone to inhibit restenosis after coronary stenting in patients with diabetes mellitus type. *Diabetes Care.* 2006; 29(1):101.

[8] Choi D, Kim SK, Choi SH, et al. Preventative effects of rosiglitazone on restenosis after coronary stent implantation in patients with diabetes mellitus type. *Diabetes Care* 2004; 27(11):2654.

[9] Rodriguez AE, Granada JF, Rodriguez-Alemparte M, et al. Oral rapamycin after coronary bare-metal stent implantation to prevent restenosis: the Prospective, Randomized Oral Rapamycin in Argentina (ORAR II) Study. *J Am Coll Cardiol.* 2006 Apr 18;47(8):1522-9.

[10] Hausleiter J1, Kastrati A, Mehilli J, Vogeser M, et al. Randomized, double-blind, placebo-controlled trial of oral sirolimus for restenosis prevention in patients with in-stent restenosis: the Oral Sirolimus to Inhibit Recurrent In-stent Stenosis (OSIRIS) trial. *Circulation.* 2004 Aug 17;110(7):790-5.

[11] Jørgensen B1, Simonsen S, Endresen K, et al. Restenosis and clinical outcome in patients treated with amlodipine after angioplasty: results from the Coronary AngioPlasty Amlodipine REStenosis Study (CAPARES). *J Am Coll Cardiol.* 2000 Mar 1;35(3):592-9.

[12] Bestehorn HP, Neumann FJ, Büttner HJ, et al. Evaluation of the effect of oral verapamil on clinical outcome and angiographic restenosis after percutaneous coronary intervention: the randomized, double-blind, placebo-controlled, multicenter Verapamil Slow-Release for Prevention of Cardiovascular Events After Angioplasty (VESPA) Trial. *J Am Coll Cardiol* 2004;43:2160 –5.

[13] Versaci F, Gaspardone A, Tomai F, et al. Immunosuppressive Therapy for the Prevention of Restenosis after Coronary Artery Stent Implantation (IMPRESS Study). *J Am Coll Cardiol* 2002; 40:1935.

[14] Ribichini F, Tomai F, Ferrero V, et al. Immunosuppressive oral prednisone after percutaneous interventions in patients with multi-vessel coronary artery disease. The IMPRESS-2/MVD study. *EuroIntervention* 2005;2:173-80

[15] Ribichini F, Tomai F, Pesarini G, et al. Long-term clinical follow-up of the multicentre, randomized study to test immunosuppressive therapy with oral prednisone for the prevention of restenosis after percutaneous coronary interventions: Cortisone plus BMS or DES veRsus BMS alone to EliminAte Restenosis (CEREA-DES). *Eur Heart J* 2013; 34:1740.

[16] Tardif JC, Cote G, Lesperance J, et al. Probucol and multivitamins in the prevention of restenosis after coronary angioplasty. Multivitamins and Probucol Study Group. *N Engl J Med* 1997;337:365-72.

[17] Tardif JC, Gregoire J, Schwartz L, et al. Effects of AGI-1067 and probucol after percutaneous coronary interventions. *Circulation* 2003;107:552-58.

[18] Tardif JC. Antioxidants and atherosclerosis: emerging drug therapies. *Curr Atheroscler Rep.* 2005;7(1):71-7.

[19] Koo BK, Kim YS, Park KW, et al. Effect of celecoxib on restenosis after coronary angioplasty with a Taxus stent (COREA-TAXUS trial): an open-label randomised controlled study. *Lancet* 2007; 370:567.

[20] Weintraub WS, Boccuzzi SJ, Klein JL, et al. Lack of effect of lovastatin on restenosis after coronary angioplasty. Lovastatin Restenosis Trial Study Group. *N Engl J Med* 1994; 331:1331.

[21] Serruys PW, Foley DP, Jackson G, et al. A randomized placebo-controlled trial of fluvastatin for prevention of restenosis after successful coronary balloon angioplasty;

final results of the fluvastatin angiographic restenosis (FLARE) trial. *Eur Heart J* 1999; 20:58.

[22] 22. Tamai H, Katoh 0, Suzuki S, et al. Impact of tranilast on restenosis after coronary angioplasty: tranilast restenosis following angioplasty trial (TREAT). *Am Heart J* 1999; 138:968-975.

[23] Holmes DR, Jr, Savage M, LaBlanche JM, et al. Results of Prevention of Restenosis with Tranilast and its Outcomes (PRESTO) trial. *Circulation* 2002;106:1243-1250.

[24] MERCATOR Study Group. Does the new angiotensin converting enzyme inhibitor cilazapril prevent restenosis after percutaneous transluminal coronary angioplasty? Results of the MERCATOR study: a multicenter, randomized, double-blind placebo-controlled trial. Multicenter European Research Trial with Cilazapril after Angioplasty to Prevent Transluminal Coronary Obstruction and Restenosis (MERCATOR) Study Group. *Circulation* 1992;86:100–10.

[25] Ellis SG, Lincoff AM, Whitlow PL, et al. Evidence that angiotensin-converting enzyme inhibitor use diminishes the need for coronary revascularization after stenting. *Am J Cardiol* 2002; 89:937.

[26] Koch W, Mehilli J, von Beckerath N, et al. Angiotensin I-converting enzyme (ACE) inhibitors and restenosis after coronary artery stenting in patients with the DD genotype of the ACE gene. *J Am Coll Cardiol* 2003; 41:1957.

[27] (ACE (I/D) polymorphism and response to treatment in coronary artery disease: a comprehensive database and meta-analysis involving study quality evaluation *BMC Medical Genetics* 2009, 10:50 doi:10.1186/1471-2350-10-50).

[28] Lange H, Suryapranata H, De Luca G, et al. Folate therapy and in-stent restenosis after coronary stenting. *N Engl J Med* 2004; 350:2673.

[29] De Luca G, Suryapranata H, Gregorio G, et al. Homocysteine and its effects on in-stent restenosis. *Circulation* 2005; 112:e307.

[30] Johansen O, Brekke M, Seljeflot I, et al. N-3 fatty acids do not prevent restenosis after coronary angioplasty: results from the CART study. Coronary Angioplasty Restenosis Trial. *J Am Coll Cardiol* 1999; 33:1619.

[31] Do fish oils prevent restenosis after coronary angioplasty? Leaf A, Jorgensen MB, Jacobs AK, Cote G, Schoenfeld DA, Scheer J, Weiner BH, Slack JD, Kellett MA, Raizner AE. *Circulation* 1994;90(5):2248.

[32] Serruys PW, Foley DP, Höfling B, et al. Carvedilol for prevention of restenosis after directional coronary atherectomy: final results of the European carvedilol atherectomy restenosis (EUROCARE) trial. *Circulation* 2000; 101:1512.

[33] Okamoto S, Inden M, Setsuda M, et al. Effects of trapidil (triazolopyrimidine), a platelet-derived growth factor antagonist, in preventing restenosis after percutaneous transluminal coronary angioplasty. *Am Heart J* 1992; 123:1439.

[34] Maresta A, Balducelli M, Cantini L, et al. Trapidil (triazolopyrimidine), a platelet-derived growth factor antagonist, reduces restenosis after percutaneous transluminal coronary angioplasty. Results of the randomized, double-blind STARC study. Studio Trapidil versus Aspirin nella Restenosi Coronarica. *Circulation* 1994; 90:2710.

[35] Serruys PW, Foley DP, Pieper M, et al. The TRAPIST Study. A multicentre randomized placebo controlled clinical trial of trapidil for prevention of restenosis after coronary stenting, measured by 3-D intravascular ultrasound. *Eur Heart J* 2001; 22:1938.

[36] Emanuelsson H, Beatt KJ, Bagger JP, et al. Long-term effects of angiopeptin treatment in coronary angioplasty. Reduction of clinical events but not angiographic restenosis. European Angiopeptin Study Group. *Circulation* 1995; 91:1689.

[37] von Essen R, Ostermaier R, Grube E, et al. Effects of octreotide treatment on restenosis after coronary angioplasty: results of the VERAS study. VErringerung der Restenoserate nach Angioplastie durch ein Somatostatin-analogon. *Circulation* 1997; 96:1482.

[38] Kholodgi FD, John M, Khurana C, et al. Sustained reduction of in stent neointimal growth with the use of the novel systemic nanoparticle of paclitaxel. *Circulation* 2002;106:1195-8.

[39] Westedt U, Kalinowski M, Wittmar M, et al. Poly(vinyl alcohol)-graft-poly (lactide-co-glycolide) nanoparticles for local delivery of paclitaxel for restenosis treatment. *J Control Release* 2007;119(1):41-51.

[40] Margolis J, McDonald J, Heuser R, et al. Systemic nanoparticle paclitaxel (nab-paclitaxel) for in-stent restenosis I (SNAPIST-I): a first-in-human safety and dose-finding study. *Clin Cardiol* 2007;30(4):165-70.

[41] Santiago FS, Khachigian LM. Evolution of nucleic acids as gene specific targeting agents. *J Mol Med* 2001;79(12):695-706.

[42] Van Belle E, Tio FO, Couffinhal T, et al. Stent endothelialisation: Time course, impact of local catheter delivery, feasibility of recombinant protein administration, and response to cytokine expedition. *Circulation* 1997: 95: 438-448.

In: Coronary Artery Restenosis
Editor: Amir S. Lotfi
ISBN: 978-1-63321-346-3

Chapter 12

Interventional Treatment of Restenosis

Larry S. Dean, MD*
Professor of Medicine and Surgery
University of Washington School of Medicine, US

Abstract

Coronary stents were introduced into clinical practice in the mid 1990s. Major advances in stent and device technology have enabled interventional cardiologist to treat complex coronary lesions. However restenosis continues to be a limitation impacting interventional cardiologist. In this chapter interventional approaches to treat coronary restenosis will be reviewed.

Introduction

Since the first description of coronary intervention by Gruentzig in 1977 [1] the procedure has been hampered by recurrence, either clinically defined typically by target vessel revascularization or angiographically as more than a 50% stenosis in the treated vessel. Initially the mechanisms were poorly understood but later known to result from intimal proliferation and a combination of elastic recoil and negative remodeling which are addressed in more detail in other chapters. Although it took many years to address these mechanisms, many of those years were spent trying to find a single approach to treat, in retrospect, a very complex process. To understand subsequent approaches to restenosis it is first necessary to briefly review the basic mechanism for vessel failure. For a more detailed review please see other appropriate chapters.

* Corresponding Author: Larry S. Dean, MD, Professor of Medicine and Surgery, University of Washington School of Medicine, US 1959 NE Pacific St. Seattle, WA 98195 lsdean@uw.edu.

Review of the Mechanisms of Restenosis

Following the barotrauma of balloon angioplasty elastic recoil of the treated segment begins almost immediately leading to early loss of a portion of the acute gain. The trauma also sets up the biologic process of wound healing that ultimately leads to intimal proliferation and scarring which produces contracture of the vessel known as negative remodeling. Although repeat balloon angioplasty (BA) was initially the only available treatment for vessel failure, many non-balloon based therapies were developed and tried over the early years, all leading to late failure of varying degrees. This dramatically changed with the advent of coronary stents. However the use of stents led to a "new disease" process with late loss of the initial gain due to instent restenosis (ISR).

Patterns of Restenosis

While this has been reviewed elsewhere it is important to remember that previous reports have suggest the pattern of ISR has an important impact on subsequent outcome, especially when target lesion revascularization (TLR) is assessed as the outcome variable with more focal instent lesions generally having lower recurrence rates [2,3]. This has been the case with both BMS and DES ISR.

Approaches to ISR

The single best approach to the interventional treatment of restenosis remains somewhat unclear especially ISR following DES restenosis. Many approaches, over the history of intervention have been tried but despite this the dominant choice remains elusive and several options remain as outlined in Figure 1. Interestingly it is unlikely we will ever have a device and or drug that result in an outcome of no restenosis or TLR. Why might this be? Because, as I was reminded many years ago by a prominent internationalist, restenosis is a form of wound healing and in order to survive as a species we must have multiple pathways to call on to heal a wound. Therefore it is likely that as we suppress one pathway another will be up regulated to heal the wound. It is also interesting to note that ISR in BMS may respond differently than that seen in DES restenosis [4]. The reasons for this are not clear but there is some evidence that the pathology of the restenotic process may be different [5]. What follows is a general review of the various approaches to ISR however it does not include a discussion of the use of bypass surgery as an option, which is beyond the scope of this review. That said it remains a viable option in the symptomatic patient with either multiple episodes of ISR or in those with multi-vessel disease and restenosis.

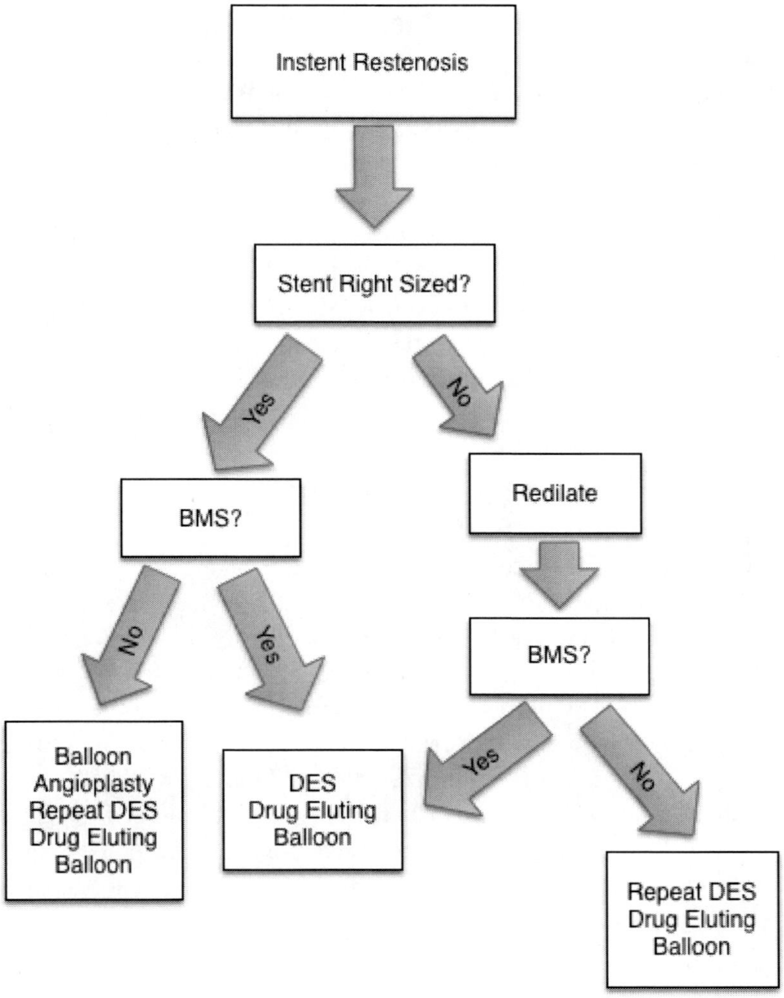

Figure 1. General approach to instent restenosis.

Repeat Balloon Intervention

The literature surrounding BA of restenosis following prior BA is becoming very aged but clearly showed superiority of BMS in restenotic lesions following BA [6]. The use of BA following ISR was an early approach to ISR [7] but re-stenting with BMS in patients with BMS restenosis has been shown to yield improved results when compared to BA alone [8]. In this study of 52 patients with ISR following BMS stenting, while the initial result was good, the restenosis rate at 6 months was very high at 54%. Contemporary use of BA alone for ISR should probably be relegated to individual patient and lesion characteristics, e.g. focal ISR in a patient at higher risk of bleeding complications with prolonged DAPT or evidence of stent under expansion by IVUS.

Bare Metal Stenting

There are several studies examining the outcomes of BMS use for instent restenosis in patients who have received a previous BMS [2,9]. With the advent of DES most studies are comparisons of BMS vs. DES and uniformly show superiority of DES over BMS for BMS restenosis [10-12]. In the Dibra, et al. [10] meta-analysis of 1230 patients, TLR and angiographic restenosis were both markedly lower with the use of DES vs. BMS (OR 0.35, 95% CI 0.25 to 0.49; $p < 0.001$ and OR 0.36, 95% CI 0.27 to 0.49; $p < 0.001$, respectively). Therefore the use of BMS to treat either BMS or DES ISR should probably be relegated to the unusual clinical scenario of a patient who is not a candidate for dual antiplatelet therapy due to concerns over an excessive risk of bleeding.

Athroablation

Athroablative techniques include rotational and laser atherectomy. While both deliver acceptable acute angiographic results, they have not been shown to have a significant impact on clinical outcome in patients with BMS restenosis [13,14]. In the randomized ARTIST trial [13] 298 patients with ISR were treated with rotational atherectomy vs. BA with minimal luminal diameter at 6 months being the primary endpoint. Restenosis rates were lower in the BA group at 51% vs. 65%, $p = 0.039$, in the rotational atherectomy group. Six-month event free survival was also higher in the BA group (91.3% vs. 79.6%, $p = 0.0052$, respectively).

Interestingly both rotational and laser atherectomy have been used in restenosis due to poorly expanded stents that cannot be expanded by balloon angioplasty techniques [15-17]. It must be remembered that there is little long-term data regarding outcome to support this approach.

Vascular Brachytherapy

Prior to the advent of DES this was the preferred approach to the treatment of BA and BMS restenosis [18-22]. The START trial [18] randomized 476 patients to receive either beta radiation or placebo as treatment of ISR. The primary endpoint was clinically driven target vessel revascularization which was 28.7% in the placebo group and 19.1% in the beta radiation group, $p = 0.024$. Eight month binary restenosis rate was reduced to 28.8% in the treated group vs. 45.2% in the placebo arm, $p = 0.001$. Its utility in treating DES ISR is not well evaluated [23].

Following the availability of DES subsequent studies clearly showed the superiority of DES for BMS restenosis vs. vascular brachytherapy (VBT) [24-27]. The SISR trial [28] showed clear superiority of sirolimus eluting stenting compared to brachytherapy, either gamma or beta radiation, with target vessel failure reduced from 21.6% to 12.4% in the DES arm of the trial. From a technical and logistical standpoint the use of a beta radiation source is easier than a gamma source in most catheterization labs.

The use of VBT may have some utility in patients who have had ISR and failed stenting with a DES. The data to support the use of VBT in this patient population, however, is quite limited and the appropriate approach to such patients remains unknown. [29] One must also recall that coronary bypass remains a viable option in patients with multiple episodes of ISR.

Drug Eluting Stents

The data on approaches to DES restenosis is unfortunately incomplete with only a small number of randomized trials assessing the question [30-32]. Most data attempting to address this question, that is, the best approach to DES restenosis has been evaluated via small studies and registries [33-36]. By in large the studies have shown that DES appears superior to either BMS or BA for DES ISR. In the ISAR-DESIRE 2 trial [30] patients with sirolimus eluting stent (SES) ISR were randomized to receive either repeat SES stenting or paclitaxel-eluting stent (PES) implantation. The primary endpoint was late lumen loss, which was similar between SES and PES stenting (0.40 $\pm$ 0.65 mm vs. 0.38 $\pm$ 0.59 mm; p = 0.85). In addition, binary restenosis (19.6% vs. 20.6%; p = 0.69) and target lesion revascularization (16.6% vs. 14.6%; p = 0.52) were also similar. Safety outcomes showed rates of death/myocardial infarction (6.1% vs. 5.8%; p = 0.86) and stent thrombosis (0.4% vs. 0.4%; p = 0.99) to be similar as well. There was a higher than expected late loss in the SES arm suggesting the possibility of drug resistance with repeated us of the same drug.

The studies of DES ISR, in general, suggest that the subsequent rate of repeat ISR is higher than rates for de novo lesions. Outcome, as also seen in patients with BMS, is impacted by the pattern of ISR being worse in patients with diffuse or occlusive ISR [37]. It also appears that overall MACE is higher for DES ISR than for either BA or BMS restenosis [34,38,39]. In the e-SELECT registry [34] among 1,590 patients treated with a SES for ISR, the 1 year MACE rate was 5.7% in the BMS and 9.5% it the DES group, p = 0.016. This was driven by a higher ischemia driven TLR rate in the DES group (6.9% vs. 3.1%, p = 0.003 respectively). Independent predictors of MACE in the DES group were diabetes mellitus, post procedure residual diameter stenosis of > 20%, and treatment of bifurcation lesions with $\geq$ 2 stents. Predictors of TLR were post procedure diameter stenosis of > 20%, diabetes and total lesions treated.

The question of whether to use the same DES or a different one has not been completely answered but there are some randomized [30] and non-randomized data [40] that have evaluated such an approach. In the RIBS III trial, 363 consecutive patients with DES ISR were stented with either the same drug, BA or BMS (89 patients) vs. a different drug (274 patients) [40]. Clinical follow up at 12 months showed a lower MACE rate in the different drug group (8.9% vs. 19.1%, p = 0.01) driven by a lower TLR rate in that group, 6.3% vs. 13.5%, p = 0.03. The problem with this study is that the control arm was "contaminated" by patients receiving different therapies making it difficult to draw firm conclusions.

Many have assumed that using a stent with a different drug at least makes logical sense but the data supporting such an approach is, as pointed out, limited and inconsistent. [30,31]

Drug Eluting Balloons

One of the more exciting developments in the mechanical treatment of ISR has been the development of drug eluting balloons. Not only does the idea of using a non-stent approach to restenosis have great interest the data supporting such an approach has been impressive so far. The use of DES to treat the problem, while potentially effective, leaves yet another device in the vessel. Multiple episodes lead to multiple devices and if nothing else, leave the vessel appearing almost violated. Obviously drug-eluting balloons are more elegant, leaving nothing behind but a drug to treat the restenotic process.

In the ISAR Desire 3 study [41] patients were randomized to 3 treatment arms comparing paclitaxel eluting balloon (PEB,) paclitaxel eluting stent (PES) and balloon angioplasty with a non-inferiority endpoint of percent diameter stenosis at 6 to 8 months in patients with ISR in a previously placed limus-eluting stent. The study confirmed that PEB was indeed non-inferior to PES (diameter stenosis of 38.0% vs. 37.4% respectively) confirming the approach of PEB instead of PES (Figure 2). With respect to clinical outcomes, MACE at 1 year was reduced in both the PEB and PES groups when compared to BA, 23.5% vs. 19.5% vs. 46.2% respectively, $p < 0.0001$ for both PEB and PES compared to BA. There was no difference in MACE between PEB and PES. Of note these results my not be generalizable to ISR in non limus-eluting stents.

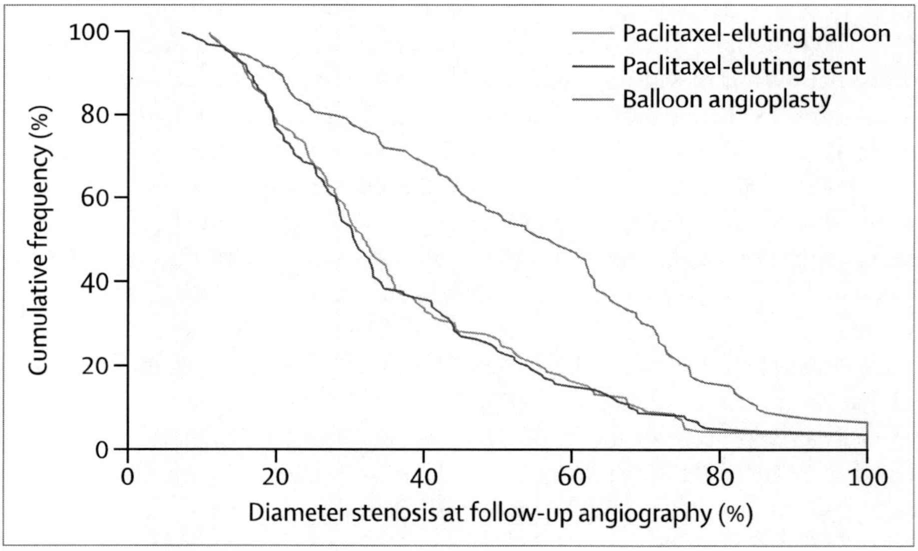

Figure 2. Cumulative frequency distribution curves for diameter stenosis by treatment group (Lancet 2013;381:461-7, used with permission).

A similar study, the PECAD-DES trial, compared PEB angioplasty or uncoated balloon angioplasty and found superiority of the PEB with respect to a primary endpoint of late lumen loss at the target lesion at 6 months (0.43 vs. 1.03 mm, $p<0.001$ respectively). Secondary endpoints included TLR and at follow up the TLR rate of 15.3% vs. 36.8%, $p=0.005$, respectively [42].

In the recently published RIBS V trial of PEB vs. everolimus eluting stents (EES) in patients with BMS ISR both PEB and EES were effective in increasing the primary endpoint of in-segment minimal lumen diameter at 9-month follow-up. However EES was more effective than PEB in this regard (2.36 $\pm$ 0.6 mm vs. 2.01 $\pm$ 0.6 mm, $p<0.001$ respectively). MACE was similar between the groups but there was a trend toward less frequent TLR in the EES group (6% vs. 1%, p = 0.09). [43]

There may be a differential effect of PEB on ISR depending on its use in BMS vs. DES with better outcomes in patients with BMS ISR as recently reported. [42,44] A recent systematic review and meta analysis containing 801 patients also suggest superiority, with respect to MACE, of PEB over BA and PES. [45](Figure 3). In addition both TLR and restenosis ($\geq$ 50% diameter stenosis) were reduced with the PEB.

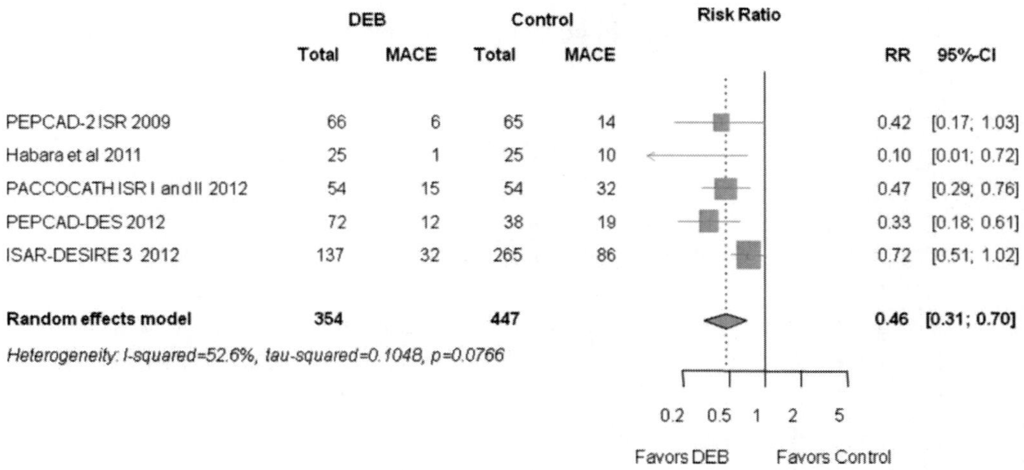

Figure 3. Forest plot of risk ratios (RR) for major adverse cardiac events.

Recommendations: As seen in the table the approach to ISR depends to some degree on the stent type but that said our best single approach, at the present time, to ISR is re-stenting with a DES. Data that continues to grow in volume seems to point to the utility of DEB as an option although that technology is not available in all countries at this time and currently has been evaluated using paclitaxel only.

Table. Relative impact of various interventional mechanical therapies on restenosis

ISR therapies	BA restenosis	BMS restenosis	DES restenosis
BA	+	+	+
Athroablation	+	+	+
VBT	++	++	+
BMS	+++	++	+
DES	++++	+++	++
DEB	-	+++	+++*

ISR = instent restenosis, BA = balloon angioplasty, Athroablation = rotational and laser atherectomy, VBT = vascular brachytherapy, BMS = bare metal stent, DES = drug eluting stent, DEB = drug eluting balloon.

* Paclitaxel only.

Conclusion

Coronary restenosis following percutaneous intervention has been an issue of some magnitude since the introduction of the procedure. Many things have been tried and many have failed to significantly impact the process. The greatest impact so far on restenosis, commonly referred to as the Achilles heel of angioplasty, occurred with the advent of coronary stenting. This addressed the issue of elastic vessel recoil that occurred after BA alone. Restenosis was further an importantly impacted with the development of drug eluting stents. However restenosis still occurs, albeit at a lower rate, and the best approach to restenosis in DES remains not yet fully addressed. Part of the problem is the endpoint used to show efficacy is typically a non-clinical endpoint due to the low event rates generally seen following contemporary coronary intervention. Perhaps the DEB is the answer but based on the body's ability to heal itself we will likely be discussing this for many years to come.

References

[1] Gruentzig AR, Senning A, Siegenthaler WE. Non operative dilatation of coronary-artery stenosis. Percutaneous transluminal coronary angioplasty. *N Engl J Med* 1979;301:61-8.

[2] Mehran R, Dangas G, Abizaid AS, et al. Angiographic Patterns of In-Stent Restenosis: Classification and Implications for Long-Term Outcome. *Circulation* 1999;100:1872-8.

[3] Cosgrave J, Melzi G, Biondi-Zoccai GG, et al. Drug-eluting stent restenosis the pattern predicts the outcome. *J Am Coll Cardiol* 2006;47:2399-404.

[4] Almalla M, Pross V, Marx N, Hoffmann R. Effectiveness of everolimus-eluting stents in the treatment of drug-eluting stent versus bare-metal stent restenosis. *Coronary artery disease* 2012;23:492-6.

[5] Byrne RA, Joner M, Tada T, Kastrati A. Restenosis in bare metal and drug-eluting stents: distinct mechanistic insights from histopathology and optical intravascular imaging. *Minerva cardioangiologica* 2012;60:473-89.

[6] Erbel R, Haude M, Hopp HW, et al. Coronary-artery stenting compared with balloon angioplasty for restenosis after initial balloon angioplasty. Restenosis Stent Study Group. *N Engl J Med* 1998;339:1672-8.

[7] Macander PJ, Roubin GS, Agrawal SK, Cannon AD, Dean LS, Baxley WA. Balloon angioplasty for treatment of in-stent restenosis: feasibility, safety, and efficacy. *Catheterization and cardiovascular diagnosis* 1994;32:125-31.

[8] Eltchaninoff H, Koning R, Tron C, Gupta V, Cribier A. Balloon angioplasty for the treatment of coronary in-stent restenosis: immediate results and 6-month angiographic recurrent restenosis rate. *J Am Coll Cardiol* 1998;32:980-4.

[9] Bauters C, Banos JL, Van Belle E, Mc Fadden EP, Lablanche JM, Bertrand ME. Six-month angiographic outcome after successful repeat percutaneous intervention for in-stent restenosis. *Circulation* 1998;97:318-21.

[10] Dibra A, Kastrati A, Alfonso F, et al. Effectiveness of Drug-Eluting Stents in Patients With Bare-Metal In-Stent Restenosis: Meta-Analysis of Randomized Trials. *J Am Coll Cardiol* 2007;49:616-23.

[11] Appleby CE, Khattar RS, Morgan K, et al. Drug eluting stents for the treatment of bare metal in-stent restenosis: long-term outcomes in real world practice. EuroIntervention: *Journal of EuroPCR in collaboration with the Working Group on Interventional Cardiology of the European Society of Cardiology* 2011;6:748-53.

[12] Beijk MA, Claessen BE, Koch KT, et al. One-year clinical outcome after treatment of bare-metal stent in-stent restenosis with the paclitaxel-eluting stent in an unselected cohort. *Int J Cardiol* 2010;145:608-9.

[13] vom Dahl J, Dietz U, Haager PK, et al. Rotational Atherectomy Does Not Reduce Recurrent In-Stent Restenosis: Results of the Angioplasty Versus Rotational Atherectomy for Treatment of Diffuse In-Stent Restenosis Trial (ARTIST). *Circulation* 2002;105:583-8.

[14] Koster R, Kahler J, Terres W, et al. Six-month clinical and angiographic outcome after successful excimer laser angioplasty for in-stent restenosis. *J Am Coll Cardiol* 2000;36:69-74.

[15] Hadjimiltiades S, Tsikaderis D, Louridas G. Rotational ablation of an unexpandable sirolimus-eluting stent. *The Journal of invasive cardiology* 2005;17:116-7.

[16] Kobayashi Y, Teirstein P, Linnemeier T, Stone G, Leon M, Moses J. Rotational atherectomy (stentablation) in a lesion with stent underexpansion due to heavily calcified plaque. Catheterization and cardiovascular interventions: *Official journal of the Society for Cardiac Angiography & Interventions* 2001;52:208-11.

[17] Latib A, Takagi K, Chizzola G, et al. Excimer Laser LEsion Modification to Expand Non-dilatable sTents: The ELLEMENT Registry. *Cardiovascular revascularization medicine: including molecular interventions* 2014;15:8-12.

[18] Popma JJ, Suntharalingam M, Lansky AJ, et al. Randomized trial of 90Sr/90Y beta-radiation versus placebo control for treatment of in-stent restenosis. *Circulation* 2002;106:1090-6.

[19] Waksman R, Ajani AE, White RL, et al. Intravascular gamma radiation for in-stent restenosis in saphenous-vein bypass grafts. *N Engl J Med* 2002;346:1194-9.

[20] Waksman R, Raizner AE, Yeung AC, Lansky AJ, Vandertie L. Use of localised intracoronary beta radiation in treatment of in-stent restenosis: the INHIBIT randomised controlled trial. *Lancet* 2002;359:551-7.

[21] Saleem MA, Aronow WS, Ravipati G, et al. Intracoronary brachytherapy for treatment of in-stent restenosis. *Cardiology in review* 2005;13:139-41.

[22] Alli OO, Teirstein PS, Satler L, et al. Five-year follow-up of the Sirolimus-Eluting Stents vs Vascular Brachytherapy for Bare Metal In-Stent Restenosis (SISR) trial. *Am Heart J* 2012;163:438-45.

[23] Thomas MR. Brachytherapy: here today, gone tomorrow? *Heart* 2005;91 Suppl 3:iii32-4.

[24] Stone GW, Ellis SG, O'Shaughnessy CD, et al. Paclitaxel-eluting stents vs vascular brachytherapy for in-stent restenosis within bare-metal stents: the TAXUS V ISR randomized trial. JAMA: *The journal of the American Medical Association* 2006;295:1253-63.

[25] Lu Y-G, Chen Y-M, Li L, Zhao R-Z, Fu C-H, Yan H. Drug-Eluting Stents vs Intracoronary Brachytherapy for In-Stent Restenosis: *A Meta-Analysis. Clinical Cardiology* 2011;34:344-51.

[26] Bailey SR. Drug-eluting stents have made brachytherapy obsolete. *Curr Opin Cardiol* 2004;19:598-600.

[27] Mukherjee D, Moliterno DJ. Brachytherapy for in-stent restenosis: a distant second choice to drug-eluting stent placement. JAMA: *the journal of the American Medical Association* 2006;295:1307-9.

[28] Holmes DR, Jr., Teirstein P, Satler L, et al. Sirolimus-eluting stents vs vascular brachytherapy for in-stent restenosis within bare-metal stents: the SISR randomized trial. JAMA: *the journal of the American Medical Association* 2006;295:1264-73.

[29] Maluenda G, Ben-Dor I, Gaglia MA, et al. Clinical Outcomes and Treatment After Drug-Eluting Stent Failure: The Absence of Traditional Risk Factors for In-Stent Restenosis. *Circulation: Cardiovascular Interventions* 2012;5:12-9.

[30] Mehilli J, Byrne RA, Tiroch K, et al. Randomized Trial of Paclitaxel- Versus Sirolimus-Eluting Stents for Treatment of Coronary Restenosis in Sirolimus-Eluting StentsThe ISAR-DESIRE 2 (Intracoronary Stenting and Angiographic Results: Drug Eluting Stents for In-Stent Restenosis 2) Study. *Journal of the American College of Cardiology* 2010;55:2710-6.

[31] Chevalier B, Moulichon R, Teiger E, et al. One-year results of the CRISTAL Trial, a randomized comparison of cypher sirolimus-eluting coronary stents versus balloon angioplasty for restenosis of drug-eluting stents. J Interv Cardiol 2012;25:586-95.

[32] Song HG, Park DW, Kim YH, et al. Randomized trial of optimal treatment strategies for in-stent restenosis after drug-eluting stent implantation. *J Am Coll Cardiol* 2012;59:1093-100.

[33] Kutcher MA, Brennan JM, Rao SV, et al. Comparative effectiveness of drug-eluting stents on long-term outcomes in elderly patients treated for in-stent restenosis: A report from the National Cardiovascular Data Registry. Catheterization and cardiovascular interventions: *Official journal of the Society for Cardiac Angiography & Interventions* 2014;83:171-81.

[34] Abizaid A, Costa JR, Jr., Banning A, et al. The sirolimus-eluting Cypher Select coronary stent for the treatment of bare-metal and drug-eluting stent restenosis: insights from the e-SELECT (Multicenter Post-Market Surveillance) registry. *JACC Cardiovascular interventions* 2012;5:64-71.

[35] Ko YG, Kim JS, Kim BK, et al. Efficacy of drug-eluting stents for treating in-stent restenosis of drug-eluting stents (from the Korean DES ISR multicenter registry study [KISS]). *Am J Cardiol* 2012;109:607-13.

[36] Meliga E, De Benedictis M, Gagnor A, et al. New drug-eluting stent implantation for recalcitrant in-stent restenosis treated with drug-eluting stents. the Stent-in-Stent Cube (SIS(3)) registry. *The Journal of invasive cardiology* 2011;23:365-8.

[37] Latib A, Mussardo M, Ielasi A, et al. Long-term outcomes after the percutaneous treatment of drug-eluting stent restenosis. *JACC Cardiovascular interventions* 2011;4:155-64.

[38] Lee MS, Yang T, Lasala JM, et al. Two-year clinical outcomes of paclitaxel-eluting stents for in-stent restenosis in patients from the ARRIVE programme. EuroIntervention: *Journal of EuroPCR in collaboration with the Working Group on Interventional Cardiology of the European Society of Cardiology* 2011;7:314-22.

[39] Abdel-Wahab M, Nienaber CA, Mostafa AE, et al. Clinical outcome of percutaneous treatment of in-stent restenosis with drug-eluting stents: results from the first phase of

the prospective multicentre German DES.DE registry. EuroIntervention: *Journal of EuroPCR in collaboration with the Working Group on Interventional Cardiology of the European Society of Cardiology* 2011;7:201-8.

[40] Alfonso F, Perez-Vizcayno MJ, Dutary J, et al. Implantation of a drug-eluting stent with a different drug (switch strategy) in patients with drug-eluting stent restenosis. Results from a prospective multicenter study (RIBS III [Restenosis Intra-Stent: Balloon Angioplasty Versus Drug-Eluting Stent]). *JACC Cardiovascular interventions* 2012;5:728-37.

[41] Byrne RA, Neumann FJ, Mehilli J, et al. Paclitaxel-eluting balloons, paclitaxel-eluting stents, and balloon angioplasty in patients with restenosis after implantation of a drug-eluting stent (ISAR-DESIRE 3): a randomised, open-label trial. *Lancet* 2013; 381:461-7.

[42] Rittger H, Brachmann J, Sinha A-M, et al. A Randomized, Multicenter, Single-Blinded Trial Comparing Paclitaxel-Coated Balloon Angioplasty With Plain Balloon Angioplasty in Drug-Eluting Stent RestenosisThe PEPCAD-DES Study. *Journal of the American College of Cardiology* 2012;59:1377-82.

[43] Alfonso F, Pérez-Vizcayno MJ, Cárdenas A, et al. A Randomized Comparison of Drug-Eluting Balloon Versus Everolimus-Eluting Stent in Patients With Bare-Metal Stent In-Stent Restenosis: The RIBS V Clinical Trial. *Journal of the American College of Cardiology* 2014.

[44] Habara S, Iwabuchi M, Inoue N, et al. A multicenter randomized comparison of paclitaxel-coated balloon catheter with conventional balloon angioplasty in patients with bare-metal stent restenosis and drug-eluting stent restenosis. *American heart journal* 2013;166:527-33.e2.

[45] Indermuehle A, Bahl R, Lansky AJ, et al. Drug-eluting balloon angioplasty for in-stent restenosis: a systematic review and meta-analysis of randomised controlled trials. *Heart* 2013;99:327-33.

In: Coronary Artery Restenosis
Editor: Amir S. Lotfi

ISBN: 978-1-63321-346-3

Chapter 13

Saphenous Vein Graft Restenosis and Management

M. Javed Ashraf MD* and James A. Grantham MD
[1]Interventional cardiologist
Truman Medical Center
Assistant Professor of Medicine
UMKC School of Medicine, Kansas City, MO, US
[2]Interventional cardiologist
Mid America Heart Institute/Saint Luke Hospital
Associate Professor of Medicine
UMKC School of Medicine, Kansas City, MO, US

Abstract

Coronary artery bypass surgery is performed in patients to improve morbidity and mortality. Saphenous vein grafts are routinely used in patients who have multivessel coronary artery disease requiring coronary artery bypass grafting. Recurrent symptoms after the first few months of the operation can occur with the development of stenosis in a bypass graft or progression of native coronary artery disease. In this chapter the pathophysiology of vein graft stenosis, treatment, and repeat treatment is discussed.

Background

After the first successful aorto-coronary saphenous vein graft (SVG) surgery in 1964 [1], coronary artery bypass graft (CABG) surgery became one of the most frequent cardiovascular surgical procedures in the USA.

---

* Corresponding Author: M. Javed Ashraf, MD, MPH, Cardiology division, Truman Medical Center, 2301 Holmes St, Kansas City, MO 64108, Email: Javed.Ashraf@tmcmed.org, Phone: 816-404-1232

In mid 1980s [2], the internal mammary artery was adopted as a better arterial conduit to the left anterior descending artery compared to veins. However, patients with multi vessel disease still needed SVG as bypass conduits to right coronary artery, left circumflex artery, major diagonal and obtuse marginal branches. Unlike the high durability and patency rate of the internal mammary artery graft, most of the vein grafts developed severe disease or occlusion over period of time. SVG have a progressive closure rate, estimated to be 12% to 20% at the end of the first year and 50% by the end of first decade [3]. The occlusive SVG disease is mainly as a result of aggressive atherosclerotic degeneration of thin-walled veins which are exposed to the higher wall stress associated with arterial pressure after implantation [4]. Clinically recurrent angina occurs in up to 10% of patients per year due to graft failure or progression of disease in native vessels requiring need for revascularization [5]. Redo coronary artery bypass graft surgery carries substantially increased risk of complications and mortality [6].

The emergence of percutaneous coronary intervention (PCI) in early 1980s offered a less invasive revascularization alternative for native coronary arteries to CABG. The success of PCI procedure lead to an explosive growth and by mid 1990s, more patients underwent PCI than CABG, and the trend has continued since [7, 8]. SVG interventions currently account for 5–10% of total PCI procedures performed in the United States [9,10]. However, the progression of SVG disease and in stent restenosis (ISR) remains a significant concern. The pathogenesis of vein graft stenosis, clinical presentation and management are discussed in this chapter.

Pathogenesis of Vein Graft Disease

Compared with native coronary arteries, SVG undergo more rapid and aggressive atherosclerotic change resulting in vein graft stenosis. Within one year, the vein graft wall is thickened as a result of diffuse intimal hyperplasia consisting of smooth muscle cells in a proteoglycan and collagen matrix [11-13]. The proposed mechanism is SVG endothelial response to injury and hemodynamic stress on the vein graft wall from distending high pressure of the arterial circulation [4, 6].

The hemodynamic change within SVG vessel leads to increased levels of intracellular adhesion molecule (ICAM)-1, vascular adhesion molecule (VCAM)-1, and monocyte chemotactic protein (MCP)-1 in the intima [14]. Subsequently, the SVG neointima is infiltrated by various inflammatory cells especially the macrophages, with varying degrees of apoptosis and necrotic core formation [15]. Compared to coronary arteries, the increased inflammatory response and cell burden ultimately leads to enhanced intimal growth, resulting in vein graft disease [Fig 1]. SVG lesions typically show larger necrotic cores than native coronaries [16].

Response of SVG Intima after Stent Implantation

The impact of stent implantation on the saphenous vein graft histopathology is poorly understood. In native coronary arteries, drug eluting stent (DES) suppress inflammatory response and smooth muscle cell proliferation, followed by incomplete endothelialization for up to 12 months or even for longer period in certain cases. In comparison, the endothelialization is usually complete within 3 to 4 months in bare metal stent (BMS) implanted coronary vessels. The SVG intima shows very aggressive response to stenting compared to native coronary arteries. Within SVG, leukocytes, platelets, and fibrin have been shown to be present at 3-14 days after stenting [17]. This results in more delayed healing in SVG than in the native coronary arteries, mainly because of a greater delay in endothelialization of vein graft.

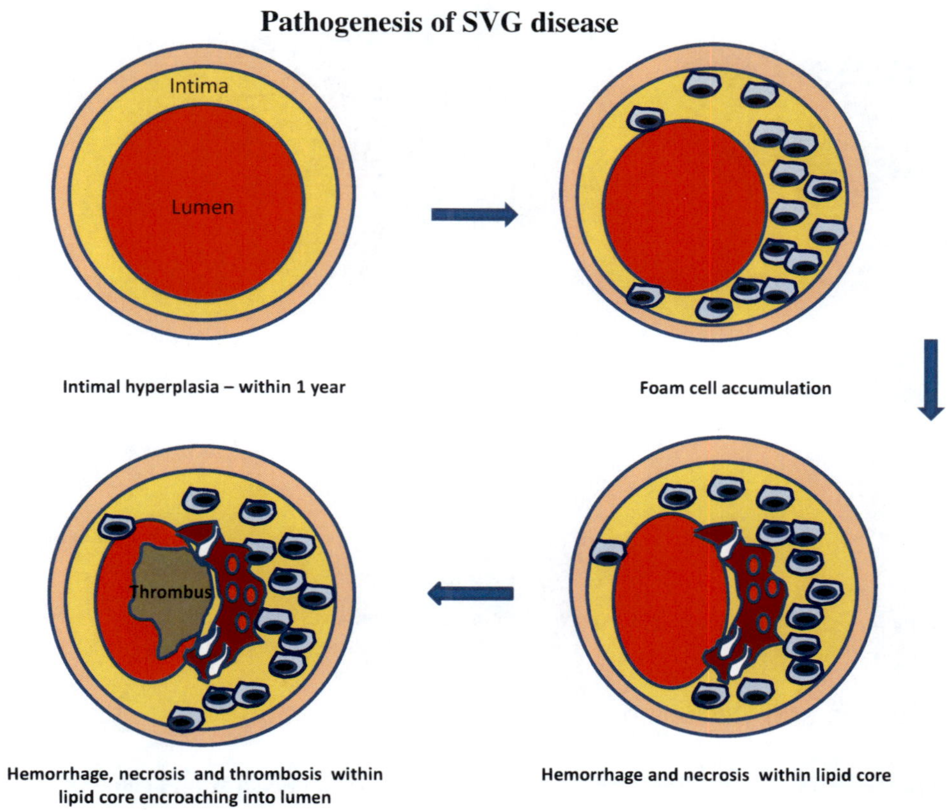

Figure 1. Pathogenesis of SVG disease.

There is a greater incidence of fibrin deposition observed in SVG stented with either DES or BMS as compared with native coronary arteries. When compared with BMS, the SVG lesions treated with DES have more uncovered stent struts and incomplete endothelialization and the trend is similar to coronary arteries [18]. As compared to De Novo lesions, the histology of SVG segment with in-stent restenosis (ISR) showed typical features of classical atherosclerosis in addition to intimal hyperplasia and contribute to increased burden of plaque [Fig. 2]. In addition to aggressive atherosclerotic plaque and fiberomuscular hyperplasia, the thrombus formation may occur several years after stent implantation in SVG. Exaggerated endothelial and intimal response after stenting of SVG ultimately causes significant in-stent restenosis in up to 30% of patients with SVG PCI. The increased rate of SVG ISR is multifactorial and either not well understood or SVG simply with its tendency to develop diffuse and aggressive atherosclerosis, makes it an ideal location for ISR. Other known risk factors for ISR in the native coronary arteries such as diabetes and diffuse disease requiring long stent, also likely to worsen the already increased SVG ISR phenomenon.

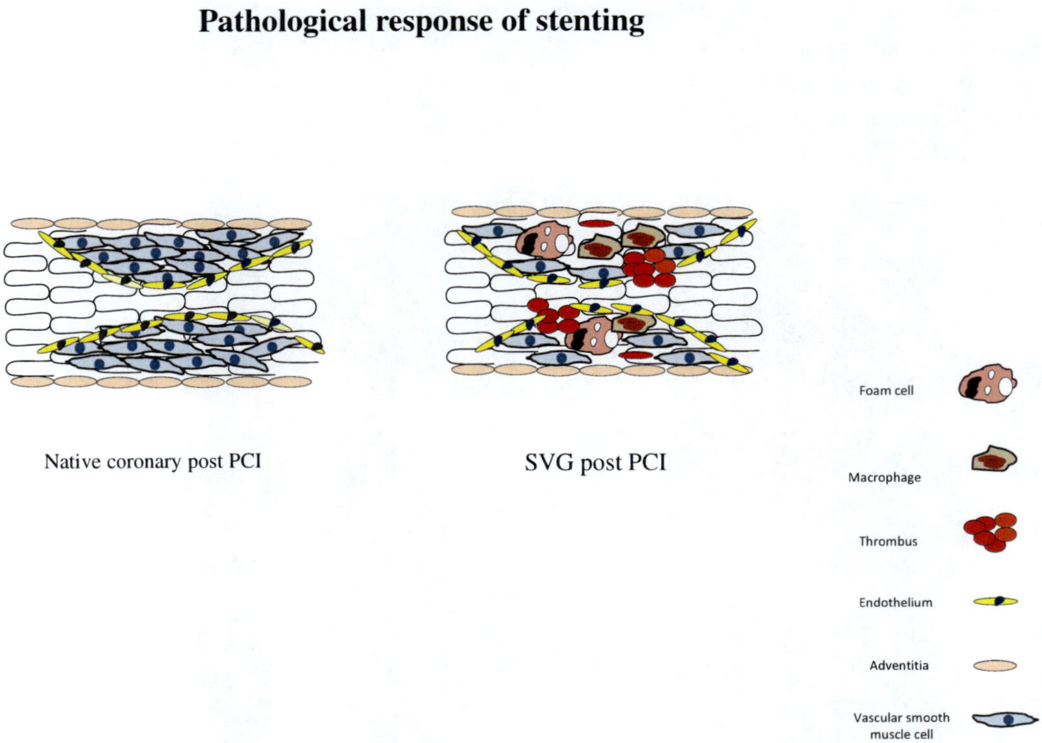

Figure 2: Pathological response of stenting in coronary artery versus SVG.

SVG Stenosis and Occlusion

There are mainly three clinical patterns of SVG stenosis and occlusion [Table 1].

1. Acute SVG occlusion occurs within days to weeks in approximately 10% of vein grafts and mostly due to surgery related technical issues such as anastomosis failure or injury to vein graft during harvesting. Other factors resulting acute SVG occlusion are acute thrombosis due to hyper coagulation state or poor distal run off [6, 19].
2. Sub-acute occlusion occurs within months to one year and usually accounts for up to 10-20% of the vein grafts failure, although in one particular study more than 70% of SVG to right coronary artery or left circumflex artery were occluded within 1 year [20]. Most important factor contributing vein graft occlusion during this period is dysfunction of SVG endothelium resulting in decreased production of nitric oxide and platelet inhibitory factors. Dysfunctional endothelium also leads to up regulation of platelet aggregation, growth factors, foam cell accumulation within endothelial cells and intimal hyperplasia, causing vein graft occlusion. The pathological process of intimal thickening starts early after CABG surgery and worsening over period of time [4, 21-26].

3. Late vein graft stenosis and occlusion is a result of progressive increase of intimal hyperplasia in the SVG after the first year of implantation. After the first year of implantation, the SVG occlude at a rate of 2% per year for next 5 years and thereafter the rate of occlusion doubles.

Table 1. Clinical patterns and pathophysiology of SVG occlusion/stenosis

Acute occlusion (10% of cases)	Days to weeks	Anastomosis failure Injury to vein graft during harvesting Poor distal run off Hyper coagulation state – acute thrombosis
Sub-acute occlusion (10-20% of cases)	Month to one year	Dysfunctional SVG endothelium Decreased production of nitric oxide Up regulation of platelet aggregation and growth factors Necrosis within lipid core
Late SVG stenosis (2% per year for 1-5 years and thereafter the occlusion rate doubles)	After one year	Progressive increase of SVG intimal hyperplasia

Following are various predictors [Table 2] for late SVG stenosis and occlusion evaluated in a number of studies [27-30].

1. History of myocardial infarction
2. Elevated triglyceride levels
3. Small graft diameter
4. Stenosis of SVG at baseline angiography
5. Low high density lipoprotein-cholesterol concentration
6. High low density lipoprotein-cholesterol concentration
7. Uncontrolled blood pressure
8. Reduced left ventricular ejection fraction
9. Female sex
10. Current smoking

Multiple distal anastomoses are predictors of acute but not for the late SVG stenosis. Similarly diabetes mellitus surprisingly does not appear to be a predictor of SVG stenosis. This is in contrast with native coronary arteries where diabetes mellitus is a strong predictor of De Novo lesion as well as for ISR.

Table 2. Predictors of late SVG stenosis and occlusion

▪ History of myocardial infarction
▪ Elevated triglyceride levels
▪ Small graft diameter
▪ Stenosis of SVG at baseline angiography
▪ Low high density lipoprotein-cholesterol concentration
▪ High low density lipoprotein-cholesterol concentration
▪ Uncontrolled blood pressure
▪ Reduced left ventricular ejection fraction
▪ Female sex
▪ Current smoking

Clinical Presentation

SVG stenosis may be silent or may present with recurrent angina months after CABG surgery. Patients occasionally may present as acute coronary syndrome. Majority of the patients will recognize their symptoms similar to those present before CABG. The cause of angina symptoms depends on the timing after the CABG surgery. Symptoms occurring soon after surgery are usually due to a technical problem with a graft causing early graft closure and these patients may present with acute coronary syndrome.

However, angina symptoms occurring months to years after CABG surgery are result of aggressive atherosclerosis disease of the SVG or progression of disease in the non-grafted native vessel. In earlier studies [6, 31] before the use of internal mammary artery (IMA), development of atherosclerosis in SVG was the main cause of recurrent angina post CABG patients. However, the data from later period after IMA implantation started, showed progression of native coronary arteries disease was common reason for late recurrent angina symptoms [32]. The rate of repeat revascularization for recurrent angina has reduced since the utilization of arterial graft [33]. In the SYNTHAX trial the repeat vascularization rate from the SVG only CABG era was between 25-31 percent compared to 11% in the CABG utilizing IMA group [34].

Management of SVG Stenosis

Patients with previous CABG and ongoing angina symptoms may benefit from repeat revascularization. The survival benefit is highest among those with angina symptoms and those with anterior wall ischemia [35-39]. Treatment of SVG stenosis depends on patient's clinical symptoms, evidence of ischemia on noninvasive tests in the distribution of diseased vein graft and angiographic evidence of a significant stenosis. Indications for revascularization in patients with SVG stenosis are to improve symptoms and possibly survival.

Vein grafts with stenosis greater than 70% are at increased risk of occlusion, therefore elective stenting of such lesions is likely to reduce the total occlusion especially when the outcomes after PCI of 100% occluded vein graft are very poor. Patients with history of previous CABG, presenting with an acute coronary syndrome have increased 30-day mortality, and therefore should be managed with invasive route similar to the ACS patients without CABG [34].

Diagnostic Modalities for SVG Stenosis

Non-invasive diagnostic testing may not be able to differentiate between ischemia due SVG stenosis or native coronary arteries. The diagnosis of SVG restenosis is usually made at the time of coronary arteriography. The role of intravascular ultrasound (IVUS) or fractional flow reserve (FFR) measurement in assessing the severity of SVG disease has not been studied in detail. Considering the similar physiological mechanism of the FFR across a native coronary artery stenosis, FFR across a SVG stenosis should be able to provide an accurate reflection of the coronary flow, at maximal hyperemia, to the distal myocardial bed supplied by the bypass graft. In one small study of patients with SVG stenosis, the accuracy of FFR was determined by comparing with corresponding myocardial perfusion imaging (MPI) studies [41]. The FFR cutoff value of 0.75 was found to be feasible with acceptable specificity and negative predictive value compared to stress MPI. Currently there is no data which had prospectively validated an FFR cutoff value to detect hemodynamically significant SVG stenosis. In the paucity of the data, it is reasonable to use the FFR cutoff value of 0.75-0.80 for hemodynamically significant stenosis.

IVUS-Guided PCI for SVG Stenosis

IVUS, being a bulky device, is not routinely used before stenting in a degenerated vein graft mainly to avoid distal embolization. However, IVUS can be performed after stenting to assess the PCI result and to evaluate the severity of intermediate lesions in the rest of graft. IVUS can reliably determine the extent of plaque tissue; identify its characteristics and whether there is thrombus in the vein graft. Accurate sizing of SVG lesions is always a practical issue as oversizing of the SVG stents can result in higher rates of peri-procedural myocardial infarction due to greater distal embolization [42, 43]. However, currently the data is lacking regarding the effectiveness of IVUS-guided PCI of SVG stenosis.

PCI versus Redo-CABG

Repeat CABG is not an ideal management strategy since many patients who develop graft disease are poor candidates for repeat surgery due to a number of reasons, including an older age and associated multiple comorbidities. As compared with initial surgery, redo-CABG surgery carries a high rate of perioperative mortality, and less complete revascularization. On the other hand, PCI of a degenerated saphenous vein grafts in comparison to native coronary arteries, is associated with a lower procedural success rate, a higher peri-procedural complication rate, and restenosis and re-occlusion rates as high as 41%

even in the DES era [44, 45]. In addition, aggressive atherosclerosis after grafting results in complete occlusion of the native coronary vessels, making percutaneous approach more difficult. [46] Therefore, the decision for repeat revascularization is not always easy. Another approach, minimally invasive CABG surgery, with less in-hospital complication may be an alternative for redo-CABG procedure, however, the data is lacking.

ACC/AHA/SCAI (American College of Cardiology Foundation/American Heart Association/Society for Cardiovascular Angiography and Interventions) 2011 PCI guidelines [47] recommend redo-CABG surgery only for patients with refractory angina and those with unsuitable anatomy for PCI, multiple diseased SVG, good distal targets and availability of IMA for grafting. Current practice is to prefer PCI over CABG in most of the patients who require revascularization for refractory angina. However, PCI of chronically occluded SVG is not recommended due to low success rates, high complication rates, and poor long-term patency rate.

The choice of revascularization therapy for refractory cardiac ischemic symptoms among patients with previous CABG should be tailored for individual patient. The factors that may favor the choice of redo-CABG include vessels unsuitable for PCI such as chronically occluded graft, number of diseased grafts, availability of the internal mammary artery, and good distal targets for bypass grafting [47]. On the other hand, factors support PCI include suitable PCI targets, symptoms due to limited ischemic burden, patent LIMA graft to the LAD artery, poor bypass graft targets and significant comorbid conditions [Table 3]

Table 3. Redo CABG versus SVG PCI – ACC/AHA 2011 guidelines

Factors favors redo CABG	Factors favors SVG PCI
• Extensive ischemic burden • Vessels unsuitable for PCI • Multiple diseased bypass grafts • Availability of the IMA for grafting • Good distal targets for bypass graft • No significant comorbidities	• Limited area of ischemia causing symptoms • Suitable PCI targets • Patent LIMA graft to the LAD • Poor CABG targets • Comorbid conditions

Initial Experience of PTCA for SVG Stenosis

With increasing population with history of CABG surgery and due to natural progression of atherosclerosis in the SVG, an increasing number of patients require repeat revascularization procedures. In the mid to late 1980's, the early success of percutaneous transluminal coronary angioplasty (PTCA) for native coronary artery disease led to the use of this technique for SVG stenosis as an alternative of redo-CABG [48]. PTCA offered good procedure success, lower procedural morbidity and mortality risks. However, in spite of very good procedural success, less in-hospital complication rate and improvement of angina symptoms, the restenosis rate requiring repeat PTCA or redo-CABG remained significantly high in the PTCA group, up to 64% in some studies [37].

PTCA versus BMS Stent for SVG Stenosis

The dramatic improvement of angiographic results and less restenosis with BMS compared to PTCA alone for native coronary arteries immediately attracted the use of stents for SVG stenosis. After success of initial land mark study “SAVED (Saphenous Vein de Novo)” of BMS versus balloon angioplasty, the intervention of SVG stenosis with stents became a standard of care. The SAVED trial [49] compared Palmaz-Schatz BMS with balloon angioplasty alone in 220 patients with SVG lesions. Repeat coronary angiography was performed at 6 months. BMS were associated with higher procedural success (92% vs. 69%, p=0.001). However, in spite of larger gains in the immediate luminal diameter in the stent group, there was only a trend of less restenosis in the BMS group (37% with BMS vs. 46% with PTCA, P=0.24).

In another randomized multicenter trial, 150 patients were randomized to either BMS or PTCA [50]. Patients were followed-up at 6 months with repeat angiography. In this trial, stenotic lesions in the body of a graft only were included. The ostial lesions, anastomotic lesions and diffusely diseased SVG segments were excluded from randomization. At 6-months follow-up, the BMS group had lower restenosis rates (19.1% vs. 32.8%, P=.069) and better event-free survival (73% vs 60%, P<.05). Patients in the BMS group also had a trend toward lower rates of death and MI.

With above data and other observational studies, PCI with BMS rapidly became a treatment of choice to establish optimal flow in the SVG intervention. It provides a better alternative for PTCA with good immediate angiographic results. There is also a greater procedural success and better gains and equivocal results regarding reduction in MACE with BMS compared with angioplasty alone. However, restenosis even after PCI with BMS remained a substantial problem, ranging from 17% to 47% [51-56]. The ISR issue becomes even more important when considering the large volume of the procedure being performed in today’s clinical practice. In an effort to reduce the ISR in SVG PCI, different PCI modalities including covered stents and brachytherapy, have been tried with variable results.

Covered Stents and SVG PCI

JOSTENT stent-graft is a distensible polytetrafluoroethylene (PTFE) membrane covering the balloon-expandable stent primarily used to treat hemodynamically significant perforation or dissection during PCI. The purposed benefit of PTFE stent-graft in SVG was to reduce peri-procedural myocardial infarction by trapping potentially embolic degenerated friable atherosclerotic debris underneath the PTFE membrane. Covered stent was also thought to reduce restenosis by acting as a barrier isolating the lumen from smooth muscle cell proliferation, and extracellular matrix production arising from the media [57]. However, the randomized trials did not prove the efficacy of covered stents for MACE or TLR.

SYMBIOT –III, a randomized Trial of a self-expanding PTFE stent Graft for SVG intervention, compared PTFE-covered Symbiot stent with BMS [58]. At 8 months follow-up, there was a trend toward increased TLR with the Symbiot stent compared to BMS (23.5% vs. 15.6%, p = 0.055), and the incidence of MACE between the covered stent and BMS was similar (30.6% vs., 26.6%, p =0.43).

In another prospective trial, RECOVERS (Randomized Evaluation of Polytetrafluoroethylene-Covered Stent in SVG), 301 patients were randomized to PTFE-covered balloon expandable stent (JoStent) or BMS [59]. The restenosis at 6 months was similar between the 2 groups (24.2% vs. 24.8%, p=0.237). The MACE incidence was higher in the covered stent group at 30 days (10.9% vs. 4.1%, p=0.047) due to increased myocardial infarction, but no difference at 6 months between the 2 groups.

A 3rd randomized study "The BARRICADE" (Barrier Approach to Restenosis: Restrict Intima to Curtail Adverse Events) [60] compared PTFE-covered balloon-expandable stent (Jo-med) with BMS in 243 patients with a long 5 year follow-up. At 5-year follow-up, target vessel failure (TVF) was higher in the covered stent group than in the BMS group (68.3% vs. 51.8%, p=0.007). The study also showed increased incidence of target vessel failure in either treatment arm at 5 year.

In summary, covered stents did not reduce restenosis rates or MACE compared with BMS. With repeated failure of trials to show efficacy and safety of covered stent during SVG intervention, there use is no longer in routine practice except in a situation of hemodynamically significant perforation.

Radiotherapy for SVG PCI

Intracoronary radiotherapy is also called as vascular brachytherapy. Gamma-radiation and beta-radiation therapy have been studied for the treatment of in-stent restenosis. Iridium-192 for gamma radiation and phosphorus- 32, strontium-90, yttrium-90, and rhenium- 188 are the radioactive isotopes for beta radiation and have been used as brachytherapy [61].

Radiation therapy interferes and breaks the double- stranded DNA bonds in the actively dividing cells of vascular media and intima, preventing their proliferation. Beta radiation penetrates 2 to 3 mm of human tissue while Gamma-radiation can penetrate deeper into the tissue up to 10 mm of human tissue. In either case, the intracoronary radiotherapy inhibits intimal and smooth muscle proliferation, delays responses after vascular injury from PTCA or other intravascular interventions.

A number of trials were done in the late 1990s and early 2000s to assess the efficacy and safety of brachytherapy treatment for ISR. Most of the data come before the drug eluting stent (DES) era in a desperate effort to reduce restenosis issue with BMS or PTCA.

Washington Radiation for In-Stent restenosis Trial for Saphenous Vein Grafts (SVG WRIST) was the first study to examine the effects of gamma radiation therapy on patients with ISR in the saphenous vein bypass grafts [62]. A total of 120 patients with diffuse ISR in SVG underwent balloon angioplasty, laser ablation or rotational atherectomy, and/or additional stents. At this stage, patients were randomized to receive gamma radiation therapy versus placebo via a catheter based local delivery system to the target lesions. At 30 days, there were no adverse events related to the radiation therapy. At 6 months, the restenosis rate was significantly lower in the irradiated group compared to control (15% vs. 43%; $p = 0.004$). The need for repeat intervention at the treatment site was significantly reduced in the irradiated group compared to control (10% vs. 48%; $p< 0.001$), and the overall major cardiac events were significantly less in the irradiated group (20% vs. 55%; $p< 0.001$).

In the follow-up study, post intervention intravascular ultrasound (IVUS) analysis was performed at 6 months. Compared to gamma irradiated group, the control patients had significant increase in intra-stent intimal hyperplasia ($p < 0.0001$) resulting in restenosis. The SVG WRIST study showed that catheter-based gamma radiation therapy for ISR in bypass grafts was safe and effective in reducing the overall restenosis rate and the need for repeat revascularization compared to conventional treatment. When compared with radiation therapy for ISR of native coronary arteries, the gamma radiation therapy in SVG had similar angiographic restenosis rates (27% vs.23%) in the WRIST series of studies. At 3 year follow-up of WRIST SVG, patients with ISR treated with IRT had a marked reduction in the need for repeat TLR at 36 months, but TVR rate was not different [63].

In spite of initial benefit from brachytherapy, the long term outcomes regarding efficacy of brachytherapy was less robust in most of the follow-up studies. The 3-year follow-up data of SCRIPPS trial also showed no benefits of brachytherapy on SVG ISR [64].

Gamma-Radiation versus Beta-Radiation

The observational studies suggest that beta and gamma-radiation have similar efficacy in the reduction of coronary in stent restenosis [65, 66]. There is no particular data for SVG ISR.

DES and SVG Intervention

Since the remarkable anti-restenotic efficacy of DES was observed in the native coronary artery disease, DES has been used for SVG PCI in an off-label fashion. According to NCDR data, PCI of SVG stenosis represented 5.7% of the total PCI volume in the USA [10]. The use of DES for SVG PCI was highest, 80%, in 2005, an era of maximum use of DES for PCI during any kind of coronary intervention. From 2005 to 2009, DES use in SVG PCI has decreased from 80% to 62%, primarily due to some conflicting results of limited data of DES use in SVG PCI. According to NCDR, patients with in-stent restenotic lesions, long diffuse stenosis in the SVG, and those needed multi grafts PCI were more likely to receive DES compared to BMS [10]. The data with regard to BMS versus DES is summarized as below.

Most of the data for SVG PCI comparing DES versus BMS come from observational studies. One large observational study, the STENT (Strategic Transcatheter Evaluation of New Therapies), reported outcomes of BMS versus DES among patients undergoing SVG PCI [67]. Those receiving DES had lower rates of TVR at 9 months (7.2% vs 10.0%, HR 0.36, 95% CI 0.22–0.61, P<.001) but the benefit was lost by 2 years (18.3% vs 16.9%, P =0.86). Similarly the benefit of combined death and MI at 9 months was not sustained at 2 year follow-up.

Data from OLYMPIA registry [68] was encouraging for interventionalists as it showed comparable 12 month clinical outcomes, including TLR rates, between SVG and native coronary arteries stented with TEXUS DES. Although it was not a randomized data, however, it was a reflection of real-world clinical practice.

There are only few randomized trials comparing DES versus BMS for SVG PCI. One initial such trial was RRISC (Reduction of Restenosis in SVG with Sirolimus-Eluting Stent),a prospective randomized trial, which reported reduction in late loss, restenosis and TLR in the sirolimus-eluting stent group compared with BMS at 6-month follow-up [69]. However, a post hoc analysis of RRISC trial at 3 years did not show difference in rates of TLR and TVR [70]. There was also higher mortality observed in the DES group at long-term follow-up.

The SOS (Stenting of Saphenous Vein Grafts) trial compared BMS with DES [71]. Eighty patients were randomized to a BMS or paclitaxel-eluting stent (PES). The trial demonstrated improved short-term angiographic and clinical outcomes with PES. After a follow-up of almost 3 years, patients with PES had a lower incidence of myocardial infarction (hazard ratio [HR]: 0.32, p = 0.01), target lesion revascularization (HR: 0.20, p = 0.004), target vessel revascularization (HR: 0.41, p = 0.03). [72] There was also decreased target vessel failure (HR: 0.34, p = 0.001) and a trend toward less stent thrombosis (HR: 0.15, p = 0.08), however, there was no difference in all-cause and cardiac mortality between the 2 groups [72].

In another a large randomized trial of 610 patients, ISAR-CABG (Prospective Randomized Trial of Drug-Eluting Stents Versus Bare Metal Stents for the Reduction of Restenosis in Bypass Grafts), there was a 50% relative reduction in the risk of TLR in the DES group at 1 year follow-up (7.2% vs. 13.1%, p= 0.02) [73].

Most of the data of SVG PCI with DES is from first generation DES. The second-generation DES are now routinely used for native coronary arteries, and similar trend has been observed for SVG intervention. A recent trial, SOS-Xience study, evaluated the use of second generation drug-eluting stents in saphenous vein graft (SVG) lesions [74]. Patients were enrolled to assess the clinical and angiographic outcomes of everolimus eluting stent (Xience V). At 12 months, the repeat vascularization rate was 30%, and 15% had ISR requiring TLR. Another study compared the clinical outcomes between first- and second-generation DES in SVG PCI. TLR, TVR and MACE were reported and there was no difference at 18-month follow-up [75].

Long term safety and efficacy was evaluated in a trial comparing DES versus BMS among patients who underwent SVG PCI between 2003 and 2008 [76]. The DES used were of first generation in this study. At 4-year follow-up, the rate of TVR was 21% in the DES group versus 27.6% in the BMS group (p = 0.004). The maximum benefit of DES was observed among diabetics and those requiring > 30 mm of stents during SVG PCI. The composite rate of myocardial infarction or death was not significantly different between the 2 groups. In another study [77] at a 7 years follow-up, the target vessel TVR was higher in the BMS group compared to the DES (either sirolimus- or paclitaxel-eluting stents) group (41% vs. 29%). There was also trend of higher MACE in BMS group (73% vs. 68%).

Apart from few randomized trials, there are several meta-analyses which compared DES with BMS for SVG PCI in the recent years [78-85]. Most of the data in these meta-analyses come from non-randomized trials. One large analysis of 7994 patients from 26 observational and 2 randomized trials compared DES versus BMS with a mean follow-up duration of 21 months [83]. DES compared with BMS in SVG were found to have decrease risk of TVR (12% vs 17%, RR 0.71, P= .0002) and MACE (19% vs 28%, RR 0.7, P<.00001). There were also trend of reduction in death and MI in the DES group.

A numbers of other meta-analyses compared DES versus BMS in SVG PCI and have demonstrated similar results of improved efficacy with DES in terms of TLR, TVR and MACE reduction and without any significant safety hazard. One important meta-analysis which included only the 4 available randomized trials [69,71-73] comparing DES versus BMS for SVG PCI [86]. At a mean follow-up of 25 months, patients with SVG PCI with DES had lower rates of repeat revascularization (OR 0.40, 95% CI 0.22–0.75). The MACE and death rates were similar between BMS and DES groups.

The overall data so far shows the DES are safe for SVG PCI and they reduce revascularization. We, therefore, recommend DES should be considered for SVG PCI, provided patient is comply with dual antiplatelet therapy and there is no need of long term anticoagulation for additional pathology or any anticipated interruption in dual antiplatelet in the near future.

Optimization of Management of SVG Disease

The percutaneous revascularization of diseased and degenerated SVG is feasible but challenging due to high rates of procedural adverse events, long-term restenosis, and ongoing SVG atherosclerosis progression outside of the treated segments. The plaque volume and severity of SVG degeneration estimated during angiogram, older age, and history of current smoking and use of glycoprotein IIb/IIIa inhibitor are significant predictors of major adverse cardiac events during 30 days after PCI of SVG [87]. The following are a number of strategies we recommend to reduce the SVG stenosis and to optimize the PCI outcomes of SVG revascularization.

1. Pharmacological Management

Aggressive lipid lowering therapy with statins reduces progression of SVG atherosclerosis disease process [88]. Low LDL level also reduce the risks of repeated myocardial infarction and coronary revascularization in post CABG patients. Similarly, aspirin has also been shown to improve short- and long-term SVG patency [89]. Currently, aspirin and statins are class I recommendation for post CABG patients. There is no data with regard to use of dual antiplatelet for prevention of SVG disease, however, dual antiplatelet therapy after SVG PCI is a class I recommendation.

Glycoprotein IIb/IIIa inhibitors have no beneficial role during SVG PCI and therefore not recommended [90, 91]. Intracoronary vasodilators such as adenosine or sodium nitroprusside) may improve angiographic flow after SVG PCI, but without improvement of cardiac outcomes [92].

2. Intervention Techniques

a) Predilation versus direct stenting

Direct stenting has a potential benefit of trapping debris, therefore reducing distal embolization compared to predilation. One study data showed less creatine kinase (CK)-myocardial isoform (MB) release (P<.001), and less non-Q-wave MI (P=.024). At 1 year follow-up, the rate of the combined death-MI-TLR was lower in the direct stenting group (P 5 .021) [93]. Similar outcomes were observed in SVG PCI study using direct stenting technique versus angioplasty using distal protection device [94]. We recommend the direct stenting approach for PCI of SVG stenosis if feasible.

b) Under sizing versus oversizing

The undersized stenting reduce the plaque intrusion through the stent struts and therefore, there is decrease likelihood of distal embolization (Fig.3). Less plaque intrusion was observed in the smaller stent group and higher CK-MB elevation as well as a trend of TLR in largest stent group at 1 year follow-up [95]. Undersized stent approach may be considered when embolic protection devices are not available or unable to deploy EPD due to anatomical reasons.

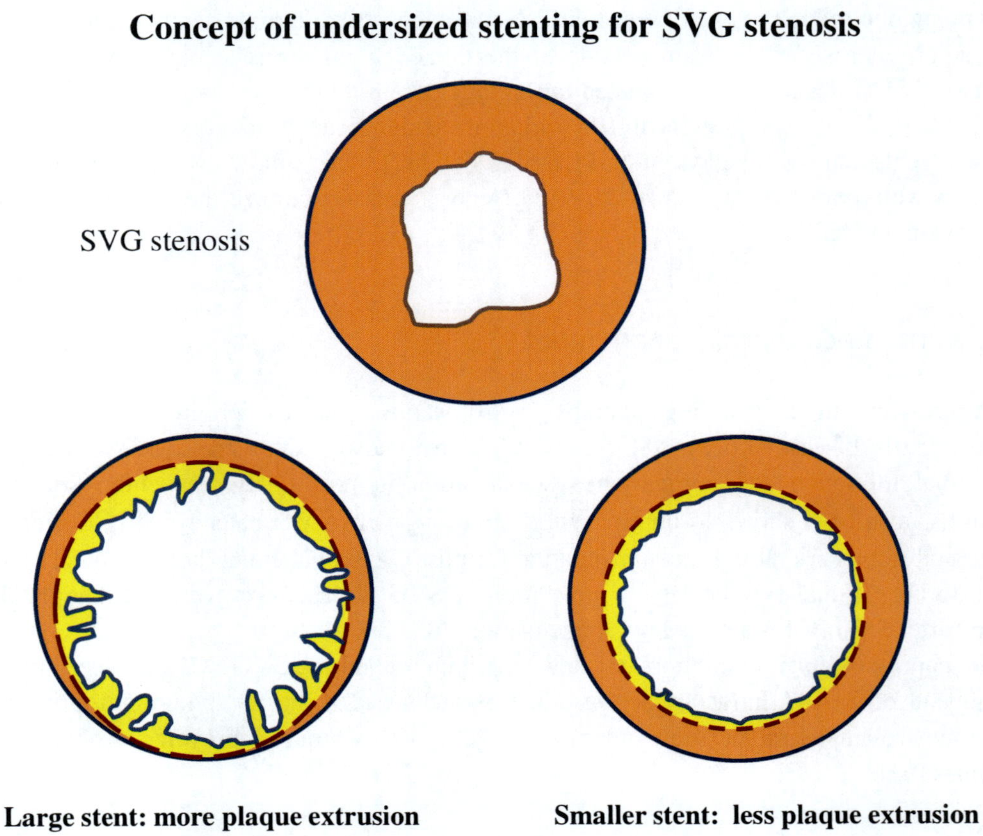

Figure 3. Concept of undersized stenting for SVG stenosis.

c) Atherectomy

Although the use of atherectomy devises during SVG interventions appears appropriate, however, there is lack of data regarding clinical outcomes and TLR [96]. Some improvement of flow and better angiographic results were observed with limited use of "directional coronary atherectomy" during PCI of focal SVG stenosis [97].

d) Embolic protection devices (EPD)

The significance of EPDs in improving the outcomes of SVG interventions is well established and recommended. However, despite the improvement in outcomes with EPDs, the rates of MACE still remains high at 30 days. There is no known data suggesting any role of EPD on SVG restenosis rate [87].

Native Coronary Vessel PCI instead of SVG PCI

As discussed above the high rates of procedural event and durability of the degenerative SVG PCI even in the DES era remains a significant concern. Therefore, the opportunity to treat native chronically total occluded (CTO) coronary vessels, negating the need to preserve the ill-fated degenerated SVG, is a therapeutic strategy worth considering [98]. To do this effectively operators must acquire sufficient advance CTO-PCI training.

Gene Therapy

The saphenous vein grafts are ideal targets for gene therapy because the explanted veins are available for ex vivo transfer of genetic material before grafting. The extracted veins can be incubated with a therapeutic vector targeting mechanisms underlying pathological process for vein occlusion including thrombosis, neo intimal hyperplasia and accelerated atherosclerosis. Similarly local delivery of therapeutic vector during PCI of diseased SVG or more favorably use of "gene-eluting" stents, might play an important future role in the prevention of vein graft disease and in-stent restenosis [99]. Pre-clinical studies have been encouraging with positive results and wait for back up in the clinical trials.

Conclusion

SVG undergo rapid and aggressive atherosclerotic change resulting in vein graft stenosis. In addition, the SVG intima shows aggressive inflammatory response to stenting compared to native coronary arteries and increases chances of restenosis. Aggressive stains and aspirin therapy has shown to improve SVG patency. Revascularization is recommended for patients with refractory angina and choice of revascularization therapy should be individualized. Redo-CABG carries more peri-procedural risks and may not be appropriate for large number of patients only because of comorbidities. The percutaneous revascularization of diseased and degenerated SVG is feasible but challenging due to high rates of procedural adverse events, long-term restenosis, and ongoing SVG atherosclerosis progression outside of the treated segments. EPD are likely to reduce peri-procedural complications during SVG intervention. There is no additional role of adding atherectomy to optimize SVG intervention in the current era. BMS and DES are safe and effective for revascularization of SVG stenosis. DES are likely to reduce restenosis compared with use of BMS for SVG intervention. We also recommend aggressive medical management and to consider PCI of chronically occluded native coronary arteries especially when SVG is occluded.

References

[1] Garrett HE, Dennis EW, DeBakey ME. Aortocoronary bypass with saphenous vein graft. Seven-year follow-up. *JAMA* 1973;223:792–794.

[2] Loop FD, Lytle BW, Cosgrove DM, et al. Influence of the internal-mammary-artery graft on 10-year survival and other cardiac events. *N. Engl. J. Med.* 1986; 314:1–6.

[3] Nwasokwa ON. Coronary artery bypass graft disease. *Ann. Intern. Med.* 1995;123:528 –545.

[4] Motwani JG, Topol EJ. Aortocoronary saphenous vein graft disease: pathogenesis, predisposition, and prevention. *Circulation*. 1998;97: 916–931.

[5] Campeau L, Lesperance J, Hermann J, Corbara F, Grondin CM, Bourassa MG. Loss of the improvement of angina between 1 and 7 years after aortocoronary bypass surgery: correlations with changes in vein grafts and in coronary arteries. *Circulation.* 1979;60:1–5.

[6] Fitzgibbon GM, Kafka HP, Leach AJ, Keon WJ, Hooper GD, Burton JR. Coronary bypass graft fate and patient outcome: angiographic follow-up of 5,065 grafts related to survival and reoperation in 1,388 patients during 25 years. *J. Am. Coll. Cardiol.* 1996;28:616–626.

[7] Gillum RF, Gillum BS, Francis CK. Coronary revascularization and cardiac catheterization in the United States: Trends in racial differences. *J. Am. Coll. Cardiol* 1997;29(7):1557–1562.

[8] Riley RF, Don CW, Powell W, et al. Trends in coronary revascularization in the United States from 2001 to 2009. Recent declines in percutaneous coronary intervention volumes. *Circ. Cardiovasc. Qual. Outcomes* 2011;4;193–197.

[9] Wilson CT, Fisher ES, Welch HG, Siewers AE, Lucas FL (2007) U.S. trends in CABG hospital volume: the effect of adding cardiac surgery programs. Health Aff (Millwood) 26: 162–168.

[10] Brilakis ES, Wang TY, Rao SV, Banerjee S, Dai D, et al. Frequency and Predictors of Drug-Eluting Stent Use in Saphenous Vein Bypass Graft Percutaneous Coronary Intervention: a report from the American College of Cardiology National Cardiovascular Data CathPCI Registry. *J. Am. Coll. Cardiol. Intv.* 2010;3(10):1068-1073.

[11] Bulkley BH, Hutchins GM. Accelerated "atherosclerosis". A morphologic study of 97 saphenous vein coronary artery bypass grafts. *Circulation* 1977;55: 163–9.

[12] Kern WH, Dermer GB, Lindesmith GG. The intimal proliferation in aortic-coronary saphenous vein grafts. Light and electron microscopic studies. *Am. Heart J.* 1972;84:771–7.

[13] Vlodaver Z, Edwards JE. Pathologic changes in aortic-coronary arterial saphenous vein grafts. *Circulation* 1971;44:719–28.

[14] Zou Y, Dietrich H, Hu Y, Metzler B, Wick G, Xu Q. Mouse model of venous bypass graft arteriosclerosis. *Am. J. Pathol.* 1998;153:1301–10.

[15] Butany JW, David TE, Ojha M. Histological and morphometric analyses of early and late aortocoronary vein grafts and distal anastomoses. *Can. J. Cardiol* 1998;14:671–7.

[16] Le May MR, Labinaz M, Marquis JF, et al. Predicators of long-term outcome after stent implantation in a saphenous vein graft. *AJC* 1999;83:681.

[17] van Beusekom HM, van der Giessen WJ, van Suylen R, Bos E, Bosman FT, Serruys PW. Histology after stenting of human saphenous vein bypass grafts: observations from surgically excised grafts 3 to 320 days after stent implantation. *JACC* 1993;21:45-54.

[18] Joner M, Finn AV, Farb A, et al. Pathology of drug-eluting stents in humans: delayed healing and late thrombotic risk. *J. Am. Coll. Cardiol.* 2006;48:193–202.

[19] Harskamp RE, Lopes RD, Baisden CE, et al. Saphenous vein graft failure after coronary artery bypass surgery: pathophysiology, management, and future directions. *Ann. Surg.* 2013; 257:824.

[20] Widimsky P, Straka Z, Stros P, Jirasek K, Dvorak J, Votava J, Lisa L, Budesinsky T, Kolesar M, Vanek T, Brucek P. One-year coronary bypass graft patency: a randomized comparison between off-pump and on-pump surgery angiographic results of the PRAGUE-4 trial. *Circulation.* 2004 Nov 30;110(22):3418-23.

[21] Kockx MM, De Meyer GR, Bortier H, et al. Luminal foam cell accumulation is associated with smooth muscle cell death in the intimal thickening of human saphenous vein grafts. *Circulation* 1996; 94:1255.

[22] Kauhanen P, Sirén V, Carpén O, et al. Plasminogen activator inhibitor-1 in neointima of vein grafts: its role in reduced fibrinolytic potential and graft failure. *Circulation* 1997; 96:1783.

[23] Yang Z, Oemar BS, Carrel T, et al. Different proliferative properties of smooth muscle cells of human arterial and venous bypass vessels: role of PDGF receptors, mitogen-activated protein kinase, and cyclin-dependent kinase inhibitors. *Circulation* 1998; 97:181.

[24] Chello M, Mastroroberto P, Perticone F, et al. Nitric oxide modulation of neutrophil-endothelium interaction: difference between arterial and venous coronary bypass grafts. *J. Am. Coll. Cardiol.* 1998; 31:823.

[25] Lüscher TF, Diederich D, Siebenmann R, et al. Difference between endothelium-dependent relaxation in arterial and in venous coronary bypass grafts. *N. Engl. J. Med.* 1988; 319:462.

[26] Hozumi T, Yoshikawa J, Yoshida K, et al. Use of intravascular ultrasound for in vivo assessment of changes in intimal thickness of angiographically normal saphenous vein grafts one year after aortocoronary bypass surgery. *Heart* 1996; 76:317.

[27] Goldman S, Zadina K, Krasnicka B, et al. Predictors of graft patency 3 years after coronary artery bypass graft surgery. Department of Veterans Affairs Cooperative Study Group No. 297. *J. Am. Coll. Cardiol.* 1997; 29:1563.

[28] Domanski MJ, Borkowf CB, Campeau L, et al. Prognostic factors for atherosclerosis progression in saphenous vein grafts: the post coronary artery bypass graft (Post-CABG) trial. Post-CABG Trial Investigators. *J. Am. Coll. Cardiol.* 2000; 36:1877.

[29] Goldman S, Zadina K, Moritz T, et al. Long-term patency of saphenous vein and left internal mammary artery grafts after coronary artery bypass surgery: results from a Department of Veterans Affairs Cooperative Study. *J. Am. Coll. Cardiol.* 2004; 44:2149.

[30] DeBakey ME, Glaeser DH. Patterns of atherosclerosis: effect of risk factors on recurrence and survival-analysis of 11,890 cases with more than 25-year follow-up. *Am. J. Cardiol.* 2000; 85:1045.

[31] Chen L, Théroux P, Lespérance J, et al. Angiographic features of vein grafts versus ungrafted coronary arteries in patients with unstable angina and previous bypass surgery. *J. Am. Coll. Cardiol.* 1996; 28:1493.

[32] Alderman EL, Kip KE, Whitlow PL, et al. Native coronary disease progression exceeds failed revascularization as cause of angina after five years in the Bypass Angioplasty Revascularization Investigation (BARI). *J. Am. Coll. Cardiol.* 2004; 44:766.

[33] Peduzzi P, Kamina A, Detre K. Twenty-two-year follow-up in the VA Cooperative Study of Coronary Artery Bypass Surgery for Stable Angina. *Am. J. Cardiol.* 1998; 81:1393.

[34] Kappetein AP, Feldman TE, Mack MJ, et al. Comparison of coronary bypass surgery with drug-eluting stenting for the treatment of left main and/or three-vessel disease: 3-year follow-up of the SYNTAX trial. *Eur. Heart J.* 2011; 32:2125.

[35] Brener SJ, Lytle BW, Casserly IP, et al. Predictors of revascularization method and long term outcome of percutaneous coronary intervention or repeat coronary bypass surgery in patients with multivessel coronary disease and previous coronary bypass surgery. *Eur. Heart J.* 2006;27: 413–8.

[36] Lytle BW, Loop FD, Taylor PC, et al. The effect of coronary reoperation on the survival of patients with stenosis in saphenous vein bypass grafts to coronary arteries. *J. Thorac. Cardiovasc. Surg.* 1993;105:605–12.

[37] Morrison DA, Sethi G, Sacks J, et al., Investigators of the Department of Veterans Affairs Cooperative Study #385, the Angina With Extremely Serious Operative Mortality Evaluation (AWESOME). Percutaneous coronary intervention versus coronary artery bypass graft surgery for patients with medically refractory myocardial ischemia and risk factors for adverse outcomes with bypass: a multicenter, randomized trial. *J. Am. Coll. Cardiol.* 2001;38:143–9.

[38] Stephan WJ, O'Keefe JH Jr, Piehler JM, et al. Coronary angioplasty versus repeat coronary artery bypass grafting for patients with previous bypass surgery. *J. Am. Coll. Cardiol.* 1996;28:1140–6.

[39] Weintraub WS, Jones EL, Morris DC, et al. Outcome of reoperative coronary bypass surgery versus coronary angioplasty after previous bypass surgery. *Circulation.* 1997;95:868 –77.

[40] Labinaz M, Kilaru R, Pieper K, et al. Outcomes of patients with acute coronary syndromes and prior coronary artery bypass grafting: results from the platelet glycoprotein IIb/IIIa in unstable angina: receptor suppression using integrilin therapy (PURSUIT) trial. *Circulation* 2002; 105:322.

[41] Aqel R, Zoghbi GJ, Hage F, et al. Hemodynamic evaluation of coronary artery bypass graft lesions using fractional flow reserve. *Cathet. Cardiovasc. Interv.* 2008; 72: 479-485.

[42] Iakovou I, Dangas G, Mintz GS, et al. Relation of final lumen dimensions in saphenous vein grafts after stent implantation to outcome. *Am. J. Cardiol.* 2004;93:963– 8.

[43] Hong YJ, Pichard AD, Mintz GS, et al. Outcome of undersized drug-eluting stents for percutaneous coronary intervention of saphenous vein graft lesions. *Am. J. Cardiol.* 2010;105:179–85.

[44] Hoffmann R, Hamm C, Nienaber CA, et al. Implantation of sirolimus-eluting stents in saphenous vein grafts is associated with high clinical follow-up event rates compared with treatment of native vessels. *Coron. Artery Dis.* 2007;18:559–64.

[45] Pucelikova T, Mehran R, Kirtane AJ, Kim YH, Fahy M, Weisz G, Lansky AJ, Moussa I, Gray WA, Collins MB, Kodali SK, Stone GW, Moses JW, Leon MB, Dangas G. Short- and long-term outcomes after stent-assisted percutaneous treatment of saphenous vein grafts in the drug-eluting stent era. *Am. J. Cardiol*. 2008 Jan 1;101(1):63-8.

[46] Bourassa MG, Enjalbert M, Campeau L, Lesperance J. Progression of atherosclerosis in coronary arteries and bypass grafts: ten years later. *Am J. Cardiol*. 1984 Jun 15;53(12):102-107.

[47] Glenn N. Levine, Eric R. Bates, James C. Blankenship, Steven R. Bailey, et al. 2011 ACCF/AHA/SCAI Guideline for Percutaneous Coronary Intervention: A Report on Practice Guidelines of the Society for Cardiovascular Angiography and Interventions/ American College of Cardiology Foundation/American Heart Association Task Force. *Circulation*. 2011 Dec 6;124(23):e574-651.

[48] Kaul TK, Fields BL, Wyatt DA, Jones CR, Kahn DR. Reoperative coronary artery bypass surgery: early and late results and management in 1300 patients. *J. Cardiovasc. Surg*. 1995 Aug;36(4):303-12.

[49] Savage MP, Douglas JS, Fischman DL, et al., for the Saphenous Vein De Novo Trial Investigators. Stent placement compared with balloon angioplasty for obstructed coronary bypass grafts. *N. Engl. J. Med* 1997;337:740 –7.

[50] Hanekamp CE, Koolen JJ, Den Heijer P, et al. Randomized study to compare balloon angioplasty and elective stent implantation in venous bypass grafts: the Vene stent study. *Catheter. Cardiovasc. Interv*. 2003;60(4):452–7.

[51] Ellis S, Savage M, Fischman D, et al. Restenosis after placement of Palmaz-Schatz stents in native coronary arteries. Initial results of a multicenter experience. *Circulation* 1992;86(6):1836 44.

[52] de Scheerder IK, Strauss BH, de Feyter PJ, et al. Stenting of venous bypass grafts: a new treatment modality for patients who are poor candidates for reintervention. *Am. Heart J*. 1992;123(4):1046–54.

[53] Piana RN, Moscucci M, Cohen DJ, et al. Palmaz- Schatz stenting for treatment of focal vein graft stenosis: immediate results and long-term outcome. *J. Am. Coll. Cardiol*. 1994;23(6):1296–304.

[54] Fenton SH, Fischman DL, Savage MP. Long-term angiographic and clinical outcome after implantation of balloon-expandable stents in aortocoronary saphenous vein grafts. *Am. J. Cardiol*. 1994;74(12): 1187–91.

[55] Wong SC, Baim DS, Schatz RA, et al. Immediate results and late outcomes after stent implantation in saphenous vein graft lesions: the multicenter US Palmaz-Schatz stent experience. *J. Am. Coll. Cardiol*. 1995;26(3):704–12.

[56] Eeckhout E, Goy JJ, Stauffer JC, et al. Endoluminal stenting of narrowed saphenous vein grafts: long term clinical and angiographic follow-up. *Cathet. Cardiovasc. Diagn*. 1994;32(2):139–46.

[57] Briguori C, De Gregorio J, Nishida T, et al. Polytetrafluoroethylene covered stent for the treatment of narrowings in aortocoronary saphenous vein grafts. *Am. J. Cardiol*. 2000;86:343– 6.

[58] Turco MA, Buchbinder M, Popma JJ, et al. Pivotal, randomized U.S. study of the Symbiot covered stent system in patients with saphenous vein graft disease: eight-month angiographic and clinical results from the Symbiot III trial. *Catheter. Cardiovasc. Interv*. 2006;68:379–88.

[59] Stankovic G, Colombo A, Presbitero P, et al. Randomized evaluation of polytetrafluoroethylene covered stent in saphenous vein grafts: the Randomized Evaluation of polytetrafluoroethylene COVERed stent in Saphenous vein grafts (RECOVERS) trial. *Circulation* 2003;108:37– 42.

[60] Stone GW, Goldberg S, O'Shaughnessy C, et al. Five-year follow-up of polytetrafluoroethylene-covered stents compared with bare-metal stents in aortocoronary saphenous vein graft: the randomized BARRICADE (Barrier Approach to Restenosis: Restrict Intima to Curtail Adverse Events) Trial. *J. Am. Coll. Cardiol.* Intv. 2011;4:300 –9.

[61] Albert W. Chan, David J. Moliterno, *Cleveland Clinci journal of Medicine*. Vol 68. Number 9 Sept 2001.

[62] Waksman R, Ajani AE, White RL, Chan RC, Satler LF, Kent KM, Pichard AD, Pinnow EE, Bui AB, Ramee S, Teirstein P, Lindsay J. Intravascular gamma radiation for in-stent restenosis in saphenous-vein bypass grafts. *N. Engl. J. Med.* 2002 Apr 18;346(16):1194-9.

[63] Rha SW, Kuchulakanti P, Ajani AE, Cheneau E, Pinnow EE, Canos DA, Torguson R, Pichard AD, Satler LF, Kent KM, Ramee S, Teirstein P, Lindsay J, Waksman R. Three-year follow-up after intravascular gamma-radiation for in-stent restenosis in saphenous vein grafts. *Catheter. Cardiovasc. Interv*. 2005 Jun;65(2):257-62.

[64] Teirstein PS, Massullo V, Jani S, et al. Three-year clinical and angiographic follow-up after intracoronary radiation: results of a randomized clinical trial. Circulation 2000; 101:360–365

[65] Waksman R, Bhargava B, White L, et al. Intracoronary beta-radiation therapy inhibits recurrence of in-stent restenosis. *Circulation* 2000; 101:1895–1898.

[66] Lansky AJ, Mehran R, Desai K, et al. Impact of gamma and beta radiation vs placebo on the changing pattern of in-stent restenosis: a matched angiographic analysis. J Am Coll Cardiol 2001; 37:29.

[67] Brodie BR, Wilson H, Stuckey T, et al. Outcomes with drug-eluting versus bare-metal stents in saphenous vein graft intervention results from the STENT (strategic transcatheter evaluation of new therapies) group. *JACC Cardiovasc Interv* 2009; 2(11):1105–12.

[68] Mendiz OA, Ahmed WH, Fava CM, et al. Clinical outcome after saphenous vein stenting with Taxus Liberte´ stent: results from the OLYMPIA Registry (TAXUS Liberte´ Postapproval Global Program). *Angiology* 2012;63(8):574–8.

[69] Vermeersch P, Agostoni P, Verheye S, et al. Randomized double-blind comparison of sirolimus-eluting stent versus bare-metal stent implantation in diseased saphenous vein grafts: six-month angiographic, intravascular ultrasound, and clinical follow-up of the RRISC trial. *J. Am. Coll. Cardiol.* 2006;48(12):2423–31.

[70] Vermeersch P, Agostoni P, Verheye S, et al., for the DELAYED RRISC Investigators. Increased late mortality after sirolimus-eluting stents versus bare-metal stents in diseased saphenous vein grafts: results from the randomized DELAYED RRISC Trial. *J. Am. Coll. Cardiol.* 2007;50:261–7

[71] Brilakis ES, Lichtenwalter C, de Lemos JA, et al. A randomized controlled trial of a paclitaxel eluting stent versus a similar bare-metal stent in saphenous vein graft lesions: the SOS (Stenting of Saphenous Vein Grafts) trial. *J. Am. Coll. Cardiol.* 2009;53:919 – 28.

[72] Brilakis ES, Lichtenwalter C, Abdel-karim AR, et al. Continued benefit from paclitaxel-eluting compared to bare-metal stent implantation in saphenous vein graft lesions during long-term follow-up of the SOS (Stenting of Saphenous Vein Grafts) trial. *J. Am. Coll. Cardiol. Intv*. 2011;4:176–82.

[73] Mehilli J, Pache J, Abdel-Wahab M, et al. Drug-eluting versus bare-metal stents in saphenous vein graft lesions (ISAR-CABG): Is Drug-Eluting-Stenting Associated with Improved Results in Coronary Artery Bypass Grafts? Lancet. 2011 Sep 17;378(9796):1071-8.

[74] Papayannis AC, Michael TT, Yangirova D, Abdel-Karim AR, Kohlhaas J, Mahmood A, Addo T, Haagen D, Makke L, Roesle M, Rangan B, Banerjee S, Brilakis ES. Optical coherence tomography analysis of the stenting of saphenous vein graft (SOS) Xience V Study: use of the everolimus-eluting stent in saphenous vein graft lesions. *J. Invasive Cardiol.* 2012 Aug;24(8):390-4.

[75] Costopoulos C, Latib A, Naganuma T, Sticchi A, Chieffo A, Figini F, Carlino M, Montorfano M, Naim C, Kawaguchi M, Giannini F, Colombo A. Comparison of first- and second-generation drug-eluting stents in saphenous vein grafts used as aorto-coronary conduits. *Am. J. Cardiol.* 2013 Aug 1;112(3):318-22.

[76] Dennis T. Ko, Helen Guo et al. Long-Term Safety and Effectiveness of Drug-Eluting Stents for the Treatment of Saphenous Vein Grafts Disease. A Population-Based Study. *J. Am. Coll. Cardiol. Intv*. 2011;4(9):965-973.

[77] Nauta ST, Van Mieghem NM, Magro M, Deckers JW, Simsek C, Van Geuns RJ, Van Der Giessen WJ, De Jaegere P, Regar E, Van Domburg RT, Serruys PW. Seven-year safety and efficacy of the unrestricted use of drug-eluting stents in saphenous vein bypass grafts. *Catheter. Cardiovasc. Interv*. 2012 May 1;79(6):912-8.

[78] Testa L, Agostoni P, Vermeersch P, et al. Drug eluting stent versus bare metal stent in the treatment of saphenous vein graft disease: a systematic review and meta-analysis. *EuroIntervention* 2010; 6(4):527–36.

[79] Joyal D, Filion KB, Eisenberg MJ. Effectiveness and safety of drug-eluting stents in vein grafts: a metaanalysis. *Am. Heart J.* 2010;159(2):159–169.

[80] Paradis JM, Belisle P, Joseph L, et al. Drug-eluting or bare metal stents for the treatment of saphenous vein graft disease: a Bayesian meta-analysis. *Circ. Cardiovasc. Interv*. 2010;3(6):565 76.

[81] Sanchez-Recalde A, Jimenez Valero S, Moreno R, et al. Safety and efficacy of drug-eluting stents versus bare-metal stents in saphenous vein grafts lesions: a meta-analysis. *EuroIntervention* 2010; 6(1):149–60.

[82] Wiisanen ME, Abdel-Latif A, Mukherjee D, et al. Drug-eluting stents versus bare-metal stents in saphenous vein graft interventions: a systematic review and meta-analysis. *JACC Cardiovasc Interv*. 2010;3(12):1262–73.

[83] Hakeem A, Helmy T, Munsif S, et al. Safety and efficacy of drug eluting stents compared with bare metal stents for saphenous vein graft interventions: a comprehensive meta-analysis of randomized trials and observational studies comprising 7,994 patients. *Catheter. Cardiovasc. Interv.* 2011;77(3): 343–55.

[84] Lupi A, Navarese EP, Lazzero M, et al. Drug-eluting stents vs. bare metal stents in saphenous vein graft disease. Insights from a meta-analysis of 7,090 patients. *Circ. J.* 2011;75(2):280–9.

[85] Mamas MA, Foley J, Nair S, et al. A comparison of drug-eluting stents versus bare metal stents in saphenous vein graft PCI outcomes: a meta-analysis. *J. Interv. Cardiol.* 2011;24(2):172–80.

[86] Alam M, Bandeali SJ, Virani SS, et al. Clinical outcomes of percutaneous interventions in saphenous vein grafts using drug-eluting stents compared to bare-metal stents: a comprehensive meta-analysis of all randomized clinical trials. *Clin. Cardiol.* 2012;35(5):291–6.

[87] Coolong A, Baim DS, Kuntz RE, et al. Saphenous vein graft stenting and major adverse cardiac events: a predictive model derived from a pooled analysis of 3958 patients. *Circulation* 2008;117:790–7.

[88] Hong YJ, Mintz GS, Kim SW, et al. Disease progression in non-intervened saphenous vein graft segments a serial intravascular ultrasound analysis. *J. Am. Coll. Cardiol.* 2009;53:1257–64.

[89] Kim FY'Marhefka G, Ruggiero NJ, Adams S, Whellan DJ. Saphenous vein graft disease: review of pathophysiology, prevention, and treatment. *Cardiol. Rev*. 2013 Mar-Apr;21(2):101-9.

[90] Mak KH, Challapalli R, Eisenberg MJ, et al. Effect of platelet glycoprotein IIb/IIIa receptor inhibition on distal embolization during percutaneous revascularization of aorto- coronary saphenous vein grafts. *Am. J. Cardiol* 1997;80:985–8.

[91] Karha J, Gurm HS, Rajagopal V, et al. Use of platelet glycoprotein IIb/IIIa inhibitors in saphenous vein graft percutaneous coronary intervention and clinical outcomes. *Am. J. Cardiol*. 2006;98:906–10.

[92] Fischell TA, Carter AJ, Foster MT, et al. Reversal of "no reflow" during vein graft stenting using high velocity boluses of intracoronary adenosine. *Cathet. Cardiovasc. Diagn*. 1998;45:360–5.

[93] Leborgne L, Cheneau E, Pichard A, et al. Effect of direct stenting on clinical outcome in patients treated with percutaneous coronary intervention on saphenous vein graft. *Am. Heart J.* 2003;146:501–6.

[94] Okabe T, Lindsay J, Torguson R, Steinberg DH, Roy P, Slottow TL, Kaneshige K, Xue Z, Satler LF, Kent KM, Pichard AD, Waksman R. Can direct stenting in selected saphenous vein graft lesions be considered an alternative to percutaneous intervention with a distal protection device? *Catheter. Cardiovasc. Interv*. 2008 Nov 15;72(6):799-803.

[95] Hong YJ, Pichard AD, Mintz GS, et al. Outcome of undersized drug-eluting stents for percutaneous coronary intervention of saphenous vein graft lesions. *Am. J. Cardiol.* 2010;105:179–85.

[96] Giugliano GR, Falcone MW, Mego D, Ebersole D, Jenkins S, Das T, Barker E, Ruggio JM, Maini B, Bailey SR. A prospective multicenter registry of laser therapy for degenerated saphenous vein graft stenosis: the COronary graft Results following Atherectomy with Laser (CORAL) trial. *Cardiovasc. Revasc. Med*. 2012 Mar-Apr;13(2):84-9.

[97] Cowley MJ, DiSciascio G. Directional coronary atherectomy for saphenous vein graft disease. *Cathet. Cardiovasc. Diagn*.1993;Suppl 1:10-6.

[98] Meliga E, García-García HM, Kukreja N, Daemen J, Tanimoto S, Ramcharitar S, van Mieghem CA, Sianos G, van der Ent M, van der Giessen WJ, de Feyter P, van Domburg R, Serruys PW. Chronic total occlusion treatment in post-CABG patients:

saphenous vein graft versus native vessel recanalization-long-term follow-up in the drug-eluting stent era. *Catheter. Cardiovasc. Interv*. 2007 Jul 1;70(1):21-5.

[99] Keith E. Robertson, Robert A. McDonald, Keith G. Oldroyd, Stuart A. Nicklin, Andrew H. Baker. Prevention of coronary in-stent restenosis and vein graft failure: Does vascular gene therapy have a role? *Pharmacology & Therapeutics* 136 (2012) 23–34.

Part IV: Future Strategies in the Treatment of Restenosis

In: Coronary Artery Restenosis
Editor: Amir S. Lotfi
ISBN: 978-1-63321-346-3

Chapter 14

Prevention of Restenosis with Stent-Based Vascular Gene Delivery: Gene Eluting Stents

Ilia Fishbein[1,2], *Michael Chorny*[1,2], *Ivan S. Alferiev*[1,2], *Richard F. Adamo*[1] *and Robert J. Levy*[1,2]
[1]Children's Hospital of Philadelphia
[2]University of Pennsylvania, PA, US

Abstract

Stent angioplasty coupled with drug elution from stents has radically changed the clinical approach and expected outcomes for millions of patients with advanced coronary artery disease. However, drug-eluting stents (DES) have several important disadvantages related to conceptual design limitations, as well as the pharmacology and release kinetics of the drugs used. Recently, synergistic research in the areas of post-angioplasty restenosis, late stent thrombosis (LST), drug-eluting stents, and cardiovascular gene therapy has shaped the concept of gene-eluting stents. Gene-eluting stents (GES) hold promise of overcoming some biological and technical problems inherent to drug-eluting stents by altering the typical inflammatory and proliferative response of vascular substrate to implanted stents through the long-term modification of gene expression programs in the injured/diseased vasculature. As the field of gene-eluting stents matures, it becomes apparent that all major design components of the gene-eluting stent (a therapeutic transgene, a gene vector, and a delivery system) are paramount for accomplishing meaningful levels of transgene expression and sustained inhibition of neointimal growth and thrombosis in the stented arteries. This chapter summarizes prior work on stent-based gene delivery for the prevention of in-stent restenosis and discusses the main optimization strategies required to move the field of gene-eluting stents into the clinical realm.

Introduction: The Problem of In-Stent Restenosis in the Era of Drug Eluting Stents

Percutaneous coronary interventions (PCIs) is a standard therapeutic approach for treating patients with symptomatic coronary artery disease. PCIs are carried out annually in more than one million patients in the USA alone [1]. A vast majority of PCI cases involve stent angioplasty performed with either bare metal stents (BMS) or drug eluting stents (DES). Although acute success rates of stent angioplasty are reasonably high, some cases are complicated later in the course of the vessel's response to stent implantation with the re-obstruction of the stented arterial segment termed "in-stent restenosis" (ISR) [2]. Introduction of DES in clinical practice in the first decade of 2000's has undeniably reduced occurrence of ISR and the need for re-intervention in comparison with BMS [3]. The remarkable success of DES in initial clinical trials, in which DES were used in single de novo lesions in the native coronary arteries [4,5] has prompted a fast expansion of DES indications to more complex lesion anatomies and to patients with significant co-morbidities, unfortunately resulting in a substantial increase of ISR rates when "real world" patient registries were analyzed and reported [6,7]. Currently, ISR rates are estimated to be higher than 10% for the patient populations with diabetes, renal failure and complex lesions including those occurring in venous grafts, ostial and bifurcation locations, small diameter (< 2 mm) arteries, etc [8-11]. Recent short- and middle-term results with the Zotarolimus-, Everolimus- and Biolumus A9-eluting stent platforms featuring highly efficient Limus-family drugs, improved stent materials and strut characteristics as well as the novel, increasingly biocompatible polymer coatings demonstrate positive trends in ISR prevalence when compared to the first generation paclitaxel- and sirolimus-eluting devices [12-14]. However, even with these newest DES, ISR is a very significant medical and healthcare problem given the sheer volume of stent angioplasty. Moreover, ISR occurring after DES implantation seems to be less manageable than the restenotic occlusion following deployment of BMS [15,16]. Therefore, new, conceptually different approaches for ISR prevention are still of high relevance even after 10 years of widespread use of DES products.

The Concept of Gene Eluting Stents (GES)

Early vascular gene delivery studies employing "arterial dwell" technique with or without use of specialized catheters [17] to locally deliver and lodge gene vectors in arterial tissue provided important initial data on suitability of different viral and non-viral vectors for vascular gene transfer and on transfectability of adventitia, media and intima (neointima) in various experimental animal species [18,19]. Additionally "pre-stent era" animal studies established numerous molecular targets for restenosis prevention that can be affected through gene therapy interventions [20]. Although few important exceptions were documented, these early vascular gene transfer studies typically showed that the reporter expression in vascular tissue is transitory even with the use of sophisticated catheters, such as Dispatch® and Infiltrator® [17]. A short duration and generally low levels of vascular tissue expression following localized gene delivery were in part attributed to the short intraluminal retention time of the delivered gene therapeutics [17].

Immobilization of gene vectors on stents embraces the best of both worlds, by combining proven advantages of DES concept with a wide range of targets manageable with gene therapy. Conceptually, modulating activity of individual genes and groups of genes has a more versatile bearing on cellular physiology and adaptation to pathological processes, such as vascular injury compared to the effects achievable with low-molecular weight drugs. Moreover, gene therapy can hypothetically attain a permanent therapeutic modification of vascular substrate without the need for re-dosing. Importantly, gene interventions, unlike the drugs used in DES can exert opposite effects on SMC and endothelium, allowing for selective inhibition of SMC proliferation and migration while maintaining and even enhancing endothelial re-growth. Moreover, while the de novo atherosclerotic process is not affected by the drugs used in currently available DES [21], the underlying atherosclerotic process can be concurrently addressed with gene therapy primarily aimed to mitigation of restenosis. Finally, a modulation of the biological activity of gene eluting stents can be achieved with systemically administered low molecular weight compounds, thus permitting turning the intervention on and off on demand and fine-tuning its therapeutic effects [22].

Compared with scaffold-less vascular gene delivery accomplished with the use of delivery catheters, stents present an advantageous physical platform for local arterial gene transfer. For example, higher local concentrations of gene vectors can be achieved in the treated artery with the stent-immobilized vectors when compared to non-immobilized vectors. Both physical vector association with a permanently implanted scaffolding device and the shielding of the metal struts from the shearing effect of blood flow contribute to better vascular wall retention of vector deposited on the adluminal surface of the stent (i.e. at a stent/tissue interface). Local uptake of the vector by arterial tissue increases as a consequence of protracted vascular residence.

Enhanced local uptake of the vector not only improves efficiency of vascular gene transfer, but also reduces the distal spread of gene vector and inadvertent inoculation of non-target tissues. Human coronary and femoral arteries are extensively branched. Therefore scaffold-less intraluminal delivery of the fluid-phase vector formulations results in immediate runoff of the vector to the circulation through the side branches. Open cell design of modern stents makes stent-based delivery of gene therapeutics feasible in arterial segments with side branches. In contrast with scaffold-less vascular gene delivery, stent-based gene transfer does not require temporary interruption of blood flow across the treated vascular segment. This circumstance is of paramount importance for coronary and carotid applications due to avoidance of procedure-related ischemic complications. Finally, stent-based gene delivery provides an optimal spatial configuration to prevent cellular proliferation and migration in the setting of ISR, since cell activation after stent deployment is typically observed in the vicinity of stent struts [23]. Physical association of gene vector with a stent establishes a transgene expression gradient that overlaps with the cell activation gradient, thus approximating vectors to the projected site of the action.

Thus, the use of gene delivery stents for atherosclerotic vascular disease offers the appealing possibility of site specific delivery of gene therapy with long lasting and controllable transgene expression that can both prevent in-stent restenosis and provide therapy for the primary atherosclerotic process.

The technological and biological requirements for GES design share several common characteristics with DES platforms. First, deliverability and strut apposition of both types of devices should not be compromised by the accommodation of a therapeutic agent depot and its matrix on the stent struts. Second, the matrix deposited on the DES and GES struts has to bear mechanical deformation associated with a change of the stent diameter during deployment without cracking, peeling and delamination. The latter may lead to erratic release kinetics of a therapeutic agent and distal embolization of polymeric debris. Third, the matrix has to be highly biocompatible, causing no more than a minimal thrombogenic and inflammatory response.

There are several important distinctions, however, in the design characteristics of DES and GES related to an intended period of active release phase. While DES have been engineered with the goal of providing sustained zero- to first-order release profile of low molecular weight drugs for the period of several months [24], this may be unnecessary for the GES since transduced arterial tissue itself presents a sustainable source of a transgene product. A minimal required duration for the arterial tissue endurance of the stent-delivered vector in a transduction competent state is not entirely clear. The medial and neointimal proliferation and centripetal migration of injury-activated vascular SMC starts no earlier than 1 week after stent deployment in human and higher animal models [25]. This circumstance argues for at least 2-3 week-long release period of a transduction competent gene vector from the stent, posing additional requirements to GES technology related to extended vector stability in vivo.

Unlike LMW anti-restenotic drugs, which are typically sufficiently lipophilic and thus well-soluble in hydrophobic matrices after solvent removal, both viral and non-viral gene vectors tend to form a separate phase when incorporated in suitable polymer coatings. Additionally, gene vectors are extremely vulnerable to the harsh chemical environments and mechanical stresses, and lose their transduction efficiency if not properly protected during matrix incorporation process.

While low molecular weight compounds used in DES do not typically elicit immune response, generation of an innate and acquired immune response toward both a vector and a therapeutic product is yet another specific problem of GES [26]. Therefore, minimizing distal spread of the vector to regional lymph nodes and spleen and preventing direct physical contact with pre-formed antibodies and antigen-presenting cells are vital for sustaining therapeutic levels of transgene expression following GES implantation.

Finally, the 1-3 orders of magnitude difference in molecular dimensions of low-molecular weight drugs and gene vectors dictates use of different matrices to enable timely release of a therapeutic agent from a GES platform. The choice of matrix and the size of the therapeutic agent further affect a predominant release mechanism (diffusion through intact polymeric matrix versus release facilitated by partial matrix degradation).

GES Prototypes

The previously described GES systems exploit several different chemical, engineering, and pharmaceutical approaches and respective designs enabling labile association of gene vectors with stent struts.

Bulk Immobilization

Initial investigations concerning gene delivery to vasculature from stent platform have utilized dispersion of gene vectors in polymer coatings cast on the surface of metallic stents. These coatings (typically 50-250 μm thick) were deposited on a primed stent surface either by a multiple dip technique or by aerosol deposition of a polymer solution containing a suspension of the vector. After solvent evaporation and polymer precipitation on the stent surface, the vector remains contained between the polymer fibers. A subsequent release of polymer-entrapped vector particles is then controlled by a limited diffusion though the polymer matrix, matrix degradation and/or dissolution of matrix in blood and tissue fluid. Depending on the vector and polymer type, these three mechanisms have varying contributions to the overall release kinetics of the vector from the polymer-coated stents. A number of synthetic polymers (PLGA [27], poly(beta-aminoester) [28-31], polyurethane [32,33], PVA [34], poly [phosphorylcholine-lauryl methacrylate] [35-41]), chemically modified natural polymers (dopamine-modified hyaluronic acid [42,43], cationized gelatin [44], styrene-modified gelatin[45], cationized pullulan [46] and naturally occurring macromolecules (collagen [47], denatured collagen [48], gelatin [28,29]) have been employed for the bulk incorporation of genetic material on stent wires.

The main advantage of bulk immobilization is the ability to integrate substantial amounts of the vector in a thick coating. Plasmid DNA quantities as high as 4 mg [33] or Ad doses up to $5x10^{10}$ particles [47] have been reported. However, several major drawbacks hindering further clinical development are inherent to this technology. For example, 80-90% of the vector load is typically released within the first 24 hours after stent deployment [28,32,34,36,37,46,49], especially in the case of non-viral systems. Part of this effect is due to the "burst release" of a sizable fraction of the vector payload, which is either deposited in the outermost layer of the polymer coating or has been adsorbed onto the polymer layer after going out of solution during the solvent evaporation step. A potential solution for limiting excessively rapid release of the vector is provided by a super-coating of a vector/polymer composite with additional layers of vector-free polymer [27-29]. Another feasible method of slowing vector release from bulk polymer coatings employs controlled cross-linking of a polymer as demonstrated by Nakayama et al. [45]. This group has developed a photoactivatable coating consisting of styrene-modified gelatin, a polymerization initiator, carboxylated camphorquinone, and a reporter Ad-LacZ adenovirus vector. Upon irradiation of dipped stents with a broad spectrum light source, gelatin chains become cross-linked forming a hydrogel that entraps adenoviral particles.

Another considerable problem related to the bulk polymer coatings is inflammation triggered by native and especially synthetic polymers in the segment of the artery underlying the polymer-coated stent [50]. The inflammatory response elicited by the polymer coating can overwhelm the therapeutic effect of a transgene. This untoward pro-inflammatory effect of polymer coatings was also observed for DES [51]. However in the case of DES, potent unselective anti-proliferation agents, such as paclitaxel and rapamycin, prevent inflammation-triggered SMC activation, albeit at expense of heightened local toxicity and impeded re-endothelialization [52]. The poly [phosphorylcholine-lauryl methacrylate] co-polymers utilized in the BiodivYsio stent [36-41]appear to possess much higher biocompatibility than any other synthetic or semi-synthetic polymer investigated for coating stents. A hydrophilic poly-phosphorylcholine (PC) moiety of this macromolecule mimics an outer phospholipid layer of cell membranes, thereby reducing platelet activation on the metal surface. A positive surface charge on the BiodivYsio stent imparted by choline residues renders the PC coating useful for electrostatic binding of negatively charged DNA plasmids, as well as Ad and AAV vectors. The latest generation of BiodivYsio stents utilizes extremely thin coatings (50 nm) precluding significant incorporation of the vector in the bulk of the polymer. Therefore, this system exemplifies a paradigm that includes both elements of bulk immobilization and the coatless surface immobilization systems as described below.

Surface Immobilization of Gene Vectors on Coatless Metal Substrate

Surface immobilization of gene vectors on the surface of endovascular stents represents a particular case of substrate mediated gene delivery, a concept put forward by the work of Shea [53,54] primarily to increase biocompatibility of bioprosthetic scaffolds. The main premise of substrate-mediated gene transfer is to use the tissue-facing surface of an implanted device to append (rather than incorporate) therapeutic gene vectors in an arranged pattern to facilitate transduction of tissue underlying bioprosthesis, thereby improving functional integration of the device. Achieving sufficient transduction of arteries with stent-tethered gene vectors requires reaching an equilibrium between two opposite tasks: binding vector to the surface of a stent *ex vivo* and releasing it upon contact with the vessel wall. This reversible tethering of gene vectors to the stent surfaces was realized using several different chemical approaches.

Vector immobilization via affinity adaptors

Studies by our group have adapted the concept of substrate-mediated delivery for use in conjunction with endovascular stents. Driven by the established data on detrimental pro-inflammatory and pro-restenotic effects of stent coatings, we designed and implemented a chemical strategy for reversible attachment to the metallic surfaces of stents of both viral and non-viral gene vectors that avoids the use of surface coating. Our method of vector immobilization is contingent upon chemical modification of the metal surface with poly(allylamine)-bisphoshonate (PAB), bridging the stent surface and gene vectors [55]. This process involves first creating a polyallylamine monolayer on the stainless steel surface of the stent that is spontaneously established due to the formation of coordination bonds between pendant bisphosphonic groups of PAB and Fe, Ni and Cr atoms and their oxides on the steel surface. This ultra-thin (less than 5 nm) permanently attached PAB monolayer is rapidly formed upon exposure of metal samples to an aqueous PAB solution. Amine groups can be further covalently modified in order to permit a covalent attachment of vector binding agents. The chemical approach entails a well-established N-hydroxysuccinime ester/amine conjugation chemical strategy targeting multiple primary amines of the polyallylamine backbone [55]. The specific bi-functional cross-linker reagent used for amine engagement, ***N***-Succinimidyl 3-(2-pyridyldithio)-propionate (SPDP), contains a thiol-reactive, pyridyldithio group. Therefore, consecutive reactions with PAB and SPDP render the stent surface thiol-reactive. Reduced (free thiol group-containing) forms of high affinity vector binding proteins such as anti-Ad knob [55], anti–DNA [56] antibodies or a recombinant D1 domain of Coxsackie-Adenovirus Receptor [55] can be attached to stent surfaces at this point. When localized in orderly fashion on stent surface, these protein molecules serve as binding adaptors enabling high-affinity binding of gene vectors to stents. Stent loading with gene vectors is achieved by simple immersion of a stent in a vector suspension, achieving vector immobilization density over 10^9 Ad particles/cm^2 of PAB-primed steel surface [55]. We further demonstrated that agents with different binding affinities can be exploited to adjust a vector capacity of the gene eluting stent and to modulate the release rate of gene therapeutics both in vitro and in vivo [55]. However, limited control over the vector release kinetics remains a disadvantage of the protein affinity binding immobilization technology. Although we have demonstrated the vector presence at the interface between stent struts and the arterial wall 24 hours post-deployment and associated reporter activity in all 3 arterial layers 7 days post-stenting [55], the duration of the vector binding to a stent *in vivo* may be far from optimal. It is challenging to prolong vector association with the stent surface using this technique, since the vector association with stents is determined by the antigen/antibody or receptor/ligand affinity, local pH, and the protein content of blood and tissue fluid, i.e. the factors that cannot be deliberately adjusted during the manufacturing process. Furthermore, the protein affinity binding technology cannot be immediately adapted to any given vector, since it implies availability of a vector-binding molecule with Kd in the range of 10^{-8}-10^{-9} M. Moreover, vector-binding strategies based on protein affinity interactions are difficult to adapt to manufacturing scale because of protein stability and species specificity issues.

Vector immobilization via hydrolyzable cross-linkers

In parallel with investigating affinity adaptor-mediated vector tethering, our research group has developed an alternative methodology for the reversible binding of recombinant replication-defective adenoviruses to metal surfaces. Importantly, this immobilization scheme completely avoids using poorly upscalable recombinant protein technology, making this new strategy more appealing for translational directions. This method is based on the use of hydrolyzable cross-linker (HC) molecules that directly append vectors to PAB-activated steel (Figure 1). Adenoviral vectors were modified by reacting NH_2 groups displayed on lysine residues of capsid proteins with a bifunctional amine/thiol reactive HC, rendering vector particles thiol-reactive. Following purification by size exclusion chromatography the thiol-reactive adenoviral vectors were directly conjugated to the thiol-derivatized stents [57]. The subsequent release of the vectors is governed by the kinetics of cross-linker hydrolysis (Figure 1) and can be modulated by the usage of HC with variable hydrolysis rates (Figure 2) [58]. A new conjugation approach required a modification of PAB chemical design to install activatable thiol groups in the side chains of polyallylamine. This novel compound, PABT, was successfully synthesized and characterized by our group [57]. The kinetics of bisphosphonate coordination with stainless steel surface and durability of polyallylamine monolayer was shown to be similar with that previously established for PAB [55]. Upon activation of latent thiols with Tris 2-carboxyethyl phosphine (TCEP), PABT-modified steel surface was shown to acquire 165±10 pmoles of thiol functions per cm^2 of modified steel surface. We also demonstrated that thiol group density can be further expanded to 739±46 pmoles/cm^2 using an additional exposure of thiol-activated metal samples to an aqueous solution of pyridyldithio (PDT)-engrafted polyethyleneimine, PEI(PDT), followed by conversion PDT groups to thiols upon reaction with dithiothreitol (DTT) (Figure 1) [57]. We further demonstrated that the "amplification" protocol resulted in a more effective Ad tethering when compared with the basic "no-amplification" protocol [57].

Synthetic, biodegradable HC are particularly promising tools for achieving a site-specific tunable release of gene therapy vectors since they can be synthesized to have a broad range of hydrolysis rates and thus the vector release rate from the surface of a stent can programmed per the formulation parameters [58].

Magnetic Targeting of Gene Vectors to Magnetizable Stents

Both bulk immobilization and surface tethering of gene vectors make use of stent-based gene delivery systems that are pre-assembled prior to the stent deployment at the diseased site. Introduction of a stent into the vasculature through the hemostatic valve of a vascular sheath and advancing it to a deployment site through the narrowed and often calcified arterial conduit entail physical damage to the stent coating and vector depot. Alternatively, stent loading with gene therapy vectors can be accomplished *in situ* after the stent has already been implanted at the chosen location. Since the deployed stent is freely accessible to blood flow, its surface can hypothetically be actively targeted with therapeutic agents delivered to systemic or regional circulation, provided the targeting forces are sufficient to capture and retain a therapeutic agent on the stent surface.

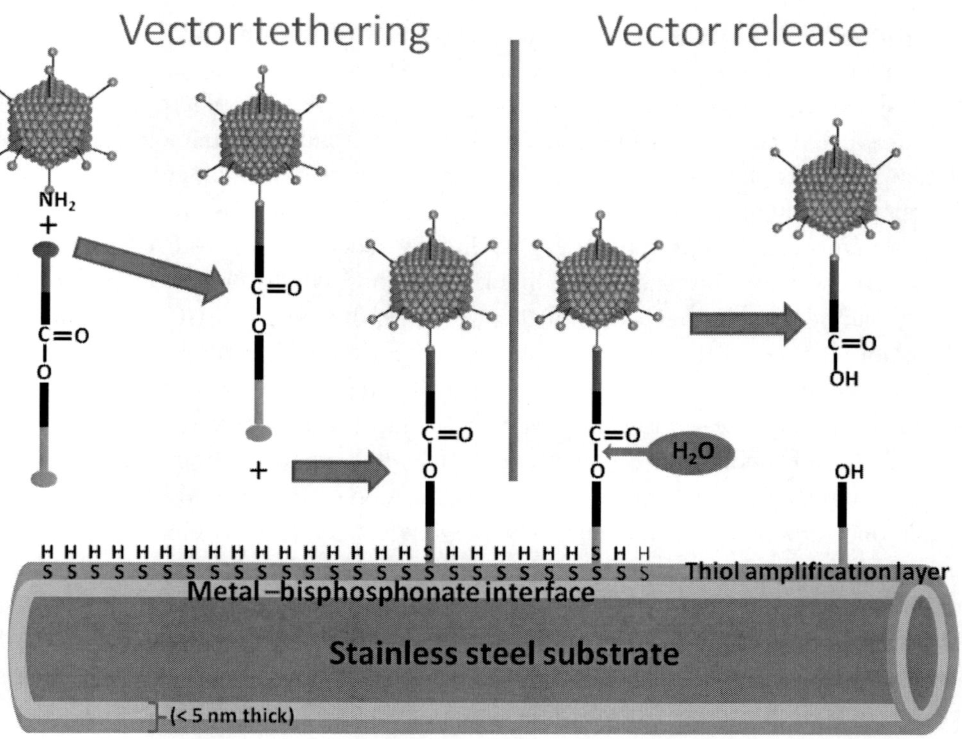

Figure 1. Reversible immobilization of adenoviral vectors on the stainless steel surfaces. A schematic representation of adenoviral vector immobilization using physical tethering to a PABT/PEI(PDT)-modified stainless steel surface via a hydrolyzable cross-linker (left) and subsequent release of the vector upon cross-linker hydrolysis (right). Adapted from [58] with permission.

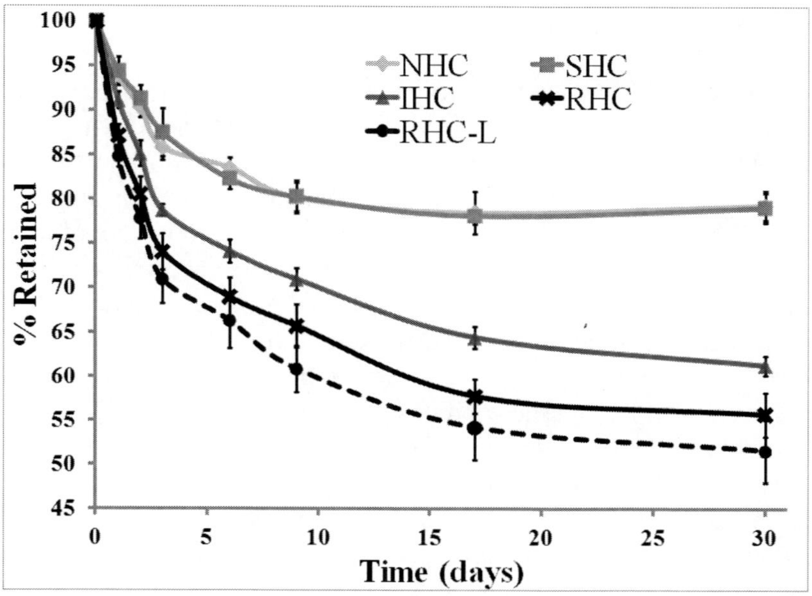

Figure 2. Release kinetics of Ad vector tethered to metal substrates with HC. Stainless steel mesh disks were formulated with ~$2x10^9$ fluorescently labeled adenovirus particles attached to the PABT/PEI(PDT)-modified surface after modification with 500 μM of non-hydrolyzable cross-linker (NHC), and hydrolyzable analogs with slow, intermediate and rapid kinetics of an in-chain ester bond hydrolysis (SHC, IHC and RHC, respectively). Additionally, a group of samples (designated as RHC-L) was formulated with the vector modified with 100 μM RHC. The release of fluorescently labeled Ad-particles was studied at the indicated time points by well-scan fluorometry at 530/555 nm. Fluorometry results are presented as means ± SEM, n =8-10. p<0.001 for all comparisons between the NHC and SHC vs IHC, RHC and RHC-L groups were determined by Anova with a post-hoc Tukey test. Reproduced from [58]with permission.

The concept of *in situ* stent loading with gene vectors was recently implemented by our group using a magnetic targeting paradigm [59]. Stents made of magnetic alloys, such as 304- and 430-grade stainless steel when positioned in uniform magnetic field (0.1 Tesla or higher) induced in MRI imagers or created by customized electromagnet assemblies generate strong highly localized magnetic forces due to steep field gradients between stent struts [59-61]. These magnetic forces enable the targeted capture of systemically or locally administered gene vectors co-formulated with iron salts (magnetite) and matrix forming excipients as magnetic nanoparticles [59-61]. In our study [59], aortic arch delivery of MNP formulation incorporating $2.5x10^9$ luciferase-encoding adenoviral vectors was carried out in rats with magnetically responsive stents implanted in the common carotid artery. The delivered vector was then transported en masse with antegrade blood flow to carotid circulation across the stented segment. During and immediately after MNP/Ad-Luc delivery a uniform magnetic field of 0.1 Tesla was established across the neck area of the rats. The localized arterial transduction confined to the stented carotid segment, was found in the treated animals 2 and 9 days post-stenting by bioluminescence imaging [59]. The observed levels of transgene expression in control rats treated with the same formulation under non-magnetic conditions and in rats delivered with free vector under the magnetic settings were 8-14 fold lower than in the magnetically targeted animals.

Magnetic Reloading of Depleted GES

The ultimate goal of stent-based vascular gene therapy is a prolonged (or even a permanent) localized expression of a transgene with established anti-restenotic effectiveness following GES implantation. Despite active research in the field for the past 15 years, it is still premature to conclude whether the goal of attaining a life-long arterial expression following a single intervention deems practical. Indeed, the duration of the transgene expression and hence the durability of the therapeutic effect is a concern, even with protracted release kinetics of gene vectors from stents, such as was observed with hydrolyzable cross-linker immobilization [58]. In most mammalian tissues, after reaching peak level, transgene expression tends to decrease over time due to promoter attenuation and mounting immune response to the vector and the transgene product. Previous reports [62,63] have documented that suppressed neointimal growth can recur if the inhibiting modality is withdrawn early. The vulnerability period for restenosis recurrence following premature treatment withdrawal in human arteries is unknown, but appears to be longer for peripheral compared to coronary vasculature. Therefore, the potential to rejuvenate therapeutic transgene expression by reloading stents with additional payloads of the same or other gene vectors is of paramount importance in designing translatable vascular gene therapy approaches to prevent restenosis, especially in peripheral vasculature. Uniform field high-gradient magnetic targeting provides a facile way of addressing reloading of depleted GES at delayed time points. In order to reload a stent *in situ*, a gene vector needs to be physically partitioned at or near the depot for sufficient time to saturate binding sites in the depot matrix with the re-delivered vectors. Magnetic field mediated targeting provides a unique physical opportunity to achieve this task.

Indeed, in our preliminary studies antegrade carotid artery delivery of a formulation comprising zinc oleate MNP co-formulated with luciferase-encoding adenoviral vector to rats previously implanted with DES harboring the same vector resulted in rejuvenation of transgene expression in the stented arterial segment (Figure 3).

Reporter Studies and Pharmacokinetics of Transgene Expression

Studies investigating reporter gene expression are instrumental for optimizing stent-based gene delivery systems in regards to transgene expression strength and durability. GFP [27,31,33,47-49,55,57,64,65], β-galactosidase [33,34,36,39,40,45] and luciferase [33,49,55,57,58] have been extensively employed to map temporal and spatial expression patterns of stent-delivered transgenes. The information provided by different reporter systems is not redundant. For example, while luciferase is typically more sensitive than the other two reporter systems, it does not readily provide a tissue level resolution. Use of GFP and β-galactosidase, on the other hand, is compatible with direct histological examination of transduced tissue, providing valuable information about transduced cell populations and their distribution in distinct compartments of the vessel wall. Native GFP fluorescence is labile and extremely sensitive to proper tissue fixation. Moreover, GFP emits light in the same part of spectrum as elastin, making unambiguous detection of GFP positive cells difficult, especially since partially disintegrated elastin accumulates in the injured media. A recent advent of high quality commercial anti-GFP antibodies makes this task easier by streamlining immunofluorescence and immunohistochemical approaches for the identification of GFP-transduced cells.

A direct comparison of the extent and duration of reporter arterial expression across the published studies is not trivial because of dissimilarities between animal models, reporter systems and reporter detection methods employed by different groups. Nevertheless, several common characteristics inherent to stent-based transduction of arterial tissue are well-conserved regardless of the specific experimental setup. First, gene transfer is highly site-specific, leading to more effective transduction of cells underlying stent struts compared to cells located between the stent wires [33,34,39,40,55,57]. Second, despite neointimal growth not occurring until 4-14 days after a stent deployment, a growing neointima is more effectively transduced than media and adventitia [33,39,49,55,57]. Third, the duration of gene expression may exceed one month following implantation of GES [39,40]. Fourth, no massive distal spread of a transgene to liver, spleen or lungs is apparent [27,33,47,55,57]. Fifth, viral vectors generally demonstrate higher efficiency than non-viral counterparts both in terms of the peak levels of arterial expression and its duration. Finally, different vector systems may have predilection for transducing specific cell populations in the arterial wall [33,39].

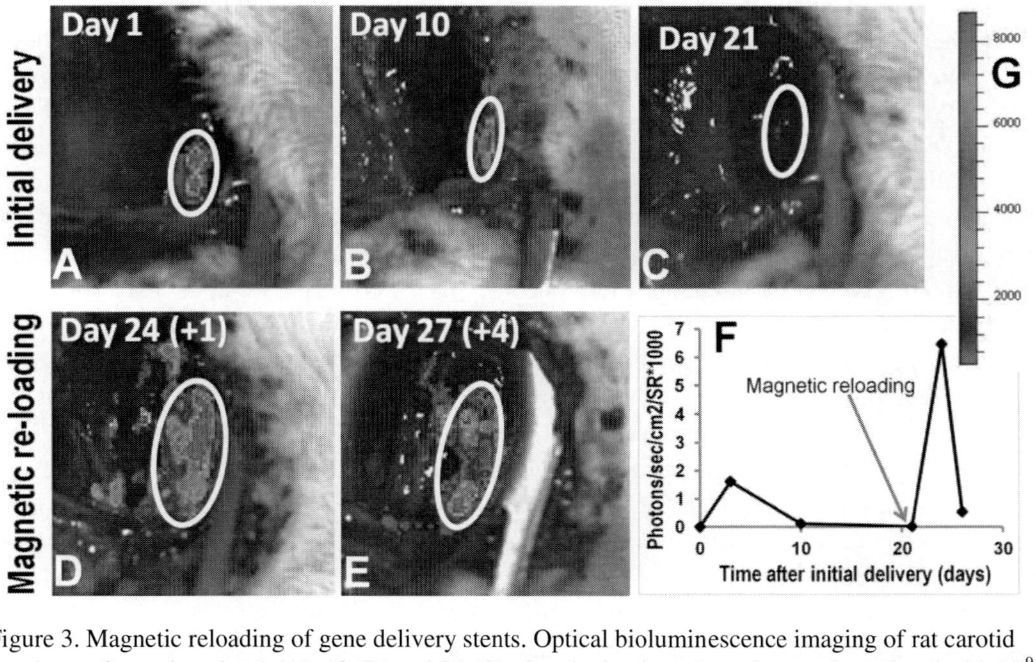

Figure 3. Magnetic reloading of gene delivery stents. Optical bioluminescence imaging of rat carotid arteries performed on day 1 (A), 10 (B) and 21 (C) after the implantation of stents formulated with 10^9 Ad-Luc particles. 23 days post-deployment the animals were treated with Ad-Luc/MNP in a dose corresponding to10^{10} viral particles via a catheter placed in the aortic arch in the presence of magnetic field (1200 Gauss). Imaging was repeated on days 24 (D) and 27 (E) after stenting (i.e. on days 1 and 4 after magnetic reloading of the stents). The time course of luciferase expression (F) is plotted based on the conversion scale (G) consistently adjusted for all time points (A-E).

Molecular Targets for the Prevention of Restenosis and Therapeutic Transgenes

In-stent restenosis is a multifactorial disease [66,67]. The stent implantation injury-related factors with proven pathogenic bearing for ISR include denudation of endothelium, direct trauma to medial SMC resulting in the initial wave of SMC apoptosis followed by subsequent SMC activation and modulation to the synthetic (proliferative) phenotype, parietal thrombus formation, unresolved inflammation and foreign body reaction to the stent and its coating. Accordingly, the number of molecular targets relevant to inhibition or stimulation of signaling pathways altered during ISR development is extremely high [66,67]. Comprehensive reviews [20,68,69] focused on gene therapy of restenosis list more than 150 genes implicated in regulation of cell proliferation, migration, ECM turnover, thrombosis and inflammation that were targeted with gene therapy interventions to alleviate restenosis. Only those therapeutic gene constructs that were investigated in conjunction with gene based delivery will be discussed here.

GES Targeting Endothelial Re-Growth

Since the seminal study by Asahara et al. [70] has demonstrated inhibition of balloon injury-induced restenosis in rats with locally administered vascular endothelial growth factor (VEGF), strategies aimed at attenuating restenosis via enhanced re-endothelialization have come into focus. In line with this concept, Walter et al. [41] have used poly [phosphorylcholine-lauryl methacrylate]-coated stents to electrostatically adsorb 200 μg plasmid DNA encoding human VEGF-2. When deployed in Fogarty balloon-denuded external iliac arteries of hypercholesterolemic rabbits, VEGF-2 plasmid eluting stents enhanced endothelial recovery in the stented arteries in comparison with the animals receiving control stents and resulted in a 60% reduction of cross-sectional arterial narrowing of the stented region 3 months after the procedure [41]. Recently Paul et al. [71] utilized a baculovirus vector expressing VEGF-A $_{(165)}$ to promote endothelial re-growth in stented canine femoral arteries. In this composite system baculovirus vectors were complexed with PAMAM dendrimers prior to incorporating the vector/PAMAM complexes into PLGA microparticles. The latter were immobilized in fibrinogen coating on the surface of bare metal stent using a layer-by-layer coating technique with recurring thrombin exposure to convert fibrinogen into fibrin. The extent of re-endothelialization of explanted stented arteries was increased at 16 weeks post-stenting in the group of Bac/VEGF-eluting stents in comparison with the BMS group (93.5 ± 5.2 vs. 72.4 ± 4.1). This accelerated restoration of endothelium was associated with a 28% reduction of neointimal area in the animals receiving GES [71]. These results are in general agreement with the previous authors' data generated in the same model and investigating both re-endothelialization and restenosis at 6 weeks after stenting with the VEGF/Angiopoietin-1 plasmid eluting stents [72]. The stents were coated with a hydrogel formed due to the ionic association of negatively charged polyacrylic acid-modified single-walled carbon nanotubes and positively charged TAT-decorated DNA nanoparticles [72].

GES Targeting SMC Proliferation, Migration and ECM Remodeling

Serine/threonine kinase, Akt1, also known as protein kinase B (PKB) is an important signaling hub integrating inputs from several pro-proliferative pathways, in particular from PI3K [73]. Akt1 activation during neointimal tissue maturation [74] as well as the anti-restenotic effectiveness of Akt1 inhibition [75] are well established. Recently Che et al. [42] implemented attachment of dopamine-conjugated hyaluronic acid (HA) to stents via stable coordination bonds established between dopamine residues and metal ions on the stent surface. The HA-coated stents were further modified with polyplexes made of siRNA to Akt1 and disulfide cross-linked PEI. A sustained release of siRNA from the stent surface was observed in vitro for at least 72 hours. In *in vivo* study, an undisclosed amount of Akt1 siRNA polyplexes was deposited on HA-coated stents. The extent of ISR in rabbit iliac arteries implanted with Akt1 siRNA-formulated stents decreased by 50% compared to the BMS-treated arteries at 4 weeks after deployment [42].

Platelet-derived growth factor (PDGF) in its homodimeric forms (PDGF-AA, PDGF-BB) and as a heterodimer (PDGF-AB) is a well established SMC mitogen [76] and pro-migratory chemoattractant [77]. All three isoforms were shown to promote SMC accumulation *in vitro* and *in vivo*, while exerting relatively weak effect on endothelial cells [78]. Therefore, LMW inhibitors of PDGF receptor tyrosine kinase activity, tyrphostins [79], as well as gene therapy modalities of inhibiting the PDGF-triggered signaling cascades [80,81] are appealing directions to selectively inhibit SMC growth without affecting endothelial cell regeneration. To this end, Li et al. [82] synthesized phosphorothioate antisense oligodeoxynucleotides (ODN) to the 15 base-long conserved coding sequence of PDGF-A gene and complexed them with PEI. This polyplex formulation was further absorbed on hydrogel-coated stents. When implanted in the coronary arteries of healthy pigs, the anti-sense eluting stents resulted in a 50% reduction of neointimal thickening in comparison with non-sense ODN-eluting and plain hydrogel stents [82]. Importantly, the endothelial lining was complete 28 days after stenting in the arterial sections from the animals treated with the antisense PDGF-A –eluting stents, while the endothelialization was patchy at the 28 days time point in the arteries of animals receiving commercial sirolimus-eluting stents [82].

Proliferative stimulation exerted by multiple growth factors and cytokines via the plasma membrane- and cytoplasm-located receptors is ultimately converged on several crucial nuclear transcription factors, activating transcription of crucial cell cycle checkpoint proteins, such as cyclins and cyclin-dependent kinases. To this end, complete re-endothelialization of stented pig coronaries and a 40% reduction of restenosis were observed with a PC-coated stent platform locally eluting 82 ± 14 μg of nuclease-resistant phosphorothioate morpholino anti-sense construct (AVI-4126) targeting expression of c-myc, a transcription factor involved in cell cycle progression [83].

As a proliferation control checkpoint, c-myc is in turn partially controlled by the activator protein-1 (AP-1) transcription factor. Synthetic decoy ODN against consensus AP-1 binding site were delivered on stents implanted in rabbit abdominal aortae, along with the stents formulated with scrambled ODN and BMS. Protein and mRNA expression of TGF-beta1 and connective tissue growth factor (CTGF), as well as neointimal thickening in abdominal aortas was significantly decreased in the AP-1 decoy ODN-eluting stents 8 weeks post-procedure as compared to both control groups targeting was coated onto DES [84].

In-stent neointima is primarily formed by the progeny of medial SMC and adventitial myofibroblasts that populate the intimal space of an injured artery. Matrix remodeling triggered by vascular trauma facilitates migration of these cell populations along the gradients of specific chemoattractants [85]. Thus, stabilization of ECM was proposed for limiting centripetal migration of SMC. In accordance with this idea, Johnson and colleagues [36] bulk-immobilized a suspension of Ad vector ($4x10^8$ pfu) encoding synthesis of the tissue inhibitor of metalloprotease-3 (TIMP3) on PC-coated stainless steel stents. At 28 days after stent implantation in pig carotid arteries, neointimal volume was reduced by 40% and 50% in the animals treated with Ad-TIMP3-decorated stents in comparison with pigs receiving BMS or Ad-LacZ immobilized stents, respectively [36].

GES Targeting Stenting-Induced Inflammation

Acute inflammatory response in the form of platelet and fibrin deposition and massive neutrophil recruitment to the site of vascular trauma via P-selectin and CD11b/CD18 engagement is triggered immediately upon stent deployment [66,86]. During the first week after stent implantation, an escalating production of IL-6, IL-8 and MCP-1 by the injured SMC and ingressing neutrophils attracts monocytes that transmigrate into arterial tissue both through the lumen and via vasa vasorum. The conversion of ingressing monocytes into macrophages denotes a stage of chronic inflammation. Macrophages are the key cell type bridging inflammation with neointimal formation, since macrophage-produced and secreted chemokines (TNF, IL-1β) and growth factors (PDGF, bFGF, IGF) stimulate luminal migration and proliferation of medial SMC as well as adventitial myofibroblasts, which collectively form neointima [66,86,87]. Therefore, curtailing initial inflammatory response represents a well-recognized anti-restenotic strategy [88,89].

In keeping with this therapeutic approach, Egashira et al. and [34] evaluated stents eluting plasmid DNA encoding N-terminus deletion mutant of MCP1. The stents deployed in the iliac arteries of hypercholesterolemic rabbits and cynomolgus monkeys resulted in approximately a 20% reduction of macrophage infiltration at the stent implantation site and a 20-30% restenosis attenuation in comparison with BMS [34].

NFkB is a master transcription factor involved in the regulation of multiple inflammatory mediators. Ohtani et al. [32] used NFkB decoy ODN (500 μg/stent) incorporated in a polyurethane coating. Stents deployed in femoral arteries of hypercholesterolemic rabbits demonstrated approximately a 30% decrease of neointimal thickening in comparison with BMS and polyurethane coated stents at 4 weeks post-stenting and a significant decrease of inflammatory marker expression at 3 and 10 days post-implantation [32].

GES Targeting Thrombus Formation in Stented Arteries

Platelets are the first cellular elements to contact the surface of newly deployed stents. Since both human patients and experimental animals undergoing stent placement are pretreated with anti-platelet and anti-coagulant drugs, acute blockage of a treated artery is seldom an issue. However, a non-occluding parietal thrombus is routinely formed at the angioplasty/stenting site. If the parietal thrombus persists, it gets populated with the migrating SMC, thus facilitating fast neointimal growth.

In an attempt to minimize platelet activation at the site of stent implantation, Takemoto et al. [44] formulated gene eluting stents incorporating plasmid DNA encoding E-NTPDase, a crucial regulator of platelet thrombus formation. This molecule is a membrane bound enzyme that locally hydrolyses ATP, thus opposing platelet aggregation. The plasmid DNA (78 ± 5 μg) was absorbed into cationized gelatin hydrogel coating on the stent struts. Implantation of E-NTPDase-eluting stents in a rabbit model of repeated femoral injury, which is characterized by a high rate of thrombus formation completely prevented the occurrence of intravascular thrombi, while 25% and 50% of femoral arteries treated with control βGal plasmid-eluting stents had compromised patency at 3 and 7 days post-stenting. Moreover, since thrombus serves as a nidus for SMC colonization, thus enhancing neointimal formation, the extent of early restenosis (at day 7) was significantly reduced in the vessels treated with E-NTPDase stents [44].

GES Targeting Nitric Oxide Production and Availability

Nitric oxide (NO), a by-product of enzymatic conversion of arginine to citrulline has recently emerged as a key signaling molecule in vascular homeostasis [90,91]. Increased NO production and availability were shown to prevent platelet aggregation [92], inhibit SMC proliferation [93,94], and migration [95], promote endothelial growth[96], and decrease expression of cell adhesion molecules by endothelium, inhibiting ingress of activated leukocytes into the arterial intima [97]. Additionally NO promotes viability of endothelial progenitor cells and enhances their capacity to reconstitute damaged endothelium [98]. The pleiotropic nature of its beneficial actions makes NO-related interventions a plausible strategy for the prevention of ISR.

Both endothelial [99,100] and inducible [101,102] forms of NO synthase (eNOS and iNOS, respectively) were investigated as genes with potential anti-restenotic activity in animal models of arterial injury/local delivery generally showing strong inhibiting effects on neointimal formation. Driven by the wide scope of anti-restenotic mechanisms bestowed by NO, we [55,57] and others [28,38,39,65] have pursued the idea of the stent-based delivery of NOS-encoding vectors.

The studies by Sharif and others [38] employed PC coated stents configured with $5x10^9$ pfu of Ad-eNOS to address the hypothesis that enhanced re-endothelialization and reduced restenosis can be achieved in a rabbit model with GES-induced eNOS overexpression. The authors demonstrated significantly enhanced restoration of the endothelial layer and reduced neointimal thickness in both normo- and hypercholesterolemic rabbits treated with Ad-eNOS stents in comparison with animals that received Ad-βGal-eluting stents or blank PC-coated stents. In an attempt to formulate a gene eluting stent devoid of immunogenic and pro-inflammatory adenoviral proteins, thus facilitating clinical translation of stent-based eNOS overexpression, the same group recently reported [39] on a Lipofectin-based lipoplex formulation containing human eNOS plasmid. Ten μg of the lipoplex formulation were uniformly deposited on PC-coated stents. The non-viral gene eluting stents deployed in iliac arteries of hypercholesterolemic rabbits achieved levels of transgene expression comparable formatting issue – line spacing to Ad-containing GES. Moreover re-endothelialization at 28 days was similarly enhanced by eNOS lipoplex eluting stents. However, no significant reduction in restenosis indices was observed in this study. The authors explain this discrepancy by the fact that liposomal formulation primarily targets the macrophage population in the diseased artery and not SMC, thus missing the vital cell type affecting restenosis.

In contrast, using a similar rabbit model for therapeutic assessment of eNOS-lipoplex eluting stents, Brito et al. [28] demonstrated a 30% reduction of restenosis accompanied by a 50% decrease of proliferation in the eNOS lipoplex-treated rabbit arteries in comparison with an empty vector control. The difference in the vector dose (10 μg vs. 25 μg) and the delivery system used (adsorption of lipoplexes on a PC-coated stent vs. stent coating with lipoplexes dispersed in a gelatin/mannitol formulation with additional lipoplex-free gelatin/PLGA supercoating) between the former and the latter studies may account for the different outcomes, highlighting the importance of proper pharmaceutical adjustments for revealing full therapeutic potential of GES.

In our studies, Ad-iNOS delivered in a rat model from PAB- or PABT-modified bare metal stents using affinity adaptors [55] or hydrolyzable cross-linkers [57] for vector tethering, respectively, resulted in a 50%-60% reduction of neointimal thickening in comparison with the BMS-implanted arteries. These effects were achieved using 10^9-10^{10} Ad-iNOS particles (10^7-10^8 pfu) appended to a stent. Our recent studies assessing NO synthesis and ROS production in cultured SMC and endothelium transduced with Ad-iNOS tethered to stainless steel disks have determined that the super-physiological levels of iNOS expression driven by the immobilized vector can lead to NOS decoupling due to deficiency of arginine and tetrahydrobiopterin [22]. Decoupled NOS is unable to generate NO, producing superoxide instead [103]. If not effectively removed by superoxide dismutases, superoxide triggers a sequence of redox reactions that result in the formation of multiple additional ROS, which can cause extensive tissue damage [103]. Therefore, pharmacological supplementation with arginine and tetrahydrobiopterin may be required to modulate the function of NOS over-expressed in the arterial wall using stent based delivery of a respective vector [22].

Which of three known isoforms of NOS is the best choice for the use in conjunction with GES is not immediately obvious. A study by Cooney et al. [100] compared the antirestenotic effectiveness of Ad-iNOS and Ad-eNOS in a model of intraluminal dwell delivery of the vectors to temporarily isolated segment of balloon-injured rabbit carotid arteries. While a 20-min incubation of both vectors (10^9 pfu) resulted in an identical extent of neointimal inhibition in comparison with Ad-βGal-treated counterparts, this was allegedly achieved by dissimilar mechanisms, since eNOS overexpression promoted and iNOS overexpression inhibited endothelial regeneration in the treated arterial segments [100]. Additional in-depth studies are required to elucidate the actual mechanisms involved in the antirestenotic effects of different NOS isoforms and their utility in the setting of GES-induced overexpression.

Conclusion

Gene eluting stents represent an interesting alternative to drug eluting stents in clinical circumstances where current DES formulations often fail to provide satisfactory results. Research related to GES has now come to a phase when the perspectives of clinical translation should always be taken into consideration. However, further work related to optimization of all three main design components of GES: a therapeutic transgene, a vector and a delivery system has to be done before stent based vascular gene therapy comes to clinical fruition.

Acknowledgments

Studies carried out as part of the experimental work discussed in this review were supported by American Heart Association Scientist Development grants (I.F. 0735110N and M.C. 10SDG4020003), U.S. National Heart, Lung, and Blood Institute grant HL 72108 (R.J.L.) and U.S. National Heart, Lung, and Blood Institute grant HL 111118 (M.C.) Support was also provided by the following Children's Hospital of Philadelphia Research Funds: The William J. Rashkind Endowment (R.J.L.), Erin's Fund (R.J.L.), and The Kibel Foundation (R.J.L.). The authors wish to acknowledge secretarial assistance of Ms. Susan Kerns.

References

[1] Go, AS; Mozaffarian, D; Roger, VL; et al. Heart disease and stroke statistics--2014 update: a report from the american heart association. *Circulation*, 2014, 129, e28-e292.

[2] Kornowski, R; Hong, MK; Tio, FO; Bramwell, O; Wu, H; Leon, MB. In-stent restenosis: contributions of inflammatory responses and arterial injury to neointimal hyperplasia. *J Am Coll Cardiol*, 1998, 31, 224-30.

[3] Wallace, EL; Abdel-Latif, A; Charnigo, R; et al. Meta-analysis of long-term outcomes for drug-eluting stents versus bare-metal stents in primary percutaneous coronary interventions for ST-segment elevation myocardial infarction. *Am J Cardiol*, 2012, 109, 932-40.

[4] Morice, MC; Serruys, PW; Sousa, JE; et al. A randomized comparison of a sirolimus-eluting stent with a standard stent for coronary revascularization. *N Engl J Med*, 2002, 346, 1773-80.

[5] Moses, JW; Leon, MB; Popma, JJ; et al. Sirolimus-eluting stents versus standard stents in patients with stenosis in a native coronary artery. *N Engl J Med*, 2003, 349, 1315-23.

[6] Liistro, F; Fineschi, M; Angioli, P; et al. Effectiveness and safety of sirolimus stent implantation for coronary in-stent restenosis: the TRUE (Tuscany Registry of Sirolimus for Unselected In-Stent Restenosis) Registry. *J Am Coll Cardiol*, 2006, 48, 270-5.

[7] Roy, P; Buch, AN; Javaid, A; et al. Impact of "off-label" utilization of drug-eluting stents on clinical outcomes in patients undergoing percutaneous coronary intervention. *Am J Cardiol*, 2008, 101, 293-9.

[8] De, Luca, G; Dirksen, MT; Spaulding, C; et al. Impact of diabetes on long-term outcome after primary angioplasty: insights from the DESERT cooperation. *Diabetes Care*, 2013, 36, 1020-5.

[9] Freixa, X; Almasood, AS; Khan, SQ; et al. Choice of stent and outcomes after treatment of drug-eluting stent restenosis in highly complex lesions. *Catheter Cardiovasc Interv*, 2013, 81, E16-22.

[10] Kim, JS; Lee, HC; Choi, BK; et al. Impact of metabolic syndrome on in-stent restenosis and clinical outcomes after percutaneous coronary stent implantation. *Diabetes Res Clin Pract*, 2010, 88, e38-41.
[11] Rathore, S; Terashima, M; Katoh, O; et al. Predictors of angiographic restenosis after drug eluting stents in the coronary arteries: contemporary practice in real world patients. *EuroIntervention*, 2009, 5, 349-54.
[12] Brener, SJ; Kereiakes, DJ; Simonton, CA; et al. Everolimus-eluting stents in patients undergoing percutaneous coronary intervention: final 3-year results of the Clinical Evaluation of the XIENCE V Everolimus Eluting Coronary Stent System in the Treatment of Subjects With de Novo Native Coronary Artery Lesions trial. *Am Heart J*, 2013, 166, 1035-42.
[13] Colmenarez, H; Fernandez, C; Escaned, J. Impact of technological developments in drug-eluting stents on patient-focused outcomes: a pooled direct and indirect comparison of randomised trials comparing first- and second-generation drug-eluting stents. *EuroIntervention, online publish-ahead-of-print*, June 17, 2013
[14] Palmerini, T; Biondi-Zoccai, G; Della, Riva, D; et al. Clinical Outcomes with Bioabsorbable Polymer-based versus Durable Polymer-based Drug-Eluting Stents and Bare Metal Stents: Evidence from a Comprehensive Network Meta-analysis. *J Am Coll Cardiol*, 2014, 63, 299-307.
[15] Dangas, GD; Claessen, BE; Caixeta, A; Sanidas, EA; Mintz, GS; Mehran, R. In-stent restenosis in the drug-eluting stent era. *J Am Coll Cardiol*, 2010, 56, 1897-907.
[16] Steinberg, DH; Gaglia, MA; Jr.; Pinto, Slottow, TL; et al. Outcome differences with the use of drug-eluting stents for the treatment of in-stent restenosis of bare-metal stents versus drug-eluting stents. *Am J Cardiol*, 2009, 103, 491-5.
[17] Sharif, F; Daly, K; Crowley, J; O'Brien, T. Current status of catheter- and stent-based gene therapy. *Cardiovasc Res*, 2004, 64, 208-16.
[18] McKay, MJ; Gaballa, MA. Gene transfer therapy in vascular diseases. *Cardiovasc Drug Rev*, 2001, 19, 245-62.
[19] Smith, RC; Walsh, K. Local gene delivery to the vessel wall. *Acta Physiol Scand*, 2001, 173, 93-102.
[20] Appleby, CE; Kingston, PA. Gene therapy for restenosis--what now, what next? *Curr Gene Ther*, 2004, 4, 153-82.
[21] Nakazawa, G; Otsuka, F; Nakano, M; et al. The pathology of neoatherosclerosis in human coronary implants bare-metal and drug-eluting stents. *J Am Coll Cardiol*, 2011, 57, 1314-22.
[22] Forbes, SP; Alferiev, IS; Chorny, M; Adamo, RF; Levy, RJ; Fishbein, I. Modulation of NO and ROS production by AdiNOS transduced vascular cells through supplementation with L-Arg and BH4: implications for gene therapy of restenosis. *Atherosclerosis*, 2013, 230, 23-32.
[23] Yutani, C; Ishibashi-Ueda, H; Suzuki, T; Kojima, A. Histologic evidence of foreign body granulation tissue and de novo lesions in patients with coronary stent restenosis. *Cardiology*, 1999, 92, 171-7.
[24] Acharya, G; Park, K. Mechanisms of controlled drug release from drug-eluting stents. *Adv Drug Deliv Rev*, 2006, 58, 387-401.
[25] Schwartz RS. Pathophysiology of restenosis: interaction of thrombosis, hyperplasia, and/or remodeling. *Am J Cardiol*, 1998, 81, 14E-7E.

[26] Nayak, S; Herzog, RW. Progress and prospects: immune responses to viral vectors. *Gene Ther*, 2010, 17, 295-304.
[27] Klugherz, BD; Jones, PL; Cui, X; et al. Gene delivery from a DNA controlled-release stent in porcine coronary arteries. *Nat Biotechnol*, 2000, 18, 1181-4.
[28] Brito, LA; Chandrasekhar, S; Little, SR; Amiji, MM. Non-viral eNOS gene delivery and transfection with stents for the treatment of restenosis. *Biomed Eng Online*, 2010, 9, 56.
[29] Brito, LA; Chandrasekhar, S; Little, SR; Amiji, MM. In vitro and in vivo studies of local arterial gene delivery and transfection using lipopolyplexes-embedded stents. *J Biomed Mater Res A*, 2010, 93, 325-36.
[30] Jewell, CM; Zhang, J; Fredin, NJ; Wolff, MR; Hacker, TA; Lynn, DM. Release of plasmid DNA from intravascular stents coated with ultrathin multilayered polyelectrolyte films. *Biomacromolecules*, 2006, 7, 2483-91.
[31] Saurer, EM; Jewell, CM; Roenneburg, DA; et al. Polyelectrolyte multilayers promote stent-mediated delivery of DNA to vascular tissue. *Biomacromolecules*, 2013, 14, 1696-704.
[32] Ohtani, K; Egashira, K; Nakano, K; et al. Stent-based local delivery of nuclear factor-kappaB decoy attenuates in-stent restenosis in hypercholesterolemic rabbits. *Circulation*, 2006, 114, 2773-9.
[33] Takahashi, A; Palmer-Opolski, M; Smith, RC; Walsh, K. Transgene delivery of plasmid DNA to smooth muscle cells and macrophages from a biostable polymer-coated stent. *Gene Ther*, 2003, 10, 1471-8.
[34] Egashira, K; Nakano, K; Ohtani, K; et al. Local delivery of anti-monocyte chemoattractant protein-1 by gene-eluting stents attenuates in-stent stenosis in rabbits and monkeys. *Arterioscler Thromb Vasc Biol*, 2007, 27, 2563-8.
[35] Ganly, S; Hynes, SO; Sharif, F; et al. Liposomal surface coatings of metal stents for efficient non-viral gene delivery to the injured vasculature. *J Control Release*, 2013, 167, 109-19.
[36] Johnson, TW; Wu, YX; Herdeg, C; et al. Stent-based delivery of tissue inhibitor of metalloproteinase-3 adenovirus inhibits neointimal formation in porcine coronary arteries. *Arterioscler Thromb Vasc Biol*, 2005, 25, 754-9.
[37] Radke, PW; Griesenbach, U; Kivela, A; et al. Vascular oligonucleotide transfer facilitated by a polymer-coated stent. Hum *Gene Ther*, 2005, 16, 734-40.
[38] Sharif, F; Hynes, SO; Cooney, R; et al. Gene-eluting stents: adenovirus-mediated delivery of eNOS to the blood vessel wall accelerates re-endothelialization and inhibits restenosis. *Mol Ther*, 2008, 16, 1674-80.
[39] Sharif, F; Hynes, SO; McCullagh, KJ; et al. Gene-eluting stents: non-viral, liposome-based gene delivery of eNOS to the blood vessel wall in vivo results in enhanced endothelialization but does not reduce restenosis in a hypercholesterolemic model. *Gene Ther*, 2012, 19, 321-8.
[40] Sharif, F; Hynes, SO; McMahon, J; et al. Gene-eluting stents: comparison of adenoviral and adeno- associated viral gene delivery to the blood vessel wall in vivo. *Hum Gene Ther*, 2006, 17, 741-50.
[41] Walter, DH; Cejna, M; Diaz-Sandoval, L; et al. Local gene transfer of phVEGF-2 plasmid by gene-eluting stents: an alternative strategy for inhibition of restenosis. *Circulation*, 2004, 110, 36-45.

[42] Che, HL; Bae, IH; Lim, KS; et al. Suppression of post-angioplasty restenosis with an Akt1 siRNA-embedded coronary stent in a rabbit model. *Biomaterials*, 2012, 33, 8548-56.

[43] Kim, TG; Lee, Y; Park, TG. Controlled gene-eluting metal stent fabricated by bio-inspired surface modification with hyaluronic acid and deposition of DNA/PEI polyplexes. *Int J Pharm*, 2010, 384, 181-8.

[44] Takemoto, Y; Kawata, H; Soeda, T; et al. Human placental ectonucleoside triphosphate diphosphohydrolase gene transfer via gelatin-coated stents prevents in-stent thrombosis. *Arterioscler Thromb Vasc Biol*, 2009, 29, 857-62.

[45] Nakayama, Y; Ji-Youn, K; Nishi, S; Ueno, H; Matsuda, T. Development of high-performance stent: gelatinous photogel-coated stent that permits drug delivery and gene transfer. *J Biomed Mater Res*, 2001, 57, 559-66.

[46] San, Juan, A; Bala, M; Hlawaty, H; et al. Development of a functionalized polymer for stent coating in the arterial delivery of small interfering RNA. *Biomacromolecules*, 2009, 10, 3074-80.

[47] Klugherz, BD; Song, C; DeFelice, S; et al. Gene delivery to pig coronary arteries from stents carrying antibody-tethered adenovirus. *Hum Gene Ther*, 2002, 13, 443-54.

[48] Perlstein, I; Connolly, JM; Cui, X; et al. DNA delivery from an intravascular stent with a denatured collagen-polylactic-polyglycolic acid-controlled release coating: mechanisms of enhanced transfection. *Gene Ther*, 2003, 10, 1420-8.

[49] Zhu, D; Jin, X; Leng, X; et al. Local gene delivery via endovascular stents coated with dodecylated chitosan-plasmid DNA nanoparticles. *Int J Nanomedicine*, 2010, 5, 1095-102.

[50] van, der, Giessen, WJ; Lincoff, AM; Schwartz, RS; et al. Marked inflammatory sequelae to implantation of biodegradable and nonbiodegradable polymers in porcine coronary arteries. *Circulation*, 1996, 94, 1690-7.

[51] Pendyala, LK; Li, J; Shinke, T; et al. Endothelium-dependent vasomotor dysfunction in pig coronary arteries with Paclitaxel-eluting stents is associated with inflammation and oxidative stress. *JACC Cardiovasc Interv*, 2009, 2, 253-62.

[52] Finn, AV; Nakazawa, G; Joner, M; et al. Vascular responses to drug eluting stents: importance of delayed healing. *Arterioscler Thromb Vasc Biol*, 2007, 27, 1500-10.

[53] Bengali Z, Shea LD. Gene Delivery by Immobilization to Cell-Adhesive Substrates. *MRS Bull*, 2005, 30, 659-62.

[54] Segura, T; Volk, MJ; Shea, LD. Substrate-mediated DNA delivery: role of the cationic polymer structure and extent of modification. *J Control Release*, 2003, 93, 69-84.

[55] Fishbein, I; Alferiev, IS; Nyanguile, O; et al. Bisphosphonate-mediated gene vector delivery from the metal surfaces of stents. *Proc Natl Acad Sci U S A*, 2006, 103, 159-64.

[56] Ma, G; Wang, Y; Fishbein, I; et al. Anchoring of self-assembled plasmid DNA/anti-DNA antibody/cationic lipid micelles on bisphosphonate-modified stent for cardiovascular gene delivery. *Int J Nanomedicine*, 2013, 8, 1029-35.

[57] Fishbein, I; Alferiev, I; Bakay, M; et al. Local delivery of gene vectors from bare-metal stents by use of a biodegradable synthetic complex inhibits in-stent restenosis in rat carotid arteries. *Circulation*, 2008, 117, 2096-103.

[58] Fishbein, I; Forbes, SP; Chorny, M; et al. Adenoviral vector tethering to metal surfaces via hydrolyzable cross-linkers for the modulation of vector release and transduction. *Biomaterials*, 2013, 34, 6938-48.

[59] Chorny, M; Fishbein, I; Tengood, JE; Adamo, RF; Alferiev, IS; Levy, RJ. Site-specific gene delivery to stented arteries using magnetically guided zinc oleate-based nanoparticles loaded with adenoviral vectors. *FASEB J*, 2013, 27, 2198-206.

[60] Chorny, M; Fishbein, I; Yellen, BB; et al. Targeting stents with local delivery of paclitaxel-loaded magnetic nanoparticles using uniform fields. *Proc Natl Acad Sci U S A*, 2010, 107, 8346-51.

[61] Polyak, B; Fishbein, I; Chorny, M; et al. High field gradient targeting of magnetic nanoparticle-loaded endothelial cells to the surfaces of steel stents. *Proc Natl Acad Sci U S A*, 2008, 105, 698-703.

[62] Carter, AJ; Aggarwal, M; Kopia, GA; et al. Long-term effects of polymer-based, slow-release, sirolimus-eluting stents in a porcine coronary model. *Cardiovasc Res*, 2004, 63, 617-24.

[63] Sirois, MG; Simons, M; Kuter, DJ; Rosenberg, RD; Edelman, ER. Rat arterial wall retains myointimal hyperplastic potential long after arterial injury. *Circulation*, 1997, 96, 1291-8.

[64] Jin, X; Mei, L; Song, C; et al. Immobilization of plasmid DNA on an anti-DNA antibody modified coronary stent for intravascular site-specific gene therapy. *J Gene Med*, 2008, 10, 421-9.

[65] Zhang, LH; Luo, T; Zhang, C; et al. Anti-DNA antibody modified coronary stent for plasmid gene delivery: results obtained from a porcine coronary stent model. *J Gene Med*, 2011, 13, 37-45.

[66] Chaabane, C; Otsuka, F; Virmani, R; Bochaton-Piallat, ML. Biological responses in stented arteries. *Cardiovasc Res*, 2013, 99, 353-63.

[67] Curcio, A; Torella, D; Indolfi, C. Mechanisms of smooth muscle cell proliferation and endothelial regeneration after vascular injury and stenting: approach to therapy. *Circ J*, 2011, 75, 1287-96.

[68] Gaffney, MM; Hynes, SO; Barry, F; O'Brien, T. Cardiovascular *gene ther*apy: current status and therapeutic potential. *Br J Pharmacol*, 2007, 152, 175-88.

[69] Rissanen, TT; Yla-Herttuala, S. Current status of cardiovascular gene therapy. *Mol Ther*, 2007, 15, 1233-47.

[70] Asahara, T; Bauters, C; Pastore, C; et al. Local delivery of vascular endothelial growth factor accelerates reendothelialization and attenuates intimal hyperplasia in balloon-injured rat carotid artery. *Circulation*, 1995, 91, 2793-801.

[71] Paul, A; Elias, CB; Shum-Tim, D; Prakash, S. Bioactive baculovirus nanohybrids for stent based rapid vascular re-endothelialization. *Sci Rep*, 2013, 3, 2366.

[72] Paul, A; Shao, W; Shum-Tim, D; Prakash, S. The attenuation of restenosis following arterial gene transfer using carbon nanotube coated stent incorporating TAT/DNA(Ang1+Vegf) nanoparticles. *Biomaterials*, 2012, 33, 7655-64.

[73] Hers, I; Vincent, EE; Tavare, JM. Akt signalling in health and disease. *Cell Signal*, 2011, 23, 1515-27.

[74] Zhou, RH; Lee, TS; Tsou, TC; et al. Stent implantation activates Akt in the vessel wall: role of mechanical stretch in vascular smooth muscle cells. *Arterioscler Thromb Vasc Biol*, 2003, 23, 2015-20.

[75] Stabile, E; Zhou, YF; Saji, M; et al. Akt controls vascular smooth muscle cell proliferation in vitro and in vivo by delaying G1/S exit. *Circ Res*, 2003, 93, 1059-65.
[76] Fager, G; Hansson, GK; Ottosson, P; Dahllof, B; Bondjers, G. Human arterial smooth muscle cells in culture. Effects of platelet-derived growth factor and heparin on growth in vitro. *Exp Cell Res*, 1988, 176, 319-35.
[77] Grotendorst, GR; Chang, T; Seppa, HE; Kleinman, HK; Martin, GR. Platelet-derived growth factor is a chemoattractant for vascular smooth muscle cells. *J Cell Physiol*, 1982, 113, 261-6.
[78] Kazlauskas, A; DiCorleto, PE. Cultured endothelial cells do not respond to a platelet-derived growth-factor-like protein in an autocrine manner. *Biochim Biophys Acta*, 1985, 846, 405-12.
[79] Fishbein, I; Waltenberger, J; Banai, S; et al. Local delivery of platelet-derived growth factor receptor-specific tyrphostin inhibits neointimal formation in rats. *Arterioscler Thromb Vasc Biol*, 2000, 20, 667-76.
[80] Deguchi, J; Namba, T; Hamada, H; et al. Targeting endogenous platelet-derived growth factor B-chain by adenovirus-mediated gene transfer potently inhibits in vivo smooth muscle proliferation after arterial injury. *Gene Ther*, 1999, 6, 956-65.
[81] Lin, ZH; Fukuda, N; Suzuki, R; et al. Adenovirus-encoded hammerhead ribozyme to PDGF A-chain mRNA inhibits neointima formation after arterial injury. *J Vasc Res*, 2004, 41, 305-13.
[82] Li, Y; Fukuda, N; Kunimoto, S; et al. Stent-based delivery of antisense oligodeoxynucleotides targeted to the PDGF A-chain decreases in-stent restenosis of the coronary artery. *J Cardiovasc Pharmacol*, 2006, 48, 184-90.
[83] Kipshidze, NN; Iversen, P; Kim, HS; et al. Advanced c-myc antisense (AVI-4126)-eluting phosphorylcholine-coated stent implantation is associated with complete vascular healing and reduced neointimal formation in the porcine coronary restenosis model. *Catheter Cardiovasc Interv*, 2004, 61, 518-27.
[84] Lin, K; Zhao, Z; Chen, L. Stent-based delivery of decoy oligodeoxynucleotides against activator protein-1 binding site decreased restenosis in rabbits. *Pharmazie*, 2013, 68, 661-7.
[85] Johnson, C; Galis, ZS. Matrix metalloproteinase-2 and -9 differentially regulate smooth muscle cell migration and cell-mediated collagen organization. *Arterioscler Thromb Vasc Biol*, 2004, 24, 54-60.
[86] Welt, FG; Rogers, C. Inflammation and restenosis in the stent era. *Arterioscler Thromb Vasc Biol*, 2002, 22, 1769-76.
[87] Sarkar, K; Sharma, SK; Sachdeva, R; Romeo, F; Garza, L; Mehta, JL., Coronary artery restenosis: vascular biology and emerging therapeutic strategies. *Expert Rev Cardiovasc Ther*, 2006, 4, 543-56.
[88] Danenberg, HD; Fishbein, I; Gao, J; et al. Macrophage depletion by clodronate-containing liposomes reduces neointimal formation after balloon injury in rats and rabbits. *Circulation*, 2002, 106, 599-605.
[89] Inoue, T; Croce, K; Morooka, T; Sakuma, M; Node, K; Simon, DI. Vascular inflammation and repair: implications for re-endothelialization, restenosis, and stent thrombosis. *JACC Cardiovasc Interv*, 2011, 4, 1057-66.
[90] Bian, K; Murad, F. Nitric oxide signaling in vascular biology. *J Am Soc Hypertens*, 2007, 1, 17-29.

[91] Pechanova, O; Simko, F. The role of nitric oxide in the maintenance of vasoactive balance. *Physiol Res*, 2007, 56 Suppl 2, S7-S16.
[92] Nong, Z; Hoylaerts, M; Van Pelt, N; Collen, D; Janssens, S. Nitric oxide inhalation inhibits platelet aggregation and platelet-mediated pulmonary thrombosis in rats. *Circ Res*, 1997, 81, 865-9.
[93] Garg, UC; Hassid, A. Nitric oxide-generating vasodilators and 8-bromo-cyclic guanosine monophosphate inhibit mitogenesis and proliferation of cultured rat vascular smooth muscle cells. *J Clin Invest*, 1989, 83, 1774-7.
[94] Groves, PH; Banning, AP; Penny, WJ; Newby, AC; Cheadle, HA; Lewis, MJ. The effects of exogenous nitric oxide on smooth muscle cell proliferation following porcine carotid angioplasty. *Cardiovasc Res*, 1995, 30, 87-96.
[95] Sarkar, R; Meinberg, EG; Stanley, JC; Gordon, D; Webb, RC. Nitric oxide reversibly inhibits the migration of cultured vascular smooth muscle cells. *Circ Res*, 1996, 78, 225-30.
[96] Papapetropoulos, A; Garcia-Cardena, G; Madri, JA; Sessa, WC. Nitric oxide production contributes to the angiogenic properties of vascular endothelial growth factor in human endothelial cells. *J Clin Invest*, 1997, 100, 3131-9.
[97] De Caterina, R; Libby, P; Peng, HB; et al. Nitric oxide decreases cytokine-induced endothelial activation. Nitric oxide selectively reduces endothelial expression of adhesion molecules and proinflammatory cytokines. *J Clin Invest*, 1995, 96, 60-8.
[98] Kong, D; Melo, LG; Mangi, AA; et al. Enhanced inhibition of neointimal hyperplasia by genetically engineered endothelial progenitor cells. *Circulation*, 2004, 109, 1769-75.
[99] Chen L, Daum G, Forough R, Clowes M, Walter U, Clowes AW. Overexpression of human endothelial nitric oxide synthase in rat vascular smooth muscle cells and in balloon-injured carotid artery. *Circ Res*, 1998, 82, 862-70.
[100] Cooney, R; Hynes, SO; Sharif, F; Howard, L; O'Brien, T. Effect of gene delivery of NOS isoforms on intimal hyperplasia and endothelial regeneration after balloon injury. *Gene Ther*, 2007, 14, 396-404.
[101] Muhs, A; Heublein, B; Schletter, J; et al. Preclinical evaluation of inducible nitric oxide synthase lipoplex *gene ther*apy for inhibition of stent-induced vascular neointimal lesion formation. *Hum Gene Ther*, 2003, 14, 375-83.
[102] Wang, K; Kessler, PD; Zhou, Z; et al. Local adenoviral-mediated inducible nitric oxide synthase gene transfer inhibits neointimal formation in the porcine coronary stented model. *Mol Ther*, 2003, 7, 597-603.
[103] Forstermann, U. Oxidative stress in vascular disease: causes, defense mechanisms and potential therapies. *Nat Clin Pract Cardiovasc Med*, 2008, 5, 338-49.

In: Coronary Artery Restenosis
Editor: Amir S. Lotfi

ISBN: 978-1-63321-346-3

Chapter 15

Future Strategies for Preventing and Treating Coronary Restenosis

Ehrin J. Armstrong and John C. Messenger*
Division of Cardiology, University of Colorado School of Medicine, CO, US

Abstract

While drug-eluting stents have improved outcomes after percutaneous coronary intervention, 4-14% of patients in modern clinical trials still develop symptomatic restenosis. Future strategies for prevention of restenosis include modifications to the stent platform, the drug polymer or drug elution system, biocompatible stent coatings, use of bioresorbable scaffolds, and optimization of local and systemic anti-restenotic agents. Novel approaches to treating restenosis include a number of ongoing trials comparing treatment strategies with currently available drug eluting stents, use of drug coated balloons, and interventional strategies to increase stent expansion. While no single technology is likely to eliminate restenosis, the combination of these prevention and treatment strategies promises to improve the long-term outcomes of percutaneous coronary intervention.

I. Introduction

Despite significant advances in drug-eluting stent technology, restenosis remains a major clinical concern, with up to 14% of patients requiring repeat revascularization in the first two years after percutaneous coronary intervention. [1-3] While prevention of restenosis is paramount, new treatment modalities also offer the opportunity to effectively treat restenosis and thereby avoid the need for a surgical bypass of otherwise recalcitrant lesions. This chapter reviews future strategies for preventing and treating restenosis. The first part of the

* Corresponding Author: John C. Messenger, MD, FACC, FSCAI, Associate Professor of Medicine, Director, Cardiac Catheterization Labs, Program Director, Interventional Cardiology Fellowship, University of Colorado School of Medicine, 12401 E. 17th Avenue, Room 522, Box B132, Aurora, CO 80045, Office 720-848-6559, Fax 720-848-7314, John.messenger@ucdenver.edu.

chapter focuses on novel stent designs that may further reduce the likelihood of restenosis after stent placement, while the second part of the chapter discusses novel treatment for coronary in-stent restenosis (ISR).

II. Prevention of Restenosis

a. Stent Platform

The stent platform provides the backbone for all stent technology, but implantation of a foreign object also provides a potential nidus for inflammation and subsequent restenosis. Development of new alloys may reduce the inflammatory reaction to stent implantation, thereby limiting restenosis. Bioresorbable scaffolds also hold the promise of providing scaffolding support during the acute healing phase, but with complete resorbtion over time, thereby allowing vessel remodeling and improved vessel geometry.

i. New Alloys

First generation drug-eluting stent (DES) platforms (e.g., Cypher®, Taxus®) were constructed of stainless steel. Although stainless steel has an excellent record of biocompatibility for medical applications, the strut thickness of these devices was significant (140 μm for Cypher® and 132 μm for Taxus Express®). Given the inverse relationship between strut thickness and restenosis in bare metal stents, [4, 5] second generation DES were designed with thinner stent struts, both to reduce restenosis and improve stent deliverability. Reduction of stainless steel strut thickness from 132μm to 97 μm in the initial Taxus® stent designs was associated with reduced rates of target lesion failure (TLF), suggesting that thinner stent struts may also reduce rates of restenosis with DES platforms. [6]

Due to the limitations of reducing stainless steel strut thickness while maintaining radial strength, newer alloys were developed for use in second generation DES. Second- and third-generation DES are based on alloys of cobalt chrome (e.g., Xience®, Promus®, Endeavor®, Resolute®) or platinum chrome (e.g., Promus Element®, Taxus Element®). The stent struts on currently available second-generation DES range from 81-91 μm in thickness, resulting in low profile stents that maintain radial force.

The relative benefits of platinum chromium alloys vs. cobalt chromium alloys are uncertain. Platinum chromium has increased radial strength relative to cobalt chromium for a given strut thickness, but clinical studies of these two stent types have suggested similar rates of restenosis. In the PLATINUM trial of everolimus-eluting platinum chromium vs. everolimus-eluting cobalt chromium DES, overall rates of target lesion revascularization (TLR) were similar (1.3% vs. 1.6%). [7] The mean lesion length in each group was only 13 mm, which likely accounted for the very low overall event rates. In a real-world unselected cohort, rates of TLRwere similar at one year (5.4% vs. 4.8%), suggesting similar rates of restenosis and clinical need for revascularization with these two stent types. [8] In the SCAAR registry, rates of restenosis with the Promus Element® stent were also similar to that of the overall DES cohort (2.8% vs. 2.7%). [9] In the most direct comparison of alloy type, a dedicated OCT study of everolimus-eluting platinum chromium vs. everolimus-eluting cobalt chromium DES found no difference in strut-level neointimal thickness six months post-implantation, suggesting that the rates of restenosis attributable to the alloy are not significantly different. [10]

Platinum chromium alloys have also been recently developed as the stent platform for paclitaxel-eluting DES. In a comparison of the Taxus Element® (platinum chromium alloy) DES with Taxus Express® (stainless steel) DES, overall TLR was 3.8% vs. 4.5% at 12 months. [11] A subgroup of patients also underwent angiography and quantitative coronary angiography at 9 months. The extent of late loss and percentage of patients with binary restenosis was not significantly different between groups. Although other proprietary alloys are under development, it is likely that current stent delivery platforms have reached a limit of optimization for strut thickness and radial strength. Technological improvements at the level of the stent platform have therefore focused more recently on bioresorbable scaffolds.

ii. Bioresorbable Scaffolds

The placement of a bioresorbable scaffold has several potential advantages, including acute structural support after angioplasty, a platform for drug elution, and the potential for the coronary artery to regain physiologic function after the stent resorbs. Although much of the research in this area has focused on the goal of minimizing very late stent thrombosis, bioresorbable scaffold technology could also limit restenosis by allowing increased positive remodeling of the vessel and normal vasoreactivity to physiologic stimuli after the scaffold resorbs. [12]

A number of bioresorbable scaffolds have been developed, with most based either on poly L-lactic acid (PLLA) or magnesium.[13] The Igaki-Tamai stent was the first bioresorbablescaffold implanted in humans and was based on a poly-L-lactic acid polymer.[14] Although the initial results were encouraging, this initial design required delivery of heated contrast within the coronary balloon, with attendant concerns regarding vessel wall injury. Further refinements of this polymer technology led to the development of a bioresorbable scaffold composed of semicrystalline PLLA, which allows the stent to be deployed on a standard delivery balloon without heating the contrast. The PLLA degrades over the course of 2-3 years into lactic acid. This stent design has also been coated with a poly D, L-lactide polymer, which elutes everolimus, thereby incorporating the advantages of DES without requiring a permanent scaffold.

The absorbable magnesium stent (AMS) has tensile strengths similar to stainless steel stents and resorbs over the course of two months. A prospective study of the AMS stent without any associated anti-restenotic drug reported a TLR rate of 45% at one year with significant late lumen loss attributable to stent recoil. [15] Subsequent redesign led to the development of the drug-eluting AMS (DREAMS) stent, which elutes paclitaxel. This stent was recently tested in 46 patients; only two patients underwent TLR in the first year of follow-up.[16] These results suggest that addition of paclitaxel to a magnesium scaffold provides adequate inhibition of restenosis. The DREAMS stent is undergoing further redesign prior to continued clinical trials.

In the ABSORB study of 30 patients who underwent placement of an everolimus-eluting PLLA bioresorbable stent, serial OCT follow up demonstrated luminal enlargement from six months to two years due to a decrease in plaque size. Vasomotion was also intact at the treated site, suggesting arterial healing at the site of plaque. [17] A subsequent iteration of the scaffold was developed to prevent early scaffold shrinkage, which was noted in the initial study. In a study of 56 patients, late lumen loss at 12 months was 0.27 ± 0.32mm by intravascular ultrasound (IVUS), and two patients underwent repeat intervention.[18] Serial IVUS confirmed scaffold resorption and also demonstrated late phase lumen expansion (Figure 1). An OCT comparison of an everolimus eluting stent (EES) vs. bioresorbable EES demonstrated no significant differences in late lumen loss.[19] Intraluminal masses, which may be associated with thrombus formation, were identified by OCT with greater frequency in the bioresorbable stents. This finding emphasizes the importance of close follow-up and an adequately sized randomized trial powered for clinical endpoints. The ABSORB II and ABSORB III trialsare currently underway, with plans to randomize patients to the Absorb® bioresorbablescaffold vs. Xience® DES. [20] The results of these studies will provide adequate power to determine the rates of restenosis with bioresorbable DES vs. current second-generation DES. This technology has already obtained CE Mark approval in Europe, where it is used clinically in selected circumstances.

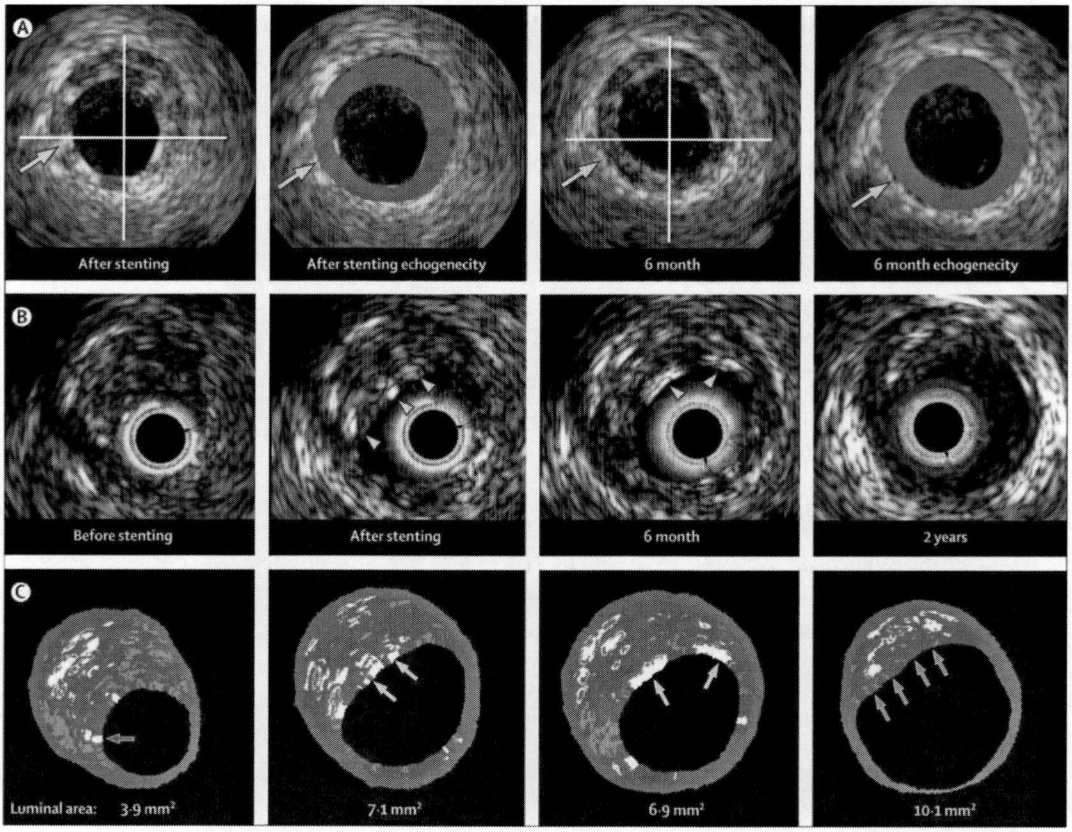

Figure 1. Serial Imaging of a Bioresorbable Scaffold. A. After bioresorbable scaffold placement, areas of echogenicity (green) are apparent and correspond to scaffold struts. Over time, this echogenicity diminished, consistent with scaffold resorption. B. Serial intravascular imaging confirms strut resorption from 6 months to 2 years. C. Intravascular ultrasound backscatter analysis demonstrates strut resorption (registered as white). At two years, the lesion is covered with a thick fibrous cap (green). The lumen area has also enlarged to 10.1 mm^2. Reprinted from The Lancet, Vol. 373. Serruys PW, Ormiston JA, Onuma Y, et al. A bioabsorbable everolimus-eluting coronary stent system (ABSORB): 2-year outcomes and results from multiple imaging methods. Pages 898-910, 2009, with permission from Elsevier.

While bioresorbable scaffolds hold significant promise for the next generation of coronary stents, rigorous clinical trials remain necessary to assess rates of restenosis with these devices. Initial concerns regarding scaffold shrinkage in the first year after deployment have been overcome with recent iterations of the device, and initial studies suggest similar angiographic outcomes to available DES. However, it is possible that restenosis will actually be higher with drug-eluting bioresorbable scaffolds, because the strut thickness of bioresorbable scaffolds is greater than that of current second-generation DES. In addition, placement of a bioresorbable scaffold requires careful vessel preparation, such that bioresorbable scaffolds may not be deliverable to heavily calcified or otherwise recalcitrant lesions. Such lesions require significant modification to ensure scaffold expansion in order to gain an adequate lumen cross-sectional area and minimize the occurrence of restenosis.

b. Drug Elution Polymer and Stent Coatings

The linking region between stent and drug controls the kinetics of anti-restenotic drug elution, which is a major determinant of restenosis inhibition. Recent technological advances have led to several innovations including biocompatible polymers, polymer-free drug elution, and the use of nanoparticles or novel coating agents. Each of these approaches could improve drug elution kinetics, while also limiting or eliminating the presence of a permanent polymer.

i. Biocompatible and Bioabsorbable Polymers

First-generation drug eluting stents used durable polymers that can potentially elicit a chronic inflammatory response. Second-generation FDA-approved DES utilize more biocompatible polymers that are less likely to elicit chronic inflammation. This use of a more biocompatible polymer, in combination with thinner stent struts, may contribute to the lower rates of restenosis observed with newer DES. However, the presence of persistent polymer after drug elution raises the concern of a possible nidus for restenosis and thrombosis. For these reasons, bioabsorbable polymers have also been developed. Most of the biodegradable polymer stents utilize poly-L lactic acid, which dissolves over the course of 1-3 years to lactic acid.

Bioabsorbable polymer DES have been studied in multiple large trials. The best studied of the bioabsorbable polymer stent systems is the Nobori® stent, which consists of a stainless steel stent with a PLLA polymer that elutes biolimus, a structural analogue of sirolimus. The Nobori® was non-inferior to the Cypher® stent in a large randomized trial (see below). The COSTAR trial randomized 1,700 patients to a Taxus® DES vs. the CoStar® DES, which elutes paclitaxel from a bioabsorbable polymer.[21] The in-segment late lumen loss was higher (0.49 vs. 0.18 mm) with the CoStar® stent; TVR was also higher (8.1% vs. 4.3%). Although this newer stent met criteria for non-inferiority compared to Taxus®, the higher event rates suggested that drug elution kinetics with the bioabsorbable polymer remain suboptimal. Other trials of bioabsorbable polymer DES include the ISAR-TEST 3 and ISAR-TEST 4 trials, which compared a bioabsorbable polymer sirolimus-eluting DES to Cypher® or Xience® DES, with similar overall results among the groups.[22, 23] Current research in this field remains focused on engineering improvements to improve rates of polymer absorption balanced with appropriate timing of drug elution.

ii. Polymer-Free Drug Elution

Novel technologies for elution of drug without use of a linking polymer utilize microabrasion of the stent or microporous structures that allow incorporation of drug onto the abluminal surface of the stent. This approach has the advantage of exposing the anti-restenotic drug only to the vessel wall, rather than the flow lumen of the stent. This approach may result in more local drug delivery and minimize the amount of drug required. Absence of a polymer may also further reduce any polymer-related inflammation that promotes late lumen loss and restenosis. Consistent with this theory, comparison of two year late lumen loss demonstrated that a polymer-free sirolimus eluting stent had less delayed late lumen loss (0.01 ± 0.42 mm) than a permanent polymer sirolimus-eluting stent (0.17 ± 0.50 mm). [24] These findings suggest that a polymer free DES may have less long-term restenosis than permanent polymer DES. However, these results are balanced against higher rates of initial restenosis in the first six months with polymer-free DES, which is likely due to an increased rate of anti-restenotic drug elution such that mid-term restenosis may be more likely to occur.

One approach to overcome the limitations of drug-elution kinetics with a polymer-free stent has been to engineer the so-called Dual-DES stent, which is a polymer-free DES that elutes both sirolimus and probucol. Probucolis an antioxidant that limits restenosis by inhibiting the extracellular related kinase (ERK) pathway, thereby inhibiting smooth muscle cell activation. [25] The high lipophilicity of probucol may also lengthen the drug release kinetics of sirolimus. The Dual-DES has been studied in two large clinical trials. In the ISAR-TEST 2 trial, 1,007 patients were randomized to implantation of the Dual DES, Cypher®, or Endeavor® DES. [26] At two-year follow-up, rates of TLR were 7.7%, 10.7%, and 14.3%. Interestingly, rates of TLR between 1 and 2 years were lower for the Dual-DES than for Cypher, again suggesting less long-term risk of restenosis with a polymer-free system. In the ISAR-TEST 5 trial, the Dual DES was tested vs. Endeavor® DES in 3,002 patients. [27] Binary in-segment restenosis was similar between both groups 13.3% vs. 13.4%), with similar late luminal loss. Overall, these results suggest that combination of a polymer-free sirolimus eluting stent with probucol has similar efficacy to current second-generation DES. Whether the polymer-free design improves long-term outcomes remains uncertain.

iii. Nanoparticles

Nanoparticles consist of phospholipid liposomes loaded internally with a drug. These nanoparticles can then be used to coat the exterior of a stent, thereby providing a platform for biocompatible drug elution. Both paclitaxel and sirolimus have been tested using nanoparticle delivery systems integrated into current stent platforms. These studies have shown optimized release kinetics and inhibition of restenosis in animal models, but none of these stents have yet been tested in clinical trials. [28-31]

iv. Novel Coating Agents

Prior to the development of DES, a number of trials were performed investigating the contribution of stent coating agents on the incidence of restenosis. For example, trials with a gold-coated stent unexpectedly demonstrated increased rates of restenosis.[32] In comparison, titanium nitride oxide coating has been shown to decrease platelet aggregation and fibrin deposition, and may therefore limit the inflammatory response after stent placement. Titanium nitride oxide stents also demonstrated less inflammatory reaction and decreased neointimal hyperplasia in a porcine angioplasty model. [33] This stent was compared in a randomized trial of 92 patients to an identical stainless steel stent without coating. [34] At six months, the titanium nitride oxide coated stent had less late loss than the uncoated stent (0.55±0.63 vs. 0.90±0.76 mm) and less binary restenosis (15% vs. 33%). A registry study of titanium nitride oxide stents vs. paclitaxel-eluting stents suggested that the titanium nitride oxide stent was associated with less TLR and decreased MACE. [35] While these results are encouraging, no randomized trials have yet compared this stent to current DES or utilized this coating in conjunction with drug elution.

c. Local Antirestenotic Agents

Currently available DES utilize inhibitors of microtubule assembly (e.g., paclitaxel) or inhibitors of the mTOR signaling pathway (e.g., sirolimus, everolimus, zotarolimus) to limit smooth muscle cell proliferation and subsequent development of restenosis after percutaneous coronary intervention. While these agents have significantly reduced rates of restenosis relative to bare metal stents, incremental improvement in these drug types could provide additional clinical benefit.

Biolimus is a sirolimus analogue that also inhibits the mTOR pathway. Compared to sirolimus, biolimus is more lipophilic. The increased lipophilicity of biolimus may translate into greater local drug delivery to target cells and more effective inhibition of smooth muscle cell proliferation. In a porcine model, biolimusalso caused less vascular inflammation compared to sirolimus-eluting stents.[36] The Nobori® stent is a stainless steel stent (strut thickness 120 μm)with a biodegradable PLLA polymer on the abluminal surface of the stent that elutes biolimus. The combination of a novel anti-restenotic combined with a biodegradable polymer may offer advantages in limiting both restenosis and chronic inflammation related to persistence of polymer after completion of drug elution. Balanced against this advantage has been the development of more biocompatible polymers in second generation DES, as well as the use of cobalt chromium and platinum chromium alloys with thinner stent struts.

The Nobori® stent has been extensively studied in comparison to both first and second generation DES. It was first compared the TaxusLiberte® in a small randomized trial. [37] At nine months, late lumen loss was significantly lower in patients randomized to the Nobori® stent (0.11 vs. 0.32 mm, p <0.001). Binary restenosis was also significantly lower with the Nobori® stent (0.7% vs. 6.2%, p=0.02). Another small randomized trial comparing the Nobori® stent to a sirolimus-eluting stent and angiographic follow-up found similar late lumen loss but significantly decreased rates of TLR with the Nobori® stent (0.5% vs. 3.9%, p=0.04). These preliminary findings were tested in the larger LEADERS trial, which randomized 1,707 patients with stable CAD or ACS to Nobori® or Cypher® stents. At nine months, TLR rates were similar (5.4% vs. 5.9%), and the overall endpoint met the criteria for non-inferiority. [38] At five-year follow-up, the Nobori® stent remained non-inferior for the primary endpoint compared to Cypher® stents.[39] In comparison, the recent SORT OUT V study failed to meet a non-inferiority endpoint of the Nobori® stent vs. Cypher® DES, with a 4.1% vs. 3.1% incidence of the primary endpoint (cardiac death, myocardial infarction, stent thrombosis, or target vessel revascularization) at one year. [40] Target lesion revascularization at 12 months was also slightly higher with the Nobori® stent (3.3%) than with the Cypher® stent (2.0%). Longer-term follow up of this study will be necessary, as the endpoints may diverge further over time.

More recent randomized trials have compared the Nobori® stent to second generation DES. The NEXT trial randomized 3,235 patients to Nobori® vs. Xience®/Promus® DES. At one year, the rate of TLR was 4.2% in both groups, thereby meeting the criteria for non-inferiority. An angiographic sub study also demonstrated similar late lumen loss (0.03 vs. 0.06 mm). The COMPARE II study also randomized patients with broad indications for PCI to the Nobori® stent or Xience®/Xience Prime® stents.[41] This trial met criteria for non-inferiority of the Nobori® stent, with TLR rates at one year of 3.7% vs. 3.1% (p=0.4). Further studies will be necessary to determine the clinical utility of the Nobori® stent relative to current FDA-approved DES.

Novolimus is a sirolimus metabolite that has also been studied as a novel mTOR inhibitor. Formulations of this agent can be delivered at a lower dose and with less polymer than comparable antirestenotic agents. In a small randomized trial, 201 patients were randomized 2:1 to a novolimus-eluting DES or the Endeavor®zotarolimus-eluting DES. [42] At 9 months, in-stent late lumen loss was significantly lower among patients randomized to novolimus-eluting DES (0.11 vs. 0.63 mm, p<0.001). There was no significant difference in rates of TLR at 9 months. A bioresorbable PLLA scaffold that elutes novolimus has also been developed and recently received CE Mark approval.

d. Gene Therapy

A number of promising preclinical studies have been conducted using gene therapy to reduce restenosis. Approaches include local plasmid-mediated delivery of nitric oxide, angiogenic agents, and use of microRNAs to limit restenosis. These approaches and others are discussed in detail in Chapter 14.

e. Agents to Promote Endothelial Cell Healing

After stent placement, endothelial cell ingrowth promotes strut coverage and limits smooth muscle cell proliferation. There are two major sources of cells for re-endothelialization: endothelial cells may proliferate locally, while circulating endothelial progenitor cells (EPCs) may home to sites of vascular injury and promote plaque stabilization. Promotion of rapid endothelial cell healing is one approach that has been evaluated with the Genous® EPC capture stent, which is coated with murine monoclonal anti-CD34 antibodies. Because CD34 is expressed by bone marrow progenitor cells, the initial concept of the Genous® stent was to promote EPC capture and therefore accelerate stent strut re-endothelialization.

The HEALING-FIM study was a pilot trial of 16 patients who underwent placement of a Genous stent. [43] At six months, late lumen loss was 0.63 ± 0.52 mm, and binary restenosis was 13%. The HEALING II study enrolled 63 patients. [44] At six months, late lumen loss was 0.78 ± 0.39 mm, and binary restenosis was 17.2%. Interestingly, the late lumen loss decreased from 6 months to 18 months, with no further cases of restenosis. A number of other large registries using the Genous® stent have been completed, including use of the stent in primary PCI.[45] The largest of these registries reported a one-year target vessel revascularization rate of 6.5% and a stent thrombosis rate of 1.1%. [46] A pilot study of the Genous® stent vs. the TaxusLiberte® also showed more late lumen loss at 12 months among patients randomized to the Genous stent (1.14±0.64 vs. 0.55±0.61 mm). A separate randomized trial was stopped early when EPC capture stents were found to have a higher rate of TLF compared to DES (17.4% vs. 7.0%). [47] Overall, these findings suggest that the Genous® stent is associated with more ISR than current DES, but that it is generally safe, with low rates of stent thrombosis.

Although EPC express CD34, other bone marrow progenitor cells, including some smooth muscle cell progenitors, also express this antigen. A CD34 capture antibody may therefore promote some increased restenosis at the expense of endothelial coverage of stent struts. One novel approach to this problem is the use of a Genous® EPC stent together with a drug-coated balloon. In a pilot trial, 120 patients were randomized to Genous stent vs. paclitaxel-coated balloon + Genous® stent. [48] Patients randomized to the addition of a paclitaxel-coated balloon has significantly decreased late lumen loss at 12 months (0.34± 0.45 vs. 0.88±0.48 mm) and lower rates of restenosis (5.1% vs. 23.2%), with no episodes of stent thrombosis.A smaller non-randomized study of a paclitaxel-coated balloon combined with the Genous® stent obtained similar results. [49]

Based on the increased late lumen loss with the Genous® stent compared to current generation DES, a new stent was designed incorporating both CD34 antibody and low-dose sirolimus (the Combo stent). This approach may minimize late lumen loss while promoting endothelial strut coverage, therefore possibly lowering the incidence of stent thrombosis. Initial implants of the Combo stent in porcine arteries confirmed that the Combo stent has less late lumen loss than the Genous® stent. The REMEDEE trial randomized183 patients to the Combo stent vs. a paclitaxel-eluting stent. The Combo stent was noninferior to a paclitaxel-eluting stent, with twelve-month in-stent late lumen loss of 0.39±0.45 vs. 0.44 ± 0.56 mm.[50] Larger trials will be necessary to determine whether this approach of dual EPC capture and local inhibition of restenosis translates into improved clinical outcomes.

f. Systemic Treatment

Prior to the development of DES, systemic treatment was studied in detail for the prevention of restenosis. Approaches included oral prednisone as well as sirolimus. [51, 52]While each of these medications showed efficacy in reducing restenosis, concerns regarding the systemic toxic effects of these drugs as well as long-term risk of malignancy with oral sirolimuslimited their clinical utility.

Cilostazol is a type III phosphodiesterase inhibitor that inhibits platelet activation as well as release of leukocyte Mac-1, an integrin that mediates leukocyte adhesion and subsequent stimulation of smooth muscle cell growth.[53] Through these mechanisms, cilostazol has been shown to limit restenosis in both experimental and animal models of restenosis. The CREST trial randomized patients to cilostazol or placebo in addition to aspirin and clopidogrel after placement of a bare metal stent. At six months, restenosis was significantly lower among patients randomized to cilostazol (22% vs. 34.5%). Restenosis was also significantly lower among important patient subgroups at increased risk for restenosis including diabetics, long lesions, and small vessels. [54]

Cilostazol has also been studied as part of a triple therapy regimen after implantation of DES in diabetic patients and patients with long lesions. In the DECLARE-DIABETES trial, 400 patients undergoing implantation of sirolimus or paclitaxel-eluting DES were randomized to addition of cilostazol on top of dual antiplatelet therapy. At six months, in-stent and in-segment late loss were significantly lower in patients assigned to triple therapy; 9 month TLR was also significantly decreased (2.5% vs. 7.0%). In the DECLARE-LONG and DECLARE-LONG II studies, late luminal loss was also significantly lower in patients with coronary lesions >25 mm who were randomized to additional therapy with cilostazol. [55, 56]A subsequent pooled analysis suggested that most of the benefit of cilostazolis associated with lesions $\geq$ 40 mm.[57] Overall, these results are promising and suggest that addition of cilostazol may have additional benefit in lowering the risk of restenosis, especially among patients at the highest risk of adverse events. However, all of the above trials were tested in the setting of either bare metal stent or earlier generation DES usage: whether cilostazol has additive benefit in the setting of newer generation DES and more potent antiplatelet therapy is unknown and requires further evaluation.

III. Treatment of Restenosis

Once a patient develops in-stent restenosis, subsequent treatment is associated with a high risk of recurrent events. Identifying the cause of the restenosis and potentially obviating placement of an additional stent are important treatment goals. For patients with refractory or recurrent in-stent restenosis, coronary artery bypass grafting should also be strongly considered.

a. Drug-Eluting Stents

Drug eluting stents have been studied for the treatment of BMS ISR and DES ISR. In general, DES have shown excellent efficacy in the treatment of BMS ISR, while the outcomes of repeat DES placement for the treatment of DES ISR are mixed. The suboptimal results with repeat DES placement have increased enthusiasm for drug-coated balloons in the treatment of DES ISR (see below).

Both sirolimus-eluting and paclitaxel-eluting DES have been studied for the treatment of BMS ISR. In the RIBS II trial, 150 patients with BMS ISR were randomized to balloon angioplasty vs. implantation of a sirolimus-eluting DES.[58] At 9-month angiographic follow-up, patients randomized to SES had significantly lower recurrent restenosis (11% vs. 39%). One year TLR was also significantly lower in the SES group (11% vs. 30%). TheISAR DESIRE trial enrolled three treatment arms for patients with BMS ISR: balloon angioplasty, a paclitaxel-eluting stent, or a sirolimus-eluting stent. At six-month angiography, both DES types were superior to balloon angioplasty.[59] TLR was lowest in the sirolimus-eluting stent group (8%), moderate in the paclitaxel-eluting stent group (19%) and highest in the balloon angioplasty group (33%). A secondary analysis of this trial suggested that sirolimus-eluting stents may be superior to paclitaxel-eluting stents for treatment of BMS ISR. No large trials have examined the use of second generation DES for the treatment of BMS ISR, but based on the excellent outcomes of these stents in de novo coronary lesions and their relative superiority to first-generation DES, it is reasonable to treat BMS ISR with a second generation DES.

Among patients with DES ISR, one approach is to consider switching anti-restenotic agents. This strategy is based on the concept that DES ISR in a given patient may be due to relative resistance to the –limus compound or to paclitaxel. Among patients with ISR from sirolimus-eluting stents, the strategy of repeat sirolimus-eluting stent or paclitaxel-eluting stent placement was tested in the ISAR-DESIRE 2 trial. At six to eight-month follow-up, there were no differences in late lumen loss, binary restenosis, or target lesion revascularization (Figure 2).[60] A more general “switch” strategy was reported in the RIBS III study, which was a cohort study of patients with DES ISR who underwent placement of a different stent type vs. alternative treatment strategy, which in most cases consisted of placing the same DES type.[61] Patients who underwent placement of a different DES type had significantly lower rates of recurrent restenosis (22% vs. 40%). Although these results are not conclusive, it is reasonable to place a different DES type when treating patients with DES ISR.

b. Drug Coated Balloons

Although DES have been efficacious in the treatment of BMS ISR and some cases of DES ISR, significant concern remains regarding placing multiple overlapping stents within a given lesion. For this reason, use of a drug-coated balloon (DCB) offers several potential advantages to DES for the treatment of ISR. All currently available DCB utilize paclitaxel, with some differences between balloon types in dose of paclitaxel and the excipient that coats paclitaxel on the balloon.

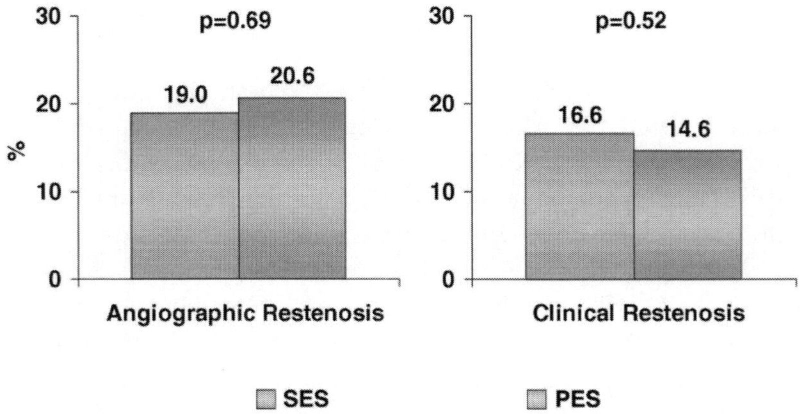

Figure 2. Use of Paclitaxel-Eluting Stents or Sirolimus-Eluting Stents to Treat Sirolimus-Eluting Stent Restenosis. Left Panel: At six to eight months, the percentage of angiographic restenosis was similar. Right Panel: Clinical restenosis at one year was also similar between groups. Reprinted from Journal of the American College of Cardiology, Vol. 55. Mehilli J, Byrne RA, Tiroch K, et al. Randomized trial of paclitaxel- versus sirolimus-eluting stents for treatment of coronary restenosis in sirolimus-eluting stents. Pages 2710-2716, 2010, with permission from Elsevier.

The initial reports of a paclitaxel-coated balloon for treatment of BMS ISR compared paclitaxel-coated balloon angioplasty to usual balloon angioplasty. In the initial study, the in-segment late lumen loss was 0.03±0.48 vs. 0.74±0.86 mm.[62] Patients randomized to paclitaxel-coated balloon also had significantly less restenosis at six months (5% vs. 43%). While these results were encouraging, DES are known to be superior to balloon angioplasty for treatment of BMS ISR. A follow-up study compared use of a paclitaxel-coated balloon or paclitaxel-coated stent for the treatment of BMS ISR.[63] At six months, binary restenosis was 7% vs. 20% (p=0.08), suggesting that paclitaxel-coated balloon angioplasty was as efficacious as and possibly superior to paclitaxel-eluting stents for the treatment of BMS ISR.

Paclitaxel-coated balloons have also been studied as a treatment for DES ISR. The ISAR-DESIRE 3 trial enrolled 402 patients with DES ISR from a previously placed –limus eluting stent (Figure 3).[64] Patients were randomized to balloon angioplasty, paclitaxel-coated balloon, or paclitaxel-eluting stent. At 6-8 month angiographic follow-up, the paclitaxel coated balloon and paclitaxel-eluting stent were associated with similar late lumen loss (0.37 vs. 0.34 mm), and significantly less late lumen loss than patients randomized to balloon angioplasty (0.70 mm). TLR trended higher for the paclitaxel-coated balloon group (22.1%) compared to paclitaxel-eluting stent group (13.5%), but was much lower than with balloon angioplasty (43.5%). These results confirmed that paclitaxel-coated balloons are associated with similar outcomes to placement of a paclitaxel-eluting stent for treatment of ISR, while obviating the need for additional stent implantation. The ongoing ISAR-DESIRE 4 trial is investigating the use of cutting or scoring balloon dilation prior to use of a DCB in order to maximize acute luminal gain at the time of angioplasty.

c. Brachytherapy

Brachytherapy in the form of gamma or ß irradiation was rigorously studied for the treatment of bare metal stent restenosis and was found to be an effective adjunctive treatment.[65, 66] The advent of DES significantly decreased the utilization of brachytherapy, both because the prevalence of ISR decreased and because DES were identified as an effective treatment of BMS ISR. However, brachytherapy may retain a clinical niche for certain patients with difficult to treat ISR. Importantly, vascular brachytherapy was compared to both paclitaxel-eluting and sirolimus-eluting DES for the treatment of BMS ISR. In the TAXUS V ISR randomized trial, 396 patients with BMS ISR were randomized to implantation a Taxus® DES or vascular brachytherapy. Vascular brachytherapy was inferior to placement of a Taxus® DES, with increased rates of angiographic restenosis, TLR, TVR, and MACE for patients randomized to vascular brachytherapy.[67] In the SISR trial, vascular brachytherapy was also inferior to placement of a Cypher® DES for treatment of BMS ISR during nine-month follow-up.[68] Interestingly, five-year results of the SISR trial showed no significant difference in outcomes between groups, suggesting that treatment of ISR with a DES may not result in an initially more favorable angiographic outcome, but that vascular brachytherapy is associated with more durable inhibition of restenosis.[69]

d. Maximizing Luminal Gain and Stent Expansion

Both rotational atherectomy and laser atherectomy were extensively studied for the treatment of in-stent restenosis during the BMS era. Overall, results of these studies failed to demonstrate any additional benefit of these technologies in treatment of restenosis. However, these technologies remain useful for specific cases of restenosis due to stent under expansion, which remains a common cause of ISR.[70] In a subset of cases, bulky calcification may limit adequate stent expansion, thereby predisposing to both restenosis and stent thrombosis. While a non-dilatable plaque is ideally modified prior to stent implantation, stent under expansion may occur at the time of stent implantation. Plaque modification and/or modification of the initial stent may therefore be necessary to achieve adequate stent expansion and obviate the need for distal surgical bypass. Both rotational and laser atherectomy may be useful for treatment of this specific clinical problem.

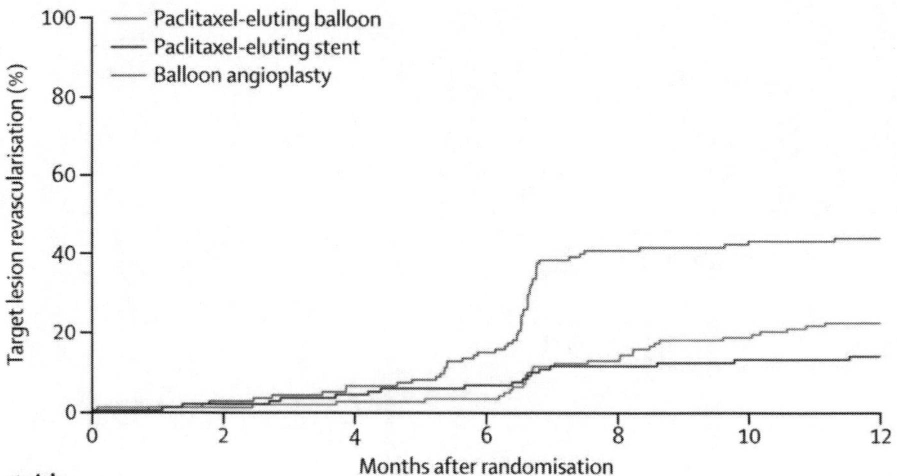

Number at risk							
Paclitaxel-eluting balloon	137	136	134	133	120	110	104
Paclitaxel-eluting stent	131	126	122	118	110	107	105
Balloon angioplasty	134	129	122	110	75	71	70

Figure 3. Use of Paclitaxel-Coated Balloon Paclitaxel-Eluting Stent, or Balloon Angioplasty to Treat Drug-Eluting Stent Restenosis.
During follow-up, the rates of target lesion revascularization were similar for patients treated with paclitaxel-coated balloon or a paclitaxel-eluting stent. Both treatment modalities were associated with significantly lower rates of target lesion revascularization compared to balloon angioplasty. Reprinted from The Lancet, Vol. 381. Byrne RA, Neumann FJ, Mehilli J, et al. Paclitaxel-eluting balloons, paclitaxel-eluting stents, and balloon angioplasty in patients with restenosis after implantation of a drug-eluting stent (ISAR-DESIRE 3): a randomized, open-label trial. Pages 461-467, 2013, with permission from Elsevier.

i. Rotational Atherectomy

Two randomized studies have examined the use of rotational atherectomy for the treatment of ISR. In the single-center ROSTER study, patients with ISR were randomized to rotational atherectomy + low pressure balloon angioplasty vs. high pressure balloon angioplasty with bailout stenting.[71] At 12-month follow-up, the rate of TLR was 32% in the rotational atherectomy group and 45% in the balloon angioplasty group (p=0.042). The larger, multicenter ARTIST trial randomized 298 patients with ISR to rotational atherectomy with balloon angioplasty vs. balloon angioplasty.[72] Unexpectedly, the rates of recurrent restenosis were higher in patients randomized to rotational atherectomy (65% vs. 51%). The authors speculated that higher pressure balloon inflation in the angioplasty only group resulted in greater acute luminal gain compared to a strategy of rotational atherectomy + low pressure balloon inflation, and hence a lower rate of restenosis. These results have tempered enthusiasm for use of rotational atherectomy in the treatment of ISR, although cases of ISR due to significant stent underexpansion from calcium could still potentially benefit from rotational atherectomy on a case-by-case basis.[73]

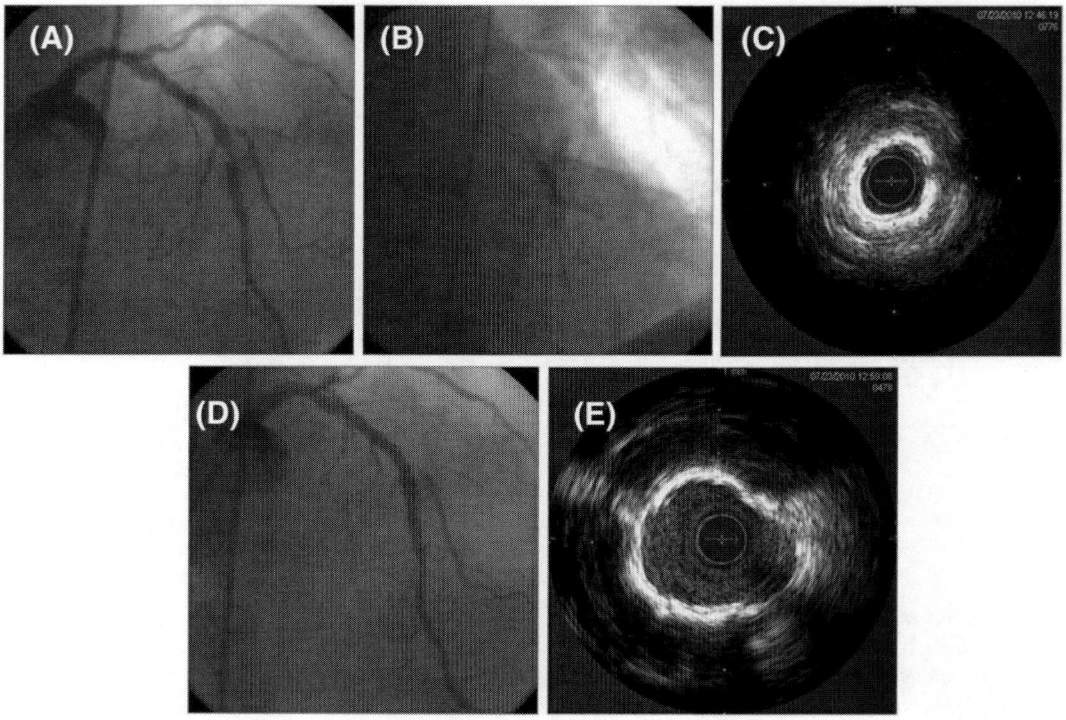

Figure 4. Use of Excimer Laser with Contrast Injection to Expand a Non-Dilatable Stent. A. A previously implanted stent in the mid LAD could not be expanded, leading to underexpansion. B. Repeat attempts at high-pressure balloon inflation could not expand the stent. C. Intravascular ultrasound confirmed a highly calcified lesion. D. After excimer laser atherectomy with contrast injection, the stent was successfully dilated. E. Follow-up intravascular ultrasound confirmed improved stent expansion. Reprinted from Cardiovascular Revascularization Medicine. Latib A, Takagi K, Chizzola G, et al. Excimer laser lesion modification to expand non-dilatable stents: the ELLEMENT registry. Epub ahead of print, 2013, with permission from Elsevier.

ii. Laser Atherectomy

Excimer laser-assisted angioplasty delivers local tissue ablation to the site of ISR, and therefore may significantly debulk ISR with associated increased acute luminal gain. Despite initial enthusiasm for this approach, clinical studies of excimer laser atherectomy followed by balloon angioplasty reported high rates of recurrent restenosis. Excimer laser angioplasty has not been studied extensively in combination with DES or drug-coated balloons; it is therefore uncertain whether neointimaldebulking followed by modern adjunctive therapies would provide marginal benefit in the incidence of restenosis.

Occasionally, ISR results from severe stent under-expansion due to a calcified plaque that could not be adequately dilated at the time of initial stent placement. In these situations, operators have reported using excimer laser to modify the plaque behind the stent struts and allow adequate stent expansion. [74] One novel approach to this problem is to inject a small volume of contrast during laser atherectomy. This results in increased cavitation and local expansion at the site of the laser (Figure 4). [75] In a recent registry, the authors reported that this approach to plaque modification can significantly increase stent expansion and achieve adequate luminal gain in order to minimize the risk of recurrent restenosis. While this is a niche application of the technology, it may be useful in specific circumstances of refractory ISR due to stent under expansion.

Conclusion

In-stent restenosis remains a difficult clinical problem to both prevent and treat. This chapter has highlighted a number of emerging technologies developed to minimize the incidence of restenosis, including novel stent alloys, improved drug elution kinetics, and bioresorbable stents. While each of these technologies may in theory provide additive benefit in preventing restenosis, rigorous clinical trials remain necessary to prove efficacy. Among patients who develop in-stent restenosis, DE Shave been particularly efficacious, especially for the treatment of BMS ISR. Although not yet approved for use in the USA, the application of drug coated balloons for treatment of ISR offers the potential to obviate the need for additional stent placement. While ISR can never be prevented completely, the emergence of these novel preventative and treatment strategies may continue to improve the outcomes for percutaneous coronary interventions and minimize the need for repeat procedures.

References

[1] Planer, D; Smits, PC; Kereiakes, DJ; et al. Comparison of everolimus- and paclitaxel-eluting stents in patients with acute and stable coronary syndromes: pooled results from the SPIRIT (A Clinical Evaluation of the XIENCE V Everolimus Eluting Coronary Stent System) and COMPARE (A Trial of Everolimus-Eluting Stents and Paclitaxel-Eluting Stents for Coronary Revascularization in Daily Practice) Trials. *JACC Cardiovascular interventions*, 2011, 4, 1104-15.

[2] Serruys, PW; Morice, MC; Kappetein, AP; et al. Percutaneous coronary intervention versus coronary-artery bypass grafting for severe coronary artery disease. *The New England journal of medicine*, 2009, 360, 961-72.

[3] Yeung, AC; Leon, MB; Jain, A; et al. Clinical evaluation of the Resolute zotarolimus-eluting coronary stent system in the treatment of de novo lesions in native coronary arteries: the RESOLUTE US clinical trial. *Journal of the American College of Cardiology*, 2011, 57, 1778-83.

[4] Pache, J; Kastrati, A; Mehilli, J; et al. Intracoronary stenting and angiographic results: strut thickness effect on restenosis outcome (ISAR-STEREO-2) trial. *Journal of the American College of Cardiology*, 2003, 41, 1283-8.

[5] Kastrati, A; Mehilli, J; Dirschinger, J; et al. Intracoronary stenting and angiographic results, strut thickness effect on restenosis outcome (ISAR-STEREO) trial. *Circulation*, 2001, 103, 2816-21.

[6] Weissman, NJ; Turco, MA; Ormiston, JA; et al. Improved strut coverage and less late incomplete apposition with thin-strut TAXUS Liberte vs. TAXUS Express: the importance of stent platform design for drug-eluting stents. *Cardiovascular revascularization medicine: including molecular interventions*, 2011, 12, 247-57.

[7] Stone, GW; Teirstein, PS; Meredith, IT; et al. A prospective, randomized evaluation of a novel everolimus-eluting coronary stent: the PLATINUM (a Prospective, Randomized, Multicenter Trial to Assess an Everolimus-Eluting Coronary Stent System [PROMUS Element] for the Treatment of Up to Two de Novo Coronary Artery Lesions) trial. *Journal of the American College of Cardiology*, 2011, 57, 1700-8.

[8] De la Torre Hernandez, JM; Garcia Camarero, T; Lerena, P; et al.A real all-comers randomized trial comparing Xience Prime and Promus Element stents. *The Journal of invasive cardiology*, 2013, 25, 182-5.

[9] Sarno, G; Lagerqvist B; Carlsson J; et al. Initial clinical experience with an everolimus eluting platinum chromium stent (Promus Element) in unselected patients from the Swedish Coronary Angiography and Angioplasty Registry (SCAAR). *International journal of cardiology*, 2013, 167, 146-50.

[10] Guagliumi, G;Capodanno, D;Ikejima, H; et al. Impact of different stent alloys on human vascular response to everolimus-eluting stent: an optical coherence tomography study: the OCTEVEREST. Catheterization and cardiovascular interventions: *official journal of the Society for Cardiac Angiography & Interventions*, 2013, 81, 510-8.

[11] Kereiakes, DJ; Cannon, LA; Feldman, RL; et al. Clinical and angiographic outcomes after treatment of de novo coronary stenoses with a novel platinum chromium thin-strut stent: primary results of the PERSEUS (Prospective Evaluation in a Randomized Trial of the Safety and Efficacy of the Use of the TAXUS Element Paclitaxel-Eluting Coronary Stent System) trial. *Journal of the American College of Cardiology*, 2010, 56, 264-71.

[12] Garg, S; Bourantas, C; Serruys, PW. New concepts in the design of drug-eluting coronary stents. *Nature reviews Cardiology*, 2013, 10, 248-60.

[13] Bourantas, CV; Zhang, Y; Farooq, V; Garcia-Garcia, HM; Onuma, Y; Serruys, PW. Bioresorbable scaffolds: current evidence and ongoing clinical trials. Current cardiology reports 2012, 14, 626-34.

[14] Tamai, H; Igaki, K; Kyo, E; et al. Initial and 6-month results of biodegradable poly-l-lactic acid coronary stents in humans. *Circulation*, 2000, 102, 399-404.

[15] Erbel, R; Di, Mario, C; Bartunek, J; et al. Temporary scaffolding of coronary arteries with bioabsorbable magnesium stents: a prospective, non-randomisedmulticentre trial. Lancet 2007, 369, 1869-75.

[16] Haude, M; Erbel, R; Erne, P; et al. Safety and performance of the drug-eluting absorbable metal scaffold (DREAMS) in patients with de-novo coronary lesions: 12 month results of the prospective, multicentre, first-in-man BIOSOLVE-I trial. Lancet 2013, 381, 836-44.

[17] Serruys, PW; Ormiston, JA; Onuma, Y; et al. A bioabsorbable everolimus-eluting coronary stent system (ABSORB): 2-year outcomes and results from multiple imaging methods. *Lancet*, 2009, 373, 897-910.

[18] Serruys, PW; Onuma, Y; Dudek, D; et al. Evaluation of the second generation of a bioresorbableeverolimus-eluting vascular scaffold for the treatment of de novo coronary artery stenosis: 12-month clinical and imaging outcomes. *Journal of the American College of Cardiology*, 2011, 58, 1578-88.

[19] Gomez-Lara, J; Brugaletta, S; Farooq, V; et al. Head-to-head comparison of the neointimal response between metallic and bioresorbableeverolimus-eluting scaffolds using optical coherence tomography. *JACC Cardiovascular interventions*, 2011, 4, 1271-80.

[20] Diletti, R; Serruys, PW; Farooq, V; et al. ABSORB II randomized controlled trial: a clinical evaluation to compare the safety, efficacy, and performance of the Absorb everolimus-eluting bioresorbable vascular scaffold system against the XIENCE everolimus-eluting coronary stent system in the treatment of subjects with ischemic heart disease caused by de novo native coronary artery lesions: rationale and study design. *American heart journal*, 2012, 164, 654-63.

[21] Krucoff, MW; Kereiakes, DJ; Petersen, JL; et al. A novel bioresorbable polymer paclitaxel-eluting stent for the treatment of single and multivessel coronary disease: primary results of the COSTAR (Cobalt Chromium Stent With Antiproliferative for Restenosis) II study. *Journal of the American College of Cardiology*, 2008, 51, 1543-52.

[22] Mehilli, J; Byrne, RA; Wieczorek, A; et al. Randomized trial of three rapamycin-eluting stents with different coating strategies for the reduction of coronary restenosis. *European heart journal*, 2008, 29, 1975-82.

[23] Byrne, RA; Kastrati, A; Kufner, S; et al. Randomized, non-inferiority trial of three limus agent-eluting stents with different polymer coatings: the Intracoronary Stenting and Angiographic Results. Test Efficacy of 3 Limus-Eluting Stents (ISAR-TEST-4) Trial. *European heart journal*, 2009, 30, 2441-9.

[24] Byrne, RA; Iijima, R; Mehilli, J; et al. Durability of antirestenotic efficacy in drug-eluting stents with and without permanent polymer. *JACC Cardiovascular interventions*, 2009, 2, 291-9.

[25] Yang, YB; Yang, YX; Su, B; et al. Probucol mediates vascular remodeling after percutaneous transluminal angioplasty via down-regulation of the ERK1/2 signaling pathway. *European journal of pharmacology*, 2007, 570, 125-34.

[26] Byrne, RA; Kastrati, A; Tiroch, K; et al. 2-year clinical and angiographic outcomes from a randomized trial of polymer-free dual drug-eluting stents versus polymer-based Cypher and Endeavor [corrected] drug-eluting stents. *Journal of the American College of Cardiology*, 2010, 55, 2536-43.

[27] Massberg, S; Byrne, RA; Kastrati, A; et al. Polymer-free sirolimus- and probucol-eluting versus new generation zotarolimus-eluting stents in coronary artery disease: the Intracoronary Stenting and Angiographic Results: Test Efficacy of Sirolimus- and Probucol-Eluting versus Zotarolimus-eluting Stents (ISAR-TEST 5) trial. *Circulation*, 2011, 124, 624-32.

[28] Luderer, F; Lobler, M; Rohm, HW; et al. Biodegradable sirolimus-loaded poly(lactide) nanoparticles as drug delivery system for the prevention of in-stent restenosis in coronary stent application. *Journal of biomaterials applications*, 2011, 25, 851-75.

[29] Lemos, PA; Farooq, V; Takimura, CK; et al. Emerging technologies: polymer-free phospholipid encapsulated sirolimusnanocarriers for the controlled release of drug from a stent-plus-balloon or a stand-alone balloon catheter. EuroIntervention: *journal of EuroPCR in collaboration with the Working Group on Interventional Cardiology of the European Society of Cardiology*, 2013, 9, 148-56.

[30] Nakano, K; Egashira, K; Masuda, S; et al. Formulation of nanoparticle-eluting stents by a cationic electrodeposition coating technology: efficient nano-drug delivery via bioabsorbable polymeric nanoparticle-eluting stents in porcine coronary arteries. *JACC Cardiovascular interventions*, 2009, 2, 277-83.

[31] Tan, A; Farhatnia, Y; de Mel, A; Rajadas, J; Alavijeh, MS; Seifalian, AM. Inception to actualization: next generation coronary stent coatings incorporating nanotechnology. *Journal of biotechnology*, 2013, 164, 151-70.

[32] Kastrati, A; Schomig, A; Dirschinger, J; et al. Increased risk of restenosis after placement of gold-coated stents: results of a randomized trial comparing gold-coated with uncoated steel stents in patients with coronary artery disease. *Circulation*, 2000, 101, 2478-83.

[33] Windecker, S; Mayer, I; De, Pasquale, G; et al. Stent coating with titanium-nitride-oxide for reduction of neointimal hyperplasia. *Circulation*, 2001, 104, 928-33.

[34] Windecker, S; Simon, R; Lins, M; et al. Randomized comparison of a titanium-nitride-oxide-coated stent with a stainless steel stent for coronary revascularization: the TiNOX trial. *Circulation*, 2005, 111, 2617-22.

[35] Karjalainen, PP; Annala, AP; Ylitalo, A; Vahlberg, T; Airaksinen, KE. Long-term clinical outcome with titanium-nitride-oxide-coated stents and paclitaxel-eluting stents for coronary revascularization in an unselected population. *International journal of cardiology*, 2010, 144, 42-6.

[36] Pendyala, LK; Matsumoto, D; Shinke, T; et al. Nobori stent shows less vascular inflammation and early recovery of endothelial function compared with Cypher stent. *JACC Cardiovascular interventions*, 2012, 5, 436-44.

[37] Chevalier, B; Silber, S; Park, SJ; et al. Randomized comparison of the NoboriBiolimusA9-eluting coronary stent with the TaxusLiberte paclitaxel-eluting coronary stent in patients with stenosis in native coronary arteries: the NOBORI 1 trial--Phase 2. *Circulation Cardiovascular interventions*, 2009, 2, 188-95.

[38] Windecker, S; Serruys, PW; Wandel, S; et al. Biolimus-eluting stent with biodegradable polymer versus sirolimus-eluting stent with durable polymer for coronary revascularisation (LEADERS): a randomised non-inferiority trial. *Lancet*, 2008, 372, 1163-73.

[39] Serruys, PW; Farooq, V; Kalesan, B; et al. Improved safety and reduction in stent thrombosis associated with biodegradable polymer-based biolimus-eluting stents versus durable polymer-based sirolimus-eluting stents in patients with coronary artery disease, final 5-year report of the LEADERS (Limus Eluted From A Durable Versus ERodable Stent Coating) randomized, noninferiority trial. *JACC Cardiovascular interventions*, 2013, 6, 777-89.

[40] Christiansen, EH; Jensen, LO; Thayssen, P; et al. Biolimus-eluting biodegradable polymer-coated stent versus durable polymer-coated sirolimus-eluting stent in unselected patients receiving percutaneous coronary intervention (SORT OUT V): a randomised non-inferiority trial. *Lancet*, 2013, 381, 661-9.

[41] Smits, PC; Hofma, S; Togni, M; et al. Abluminal biodegradable polymer biolimus-eluting stent versus durable polymer everolimus-eluting stent (COMPARE II): a randomised, controlled, non-inferiority trial. *Lancet*, 2013, 381, 651-60.

[42] Serruys, PW; Garg, S; Abizaid, A; et al. A randomised comparison of novolimus-eluting and zotarolimus-eluting coronary stents: 9-month follow-up results of the EXCELLA II study. EuroIntervention: *journal of EuroPCR in collaboration with the Working Group on Interventional Cardiology of the European Society of Cardiology*, 2010, 6, 195-205.

[43] Aoki, J; Serruys, PW; van, Beusekom, H; et al. Endothelial progenitor cell capture by stents coated with antibody against CD34; the HEALING-FIM (Healthy Endothelial Accelerated Lining Inhibits Neointimal Growth-First In Man) Registry. *Journal of the American College of Cardiology*, 2005, 45, 1574-9.

[44] den, Dekker, WK; Houtgraaf, JH; Onuma, Y; et al. Final results of the HEALING IIB trial to evaluate a bio-engineered CD34 antibody coated stent (GenousStent) designed to promote vascular healing by capture of circulating endothelial progenitor cells in CAD patients. *Atherosclerosis*, 2011, 219, 245-52.

[45] Low, AF; Lee, CH; Teo, SG; et al. Effectiveness and safety of the genous endothelial progenitor cell-capture stent in acute ST-elevation myocardial infarction. *The American journal of cardiology*, 2011, 108, 202-5.

[46] Silber, S; Damman, P; Klomp, M; et al. Clinical results after coronary stenting with the Genous Bio-engineered R stent: 12-month outcomes of the e-HEALING (Healthy Endothelial Accelerated Lining Inhibits Neointimal Growth) worldwide registry. EuroIntervention: *journal of EuroPCR in collaboration with the Working Group on Interventional Cardiology of the European Society of Cardiology*, 2011, 6, 819-25.

[47] Klomp, M; Beijk, MA; Varma, C; et al. 1-year outcome of TRIAS HR (TRI-stent adjudication study-high risk of restenosis) a multicenter, randomized trial comparing genous endothelial progenitor cell capturing stents with drug-eluting stents. *JACC Cardiovascular interventions*, 2011, 4, 896-904.

[48] Wohrle, J; Birkemeyer, R; Markovic, S; et al. Prospective randomised trial evaluating a paclitaxel-coated balloon in patients treated with endothelial progenitor cell capturing stents for de novo coronary artery disease. *Heart (British Cardiac Society)*, 2011, 97, 1338-42.

[49] Jim, MH; Fung, RC; Yiu, KH; Ng, AK; Siu, CW; Fan, KY. Combined Paclitaxel-Eluting Balloon and Genous Cobalt-Chromium Alloy Stent Utilization in De Novo Coronary Stenoses (PEGASUS). *Journal of interventional cardiology*, 2013, 26, 556-60.

[50] Haude, M; Lee, SW; Worthley, SG; et al. The REMEDEE trial: a randomized comparison of a combination sirolimus-eluting endothelial progenitor cell capture stent with a paclitaxel-eluting stent. *JACC Cardiovascular interventions*, 2013, 6, 334-43.

[51] Versaci, F; Gaspardone, A; Tomai, F; et al. Immunosuppressive Therapy for the Prevention of Restenosis after Coronary Artery Stent Implantation (IMPRESS Study). *Journal of the American College of Cardiology* 2002, 40, 1935-42.

[52] Hausleiter, J; Kastrati, A; Mehilli, J; et al. Randomized, double-blind, placebo-controlled trial of oral sirolimus for restenosis prevention in patients with in-stent restenosis: the Oral Sirolimus to Inhibit Recurrent In-stent Stenosis (OSIRIS) trial. *Circulation*, 2004, 110, 790-5.

[53] Inoue, T; Uchida, T; Sakuma, M; et al. Cilostazol inhibits leukocyte integrin Mac-1, leading to a potential reduction in restenosis after coronary stent implantation. *Journal of the American College of Cardiology*, 2004, 44, 1408-14.

[54] Douglas, JS; Jr. Holmes, DR; Jr. Kereiakes, DJ; et al. Coronary stent restenosis in patients treated with cilostazol. *Circulation*, 2005, 112, 2826-32.

[55] Lee, SW; Park, SW; Kim, YH; et al. Comparison of triple versus dual antiplatelet therapy after drug-eluting stent implantation (from the DECLARE-Long trial). *The American journal of cardiology*, 2007, 100, 1103-8.

[56] Lee, SW; Park, SW; Kim, YH; et al. A randomized, double-blind, multicenter comparison study of triple antiplatelet therapy with dual antiplatelet therapy to reduce restenosis after drug-eluting stent implantation in long coronary lesions: results from the DECLARE-LONG II (Drug-Eluting Stenting Followed by Cilostazol Treatment Reduces Late Restenosis in Patients with Long Coronary Lesions) trial. *Journal of the American College of Cardiology*, 2011, 57, 1264-70.

[57] Lee, SW; Lee, JY; Ahn, JM; et al. Comparison of dual versus triple antiplatelet therapy after drug-eluting stent according to stent length (from the pooled analysis of DECLARE trials). *The American journal of cardiology*, 2013, 112, 1738-44.

[58] Alfonso, F; Perez-Vizcayno, MJ; Hernandez, R; et al. A randomized comparison of sirolimus-eluting stent with balloon angioplasty in patients with in-stent restenosis: results of the Restenosis Intrastent: Balloon Angioplasty Versus Elective Sirolimus-Eluting Stenting (RIBS-II) trial. *Journal of the American College of Cardiology*, 2006, 47, 2152-60.

[59] Kastrati, A; Mehilli, J; von, Beckerath, N; et al. Sirolimus-eluting stent or paclitaxel-eluting stent vs balloon angioplasty for prevention of recurrences in patients with coronary in-stent restenosis: a randomized controlled trial. *JAMA: the journal of the American Medical Association*, 2005, 293, 165-71.

[60] Mehilli, J; Byrne, RA; Tiroch, K; et al. Randomized trial of paclitaxel- versus sirolimus-eluting stents for treatment of coronary restenosis in sirolimus-eluting stents:the ISAR-DESIRE 2 (Intracoronary Stenting and Angiographic Results: Drug Eluting Stents for In-Stent Restenosis 2) study. *Journal of the American College of Cardiology*, 2010, 55, 2710-6.

[61] Alfonso, F; Perez-Vizcayno, MJ; Dutary, J; et al. Implantation of a drug-eluting stent with a different drug (switch strategy) in patients with drug-eluting stent restenosis. Results from a prospective multicenter study (RIBS III [Restenosis Intra-Stent: Balloon Angioplasty Versus Drug-Eluting Stent]). *JACC Cardiovascular interventions*, 2012, 5, 728-37.

[62] Scheller, B; Hehrlein, C; Bocksch, W; et al. Treatment of coronary in-stent restenosis with a paclitaxel-coated balloon catheter. *The New England journal of medicine*, 2006, 355, 2113-24.

[63] Unverdorben, M; Vallbracht, C; Cremers, B; et al. Paclitaxel-coated balloon catheter versus paclitaxel-coated stent for the treatment of coronary in-stent restenosis. *Circulation*, 2009, 119, 2986-94.

[64] Byrne, RA; Neumann, FJ; Mehilli, J; et al. Paclitaxel-eluting balloons, paclitaxel-eluting stents, and balloon angioplasty in patients with restenosis after implantation of a drug-eluting stent (ISAR-DESIRE 3): a randomised, open-label trial. *Lancet*, 2013, 381, 461-7.

[65] Waksman, R; Raizner, AE; Yeung, AC; Lansky, AJ; Vandertie, L. Use of localised intracoronary beta radiation in treatment of in-stent restenosis: the INHIBIT randomised controlled trial. *Lancet*, 2002, 359, 551-7.

[66] Leon, MB; Teirstein, PS; Moses, JW; et al. Localized intracoronary gamma-radiation therapy to inhibit the recurrence of restenosis after stenting. *The New England journal of medicine*, 2001, 344, 250-6.

[67] Stone, GW; Ellis, SG; O'Shaughnessy, CD; et al. Paclitaxel-eluting stents vs vascular brachytherapy for in-stent restenosis within bare-metal stents: the TAXUS V ISR randomized trial. *JAMA: the journal of the American Medical Association*, 2006, 295, 1253-63.

[68] Holmes, DR; Jr. Teirstein, P; Satler, L; et al. Sirolimus-eluting stents vs vascular brachytherapy for in-stent restenosis within bare-metal stents, the SISR randomized trial. JAMA: *the journal of the American Medical Association*, 2006, 295, 1264-73.

[69] Alli, OO; Teirstein, PS; Satler, L; et al. Five-year follow-up of the Sirolimus-Eluting Stents vs Vascular Brachytherapy for Bare Metal In-Stent Restenosis (SISR) trial. *American heart journal*, 2012, 163, 438-45.

[70] Kang, SJ; Mintz, GS; Park, DW; et al. Mechanisms of in-stent restenosis after drug-eluting stent implantation: intravascular ultrasound analysis. *Circulation Cardiovascular interventions*, 2011, 4, 9-14.

[71] Sharma, SK; Kini, A; Mehran, R; Lansky, A; Kobayashi, Y; Marmur, JD. Randomized trial of Rotational Atherectomy Versus Balloon Angioplasty for Diffuse In-stent Restenosis (ROSTER). *American heart journal*, 2004, 147, 16-22.

[72] vom, Dahl, J; Dietz, U; Haager, PK; et al. Rotational atherectomy does not reduce recurrent in-stent restenosis: results of the angioplasty versus rotational atherectomy for treatment of diffuse in-stent restenosis trial (ARTIST). *Circulation*, 2002, 105, 583-8.

[73] Alfonso, F; Sandoval, J; Nolte, C. Calcified in-stent restenosis: a rare cause of dilation failure requiring rotational atherectomy. *Circulation Cardiovascular interventions*, 2012, 5, e1-2.

[74] Noble, S; Bilodeau, L. High energy excimer laser to treat coronary in-stent restenosis in an underexpanded stent. Catheterization and cardiovascular interventions: *official journal of the Society for Cardiac Angiography & Interventions*, 2008, 71, 803-7.

[75] Latib, A; Takagi, K; Chizzola, G; et al. Excimer Laser LEsion Modification to Expand Non-dilatable sTents: The ELLEMENT Registry. *Cardiovascular revascularization medicine: including molecular interventions*, 2013.

Editor Contact Information

Dr. Amir S. Lotfi, M.D.
Baystate Medical Center
Tufts University School of Medicine Division of Cardiology
759 Chestnut Street
Springfield, Massachusetts, USA 01199
E-mail: Amir.LotfiMD@baystatehealth.org

Index

A

acetylcholine, 28, 94
adaptation, 40, 241
adenosine, 128, 225, 234
adenovirus, 243, 247, 257, 258, 260
adhesion, 21, 214, 253, 261, 271
adjustment, 37, 39, 46, 54, 92
ADP, 96
adsorption, 254
advancement(s), 18, 24, 27, 28, 73, 169, 170
adventitia, 18, 20, 52, 100, 101, 240, 249
adverse effects, 190, 194
albumin, 196
algorithm, 54, 55
allele, 14
allergens, 11
allergic reaction, 179
allylamine, 244
alopecia, 196
alters, 71
amine(s), 244, 245
anastomosis, 216
anatomy, 163, 220
angina, 7, 9, 18, 42, 70, 71, 89, 122, 154, 156, 188, 214, 218, 220, 227, 228, 230
angiogram, 225
angioplasty, 6, 10, 12, 14, 18, 19, 20, 27, 29, 54, 57, 66, 74, 79, 90, 93, 97, 131, 140, 141, 149, 161, 191, 192, 193, 195, 196, 198, 199, 202, 206, 208, 209, 221, 226, 230, 239, 240, 253, 255, 258, 261, 265, 269, 272, 274, 275, 276, 279, 283
angiotensin converting enzyme, 194, 199
angiotensin II, 157
angiotensin receptor blockers, 90
antibody, 29, 245, 258, 259, 271, 281
anticoagulation, 114, 144, 225
antigen, 29, 242, 245, 271
antigen-presenting cell, 242
anti-inflammatory agents, 190
antioxidant, 189, 192, 195, 268
antisense, 251, 260
apoptosis, 20, 214, 250
arginine, 253, 254
arterial remodeling, 4, 29, 136
arterial spasm, 4
arteries, 18, 19, 23, 29, 157, 158, 162, 171, 215, 227, 239, 240, 241, 244, 248, 250, 251, 252, 253, 254, 259, 271
arteriography, 219
arteriosclerosis, 69, 228
asymptomatic, 12, 70, 74, 170, 188
atherosclerosis, 17, 25, 52, 85, 86, 90, 99, 102, 126, 163, 198, 215, 218, 220, 225, 227, 228, 229, 231
atherosclerotic plaque, 19, 40, 86, 152, 162, 165, 215
atherosclerotic vascular disease, 241
ATLAS, 145
atoms, 244
ATP, 253
attachment, 244, 251
autopsy, 24, 25, 26, 30, 87

B

backscattering, 49, 84, 151
bare-metal stents, 33, 34, 55, 56, 58, 66, 77, 78, 94, 97, 110, 143, 149, 164, 166, 169, 179, 209, 210, 232, 233, 234, 255, 256, 258, 283
barotrauma, 43, 70, 202
base pair, 196
basement membrane, 18
beneficial effect, 191
benefits, 48, 91, 131, 190, 192, 223, 264
benign, 12, 54, 73, 74
beta blocker, 191
biocompatibility, 243, 244, 264

biological activity, 241
biological responses, 93
bioluminescence, 247, 249
biomaterials, 280
biosynthesis, 193
biotechnology, 280
bleeding, 203, 204
blood flow, 121, 128, 178, 241, 246, 247
blood pressure, 217, 218
blood supply, 121
blood vessels, 19, 151, 171
bone marrow, 21, 270, 271
bounds, 7
brachytherapy, 54, 131, 140, 141, 149, 204, 207, 209, 210, 221, 222, 223, 274, 283
bradycardia, 189
bypass graft, 170, 173, 209, 213, 219, 220, 222, 223, 228, 229, 230, 231, 232, 233, 277

C

calcification(s), 40, 132, 135, 153, 158, 159, 160, 162, 171, 275
calcium, 26, 49, 160, 166, 191, 276
calcium channel blocker, 191
carbon nanotubes, 250
cardiac catheterization, 125, 126, 182, 228
cardiac surgery, 228
cardiovascular disease, 190
carotid arteries, 22, 29, 249, 252, 254, 258
catabolism, 189
catheter, 97, 109, 113, 132, 145, 146, 152, 157, 182, 200, 211, 222, 223, 249, 256, 280, 282
cell cycle, 22, 23, 30, 31, 251
cell death, 18, 229
cell division, 18, 22, 45
cell membranes, 244
challenges, 171, 179
channel blocker, 10, 188, 189
chemical, 242, 244, 245
chemokines, 22, 23, 252
chitosan, 258
cholesterol, 89, 217, 218
choline, 244
chromatography, 245
chromium, 72, 264, 265, 269, 278
chronic inflammatory cells, 86
chronic obstructive pulmonary disease, 125
chronic renal failure, 18
circulation, 70, 214, 241, 246, 247
citrulline, 253
classification, 33, 34, 35, 36, 37, 39, 45, 48, 57, 74, 87, 90, 96, 141, 143, 148, 149
claudication, 190
clinical presentation, 12, 42, 51, 58, 69, 70, 71, 74, 154, 156, 214
closure, 17, 105, 106, 214, 218
cobalt, 72, 264, 269
coenzyme, 193
coherence, 5, 12, 24, 30, 33, 34, 58, 63, 64, 65, 66, 77, 79, 81, 83, 84, 87, 94, 95, 96, 100, 114, 147, 151, 163, 164, 165, 166, 167, 233, 278, 279
collaboration, 58, 166, 167, 209, 210, 211, 280, 281
collagen, 18, 20, 23, 34, 39, 40, 53, 86, 214, 243, 258, 260
collateral, 128
colonization, 253
commercial, 94, 249, 251
comparative analysis, 60, 178
compliance, 99, 100, 105, 106, 108, 109, 110, 112, 115
complications, 14, 90, 105, 113, 119, 134, 141, 155, 203, 214, 227, 241
composition, 20, 21, 24, 40, 47, 60, 88, 105, 152, 154, 171
compounds, 193, 241, 242
computed tomography, 12, 124, 170, 179, 180, 181, 182, 183
connective tissue, 251
coronary angioplasty, 12, 14, 15, 29, 74, 113, 114, 115, 128, 198, 199, 200, 208, 220, 230
coronary artery bypass graft, 71, 157, 195, 213, 214, 228, 229, 230, 272
coronary artery disease, 18, 30, 58, 60, 61, 62, 63, 64, 69, 75, 91, 95, 97, 115, 122, 127, 143, 153, 157, 158, 163, 169, 181, 182, 183, 193, 198, 199, 213, 220, 223, 239, 240, 277, 279, 280, 281
coronary artery restenosis, 119, 187
coronary bypass surgery, 230
coronary heart disease, 194
coronary intervention, 10, 17, 55, 64, 65, 69, 70, 122, 128, 193, 194, 201, 208, 223, 230, 240, 263, 277
coronary thrombosis, 86, 94
corticosteroid therapy, 192
corticosteroids, 188, 191
cost, 24, 99, 100, 102, 136, 146
cost effectiveness, 146
covering, 221
CRP, 191
CT scan, 170, 172, 176
CV, 64, 65, 129, 278
cyclins, 22, 251
cyclooxygenase, 193
cytochrome, 94
cytokines, 22, 191, 251, 261
cytoplasm, 251

D

decoupling, 254
deformation, 105, 242
degradation, 20, 23, 24, 242, 243
deposition, 21, 22, 24, 46, 82, 89, 93, 100, 153, 215, 243, 252, 258, 268
deposits, 85, 166
depth, 34, 71, 152, 254
destruction, 21
detection, 78, 152, 153, 157, 158, 162, 170, 173, 179, 180, 249
diabetes, 5, 9, 13, 18, 25, 47, 56, 65, 70, 91, 155, 194, 205, 216, 217, 240, 255
diabetic patients, 9, 13, 30, 47, 48, 55, 60, 65, 67, 160, 189, 190, 191, 192, 272
diffusion, 242, 243
dilation, 115, 274, 283
discontinuity, 44
discordance, 123
disease progression, 230
dispersion, 243
displacement, 6
distribution, 5, 9, 11, 24, 39, 46, 48, 53, 59, 65, 121, 128, 139, 143, 218, 248
dopamine, 243, 251
down-regulation, 279
drug delivery, 9, 23, 24, 25, 34, 43, 188, 196, 258, 268, 269, 280
drug release, 46, 256, 268
drug resistance, 84, 93, 205
drug therapy, 187
drug-eluting stents, 8, 9, 13, 23, 25, 28, 30, 33, 49, 57, 59, 60, 61, 63, 64, 66, 77, 95, 96, 97, 100, 102, 110, 113, 145, 146, 149, 156, 164, 169, 188, 191, 193, 194, 208, 210, 224, 229, 230, 233, 234, 239, 255, 256, 263, 278, 279, 281
dyspnea, 125

E

edema, 189
elastic recoil, 3, 4, 5, 6, 17, 18, 19, 20, 23, 27, 29, 100, 115, 201, 202
elastin, 18, 19, 249
electrodeposition, 280
electron, 180, 228
emboli, 219, 225, 226, 234, 242
embolization, 219, 225, 226, 234, 242
encoding, 247, 248, 250, 252, 253
endothelial cells, 18, 21, 22, 23, 24, 25, 27, 85, 216, 251, 259, 260, 261, 270
endothelial dysfunction, 26, 27, 52, 82
endothelium, 20, 21, 22, 25, 28, 216, 217, 229, 241, 250, 253, 254
energy, 171, 283
environment(s), 196, 242
ester, 244, 247
evaporation, 243
exclusion, 245
exercise, 12, 70
extracellular matrix, 18, 21, 22, 39, 53, 57, 153, 221

F

false positive, 174
fatty acids, 199
fibers, 34, 40, 243
fibrin, 22, 46, 82, 85, 89, 100, 215, 250, 252, 268
fibrinogen, 250
fibrinolytic, 229
fibroblast growth factor, 23
fibroblasts, 18, 100
fibrosis, 21, 23
fibrous cap, 83, 86, 88, 89, 156, 160, 162, 266
filters, 179, 181
financial, 94
fish oil, 195, 199
fluorescence, 248
folate, 188, 194
folic acid, 194
Fractional flow reserve (FFR), 53, 70, 71, 120, 121, 122, 123, 124, 125, 126, 127, 129, 140, 153, 158, 160, 162, 176, 177, 178, 219
fractures, 53, 100, 135, 176, 182
frequency distribution, 206
friction, 120

G

gamma radiation, 149, 209, 222, 223, 232
gene expression, 21, 239, 248, 249
gene therapy, 227, 235, 239, 240, 241, 246, 248, 250, 251, 255, 256, 259, 261, 270
gene transfer, 240, 241, 244, 249, 257, 258, 259, 260, 261
genes, 196, 241, 250, 253
genotype, 199
geometry, 24, 120, 123, 264
glucocorticoid, 189
glucocorticoid receptor, 189
glucose, 190
growth factor, 21, 22, 23, 29, 190, 195, 199, 216, 217, 251, 252, 259, 260, 261

H

headache, 189
healing, 3, 9, 20, 24, 25, 27, 28, 40, 43, 53, 57, 61, 82, 86, 95, 96, 153, 166, 215, 229, 258, 260, 264, 265, 270, 281
heart disease, 29, 119, 127, 170, 180, 279
heart failure, 189
heart rate, 171, 176
hemodialysis, 87, 91
hemoglobin, 190
hemorrhage, 95, 154
heterogeneity, 149
high density lipoprotein, 217, 218
histological examination, 248
histology, 12, 28, 33, 34, 153, 215
homocysteine, 194
hydrolysis, 245, 246, 247
hyperemia, 11, 120, 121, 128, 219
hyperglycemia, 25
hyperlipidemia, 162
hypersensitivity, 70, 82, 84, 93, 94
hypertension, 155, 189

I

ICAM, 21, 214
IL-8, 252
imaging modalities, 28, 135, 162
immobilization, 243, 244, 245, 246, 248
immune response, 53, 242, 248, 257
immunofluorescence, 249
immunosuppressive agent, 196
immunosuppressive drugs, 196
intravascualar ultrasound (IVUS), 3, 6, 9, 19, 20, 24, 26, 27, 28, 34, 37, 44, 45, 46, 47, 48, 49, 70, 71, 79, 80, 84, 87, 88, 89, 93, 94, 95, 99, 100, 101, 102, 103, 104, 105, 106, 109, 112, 114, 115, 131, 132, 133, 134, 35, 136, 137, 139, 140, 141, 142, 147, 151, 152, 153, 154, 155, 156, 157, 158, 159, 160, 161, 162, 163, 166, 173, 176, 203, 219, 223, 260
in vitro, 106, 115, 180, 245, 251, 260
in vivo, 20, 56, 106, 115, 128, 132, 181, 182, 229, 242, 245, 251, 257, 260
infarction, 58, 71, 91, 92, 101, 123, 124, 137, 160
infection, 189
inflammation, 19, 20, 21, 22, 23, 25, 29, 40, 46, 61, 82, 84, 86, 90, 93, 95, 155, 190, 243, 250, 252, 258, 260, 264, 267, 268, 269, 280
inflammatory cells, 23, 85, 214
inflammatory mediators, 252
inflammatory responses, 255
infrared spectroscopy, 34, 52, 162
inhibition, 5, 27, 29, 45, 189, 190, 194, 196, 234, 239, 241, 250, 251, 254, 257, 261, 265, 267, 268, 269, 271, 274
initiation, 18, 21, 22
injury, 3, 4, 5, 6, 8, 17, 18, 19, 20, 21, 22, 23, 24, 27, 29, 44, 47, 100, 190, 195, 214, 216, 222, 241, 242, 250, 253, 255, 259, 260, 261, 265, 270
inoculation, 241
insertion, 194
insulin, 9, 23, 29, 190, 195
integration, 244
integrin(s), 21, 22, 271, 282
intercellular adhesion molecule, 29
interferon (IFN), 22
intima, 18, 19, 22, 23, 25, 42, 51, 57, 80, 88, 94, 101, 154, 156, 159, 164, 214, 215, 222, 227, 240, 253
iodinated contrast, 176, 177
irradiation, 141, 149, 243, 274
ischemia, 3, 4, 7, 8, 9, 10, 70, 120, 121, 122, 124, 136, 137, 157, 158, 169, 182, 188, 192, 193, 205, 218, 219, 220

K

kinase activity, 251
kinetics, 46, 239, 242, 243, 245, 247, 248, 267, 268, 277
Krebs cycle, 28

L

lactic acid, 28, 96, 265, 267, 278
laminar, 120
laser ablation, 222
leukocytes, 21, 253
ligand, 245
liposomes, 260, 268
lovastatin, 193, 198
luciferase, 247, 248, 249
lymph node, 242
lymphocytes, 85
lysine, 245

M

macromolecules, 243
macrophages, 21, 22, 25, 26, 28, 40, 78, 85, 153, 191, 214, 252, 257
magnesium, 171, 265, 278
magnetic field, 247, 249

malignancy, 271
mammalian tissues, 248
management, 37, 69, 122, 127, 132, 140, 142, 154, 158, 163, 187, 190, 193, 194, 214, 219, 227, 229, 231
mannitol, 254
mast cells, 18
matrix, 23, 39, 53, 86, 214, 242, 243, 247, 248
MCP, 22, 214, 252
MCP-1, 22, 252
mechanical stress, 242
media, 18, 19, 22, 23, 40, 100, 101, 105, 135, 152, 221, 222, 240, 249
median, 52, 87, 92
membranes, 22, 244
messenger RNA, 29
metabolic syndrome, 256
metal ion(s), 251
metalloproteinase, 257, 260
microcrystalline, 92
microparticles, 250
microscopy, 40
migration, 20, 21, 23, 24, 25, 60, 189, 190, 193, 195, 196, 241, 242, 250, 252, 253, 260, 261
mitogen, 190, 229, 251
MMP(s), 20, 23
monocyte chemoattractant protein, 21, 29, 257
morphometric, 228
mortality, 8, 12, 69, 72, 73, 137, 146, 213, 214, 219, 220, 224, 232
mortality risk, 220
MRI, 180, 247
myocardial infarction, 7, 37, 46, 52, 66, 71, 91, 92, 96, 101, 121, 123, 124, 125, 126, 131, 135, 137, 138, 147, 158, 160, 166, 192, 193, 205, 217, 218, 219, 221, 222, 224, 225, 255, 269, 281
myocardial ischemia, 119, 120, 177, 188, 230
myocyte, 195
myofibroblasts, 252

N

nanoparticles, 196, 200, 247, 250, 258, 259, 267, 268, 280
nanotechnology, 196, 280
nanotube, 259
natural polymers, 243
necrosis, 22
necrotic core, 26, 49, 89, 153, 160, 214
neoangiogenesis, 42
neoatherosclerosis, 17, 18, 25, 26, 27, 30, 40, 42, 51, 52, 53, 57, 66, 78, 82, 87, 88, 89, 90, 93, 94, 95, 153, 154, 155, 156, 161, 164, 256
neovascularization, 53, 57, 80, 86, 94, 154, 155, 156, 164
neuropathy, 196
neutropenia, 196
neutrophils, 29, 85, 252
nitric oxide, 22, 23, 197, 216, 217, 261, 270
nitric oxide synthase, 261
noninvasive tests, 218
NSAIDs, 189
nucleic acid, 196, 200

O

obesity, 189
occlusion, 9, 18, 30, 35, 37, 38, 54, 70, 71, 152, 214, 216, 217, 218, 219, 220, 227, 234, 240
omega-3, 195
opacification, 178
Optical Coherene Tomography (OCT), 3, 24, 34, 79, 87, 100, 135, 151
optical properties, 49
optimization, 102, 136, 139, 141, 146, 163, 239, 255, 263, 265
overlap, 59
oxidative stress, 258
oxygen, 21, 29

P

pathology, 3, 30, 48, 57, 77, 87, 94, 95, 202, 225, 256
pathophysiological, 34, 47
pathophysiology, 17, 20, 21, 25, 33, 34, 114, 213, 217, 229, 234
percutaneous coronary intervention, vii, 9, 10, 12, 14, 33, 34, 39, 59, 61, 63, 64, 74, 78, 79, 84, 96, 114, 122, 124, 127, 129, 134, 146, 147, 152, 163, 165, 166, 167, 177, 187, 198, 214, 228, 230, 234, 255, 256, 263, 269, 277, 281
percutaneous revascularization, 3, 37, 54, 55, 74, 157, 225, 227, 234
perforation, 221, 222
perfusion, 120, 148, 165, 169, 170, 176, 177, 179, 182, 219
phosphorus, 222
photodetector, 152
photons, 171
pioglitazone, 14, 190, 197
plaque, 14, 19, 21, 42, 43, 47, 81, 82, 83, 86, 87, 88, 89, 95, 100, 131, 132, 133, 135, 136, 139, 140, 142, 147, 156, 157, 160, 162, 167, 209, 215, 219, 225, 226, 265, 270, 275, 277

plasma membrane, 251
plasmid, 196, 250, 252, 253, 257, 258, 259, 270
plasmid DNA, 196, 250, 252, 253, 257, 258, 259
platelet aggregation, 22, 216, 217, 253, 261, 268
platelets, 21, 22, 23, 29, 85, 215
platinum, 178, 264, 265, 269, 278
polymer(s), 12, 23, 24, 27, 46, 47, 58, 59, 60, 62, 63, 64, 82, 84, 90, 93, 96, 143, 154, 161, 164, 167, 179, 196, 240, 242, 243, 257, 258, 259, 263, 265, 267, 268, 269, 270, 279, 280, 281
polymer matrix, 243
polymer structure, 258
polymerization, 243
polymorphism(s), 21, 84, 94, 194, 199
polyunsaturated fat, 195
polyunsaturated fatty acids, 195
polyurethane, 243, 252
prednisone, 191, 192, 198, 271
pressure gradient, 121, 129
prevention, 14, 74, 77, 78, 89, 90, 96, 131, 132, 188, 190, 191, 193, 195, 196, 197, 198, 199, 225, 227, 228, 234, 239, 240, 253, 263, 271, 280, 282
progenitor cells, 21, 253, 261, 270, 271, 281
pro-inflammatory, 27, 243, 244, 253
prolapse, 19, 133, 140, 157
proliferation, 19, 21, 22, 23, 24, 34, 39, 45, 46, 58, 62, 64, 86, 90, 122, 143, 147, 149, 189, 190, 191, 193, 194, 195, 196, 201, 202, 214, 221, 222, 228, 241, 242, 243, 250, 251, 252, 253, 254, 259, 260, 261, 269, 270
promoter, 248
propagation, 18
protection, 226, 227, 234
proteins, 22, 244, 245, 251, 253
proteoglycans, 22, 23, 53, 82, 89
proto-oncogene, 29
PTFE, 221, 222
purification, 245

Q

quantification, 53, 153

R

racial differences, 228
radiation, 11, 141, 143, 148, 149, 172, 176, 179, 180, 182, 204, 209, 222, 223, 232, 283
radiation therapy, 11, 148, 149, 222, 223, 232, 283
radioactive isotopes, 222
radiotherapy, 222
reactivity, 90, 96
reality, 60
receptors, 22, 229, 251
recurrence, 37, 38, 71, 90, 131, 149, 192, 201, 202, 229, 232, 248, 283
regeneration, 251, 254, 259, 261
regression, 7, 14, 25, 37, 39, 78, 139, 155
renal failure, 240
resistance, 53, 96, 105, 120, 121, 124, 128, 160, 166, 273
resolution, 7, 24, 132, 151, 152, 153, 155, 157, 158, 160, 162, 163, 170, 171, 172, 176, 179, 248
response, 3, 4, 5, 8, 9, 11, 19, 21, 23, 24, 25, 28, 29, 30, 37, 39, 40, 43, 45, 47, 48, 57, 61, 64, 65, 78, 84, 86, 94, 95, 100, 120, 122, 128, 143, 149, 163, 199, 200, 214, 215, 216, 227, 239, 240, 242, 243, 252, 267, 268, 278, 279
responsiveness, 96
restoration, 28, 119, 250, 253
rhenium, 222
ribonucleic acid, 196
risk assessment, 170, 180
risk factors, 3, 9, 39, 97, 157, 216, 229, 230
risks, 113, 127, 225, 227
rosiglitazone, 15, 190, 198

S

safety, 27, 55, 56, 61, 65, 78, 91, 92, 189, 192, 196, 197, 200, 208, 222, 224, 233, 255, 279, 280, 281
salts, 247
scatter, 107
scattering, 49, 152
second generation, 24, 27, 66, 224, 264, 269, 270, 272, 279
SES, 33, 37, 39, 40, 41, 43, 44, 45, 46, 47, 49, 52, 53, 54, 71, 72, 73, 82, 84, 89, 91, 93, 145, 205, 272
sex, 70, 217, 218
shear, 20, 24
side chain, 245
side effects, 189, 191, 192
signaling pathway, 250, 269, 279
signalling, 22, 259
signals, 20, 52, 80, 81, 83, 86, 88, 89, 132
signal-to-noise ratio, 152
siRNA, 251, 258
smoking, 157, 217, 218, 225
smooth muscle, 18, 22, 23, 29, 34, 39, 40, 45, 53, 60, 78, 85, 89, 90, 100, 153, 154, 189, 190, 191, 193, 195, 196, 214, 221, 222, 229, 257, 259, 260, 261, 268, 269, 270, 271

smooth muscle cells, 18, 22, 29, 40, 45, 53, 78, 85, 89, 90, 100, 153, 154, 189, 193, 214, 229, 257, 259, 260, 261
stability, 78, 242, 245
stabilization, 88, 252, 270
stable angina, 29, 43, 57, 70, 154, 156, 160
statin, 167
steel, 86, 244, 245, 246, 247, 252, 254, 259, 264, 265, 267, 269, 280
stimulation, 5, 23, 250, 251, 271
stress, 7, 9, 12, 18, 20, 24, 105, 140, 148, 158, 165, 177, 179, 182, 214, 219, 261
stress test, 7, 12, 18, 140, 158
stress testing, 7, 158
stroke, 255
strontium, 222
structural characteristics, 49
structure, 18, 19, 28, 49, 51, 80, 87, 92, 153, 154, 157
styrene, 243
substrate(S), 19, 239, 241, 244, 247
success rate, 220, 240
sulfate, 22, 23
superimposition, 51
supplementation, 195, 254, 256
suppression, 45, 46, 143, 230
surface component, 21
surface modification, 258
surrogates, 134
surveillance, 56
survival, 45, 92, 140, 141, 148, 165, 191, 192, 195, 204, 218, 221, 228, 229, 230
survival rate, 140, 191
susceptibility, 161
symptoms, 7, 8, 18, 70, 71, 86, 122, 140, 171, 190, 213, 218, 220
synthesis, 252, 254
synthetic polymers, 243

T

T lymphocytes, 85
technological advances, 17, 18, 187, 267
technological developments, 256
tensile strength, 265
tension, 189
TGF, 22, 23, 251
thallium, 12
therapeutic agents, 196, 246
therapeutic effects, 241
therapeutics, 29, 61, 188, 240, 241, 245
therapy, 8, 14, 54, 90, 93, 96, 128, 132, 140, 149, 159, 162, 165, 167, 187, 188, 189, 190, 191, 194, 197, 198, 199, 204, 220, 222, 223, 225, 227, 230, 234, 241, 248, 250, 256, 259, 272, 282
therapy interventions, 250
threonine, 251
thrombin, 21, 22, 250
thrombogenesis, 17, 18, 21, 23
thrombus, 21, 22, 24, 52, 82, 83, 84, 88, 89, 94, 95, 135, 155, 156, 162, 215, 219, 250, 252, 253, 266
time frame, 17
titanium, 268, 280
TNF, 22, 252
TNF-α, 22
toxic effect, 271
toxicity, 82, 84, 196, 243
transcription, 251, 252
transcription factors, 251
transduction, 242, 244, 247, 249, 259
transfection, 257, 258
transforming growth factor, 23
transgene, 239, 241, 242, 243, 247, 248, 249, 253, 255
translation, 253, 255
transplantation, 126
trauma, 9, 44, 100, 105, 202, 250, 252
triggers, 254
turnover, 20, 250
tyrosine, 22, 23, 251

U

ulcer, 51
ultrasonography, 182
underlying mechanisms, 25, 33
unstable angina and USA, 7, 39, 51, 57, 65, 69, 71, 89, 90, 91, 151, 154, 155, 156, 166, 213, 223, 230, 240, 277

V

vascular diseases, 256
vascular endothelial growth factor (VEGF), 197, 250
vascular wall, 241
vasodilator, 120
vasomotor, 28, 94, 258
vasospasm, 94, 152
vector, 227, 239, 241, 242, 243, 244, 245, 246, 247, 248, 249, 250, 252, 254, 255, 258, 259
vein, 9, 18, 70, 132, 162, 209, 213, 214, 216, 217, 218, 219, 222, 224, 227, 228, 229, 230, 231, 232, 233, 234, 235
velocity, 120, 128, 234
vessel wall damage, 17

vessels, 21, 24, 42, 60, 70, 86, 102, 105, 106, 109, 111, 122, 124, 127, 132, 136, 142, 157, 169, 170, 177, 187, 214, 215, 220, 227, 229, 230, 253, 271
viral gene, 242, 244, 253, 257
viral vectors, 240, 249, 257
visualization, 134, 170, 171, 172, 180
vitamin B1, 194
vitamin B12, 194
vitamin B6, 194
vitamin E, 195
vulnerability, 86, 162, 248

W

wavelengths, 152
wires, 243, 249
withdrawal, 248
wound healing, 23, 84, 86, 90, 202

Y

yield, 91, 158, 203
yttrium, 222

Z

zinc, 248, 259